Contemporary Issues of Care

Contemporary Issues of Care has been co-published simultaneously as *Journal of Human Behavior in the Social Environment*, Volume 14, Numbers 1/2 2006.

Monographic Separates from the *Journal of Human Behavior in the Social Environment*™

Contemporary Issues of Care, edited by Roberta R. Greene, PhD (Vol. 14, No. 1/2, 2006). *"A comprehensive and cutting-edge contribution addressing the contemporary issues of giving care that encompasses the variations and diversity of caregiving situations. It highlights the importance of culture, race, and ethnicity while viewing care as a lifespan issue." (Robyn L. Golden, LCSW, Director of Older Adult Programs, Rush University Medical Center)*

The Impact of Welfare Reform: Balancing Safety Nets and Behavior Modification, edited by Christopher R. Larrison, PhD, and Michael Sullivan, PhD (Vol. 12, No. 2/3, 2005). *An in-depth examination of the impact of the Personal Responsibility and Work Opportunity Reconciliations Act of 1996 on clients, organizational staff, program responses, philosophy of service provision, and the goals of welfare.*

Approaches to Measuring Human Behavior in the Social Environment, edited by William R. Nugent, PhD (Vol. 11, No. 3/4, 2005). *Cutting-edge examinations of how family functioning, childhood depression, neighborhoods (from children's perspectives), spirituality, and psychosocial problems within seriously mentally ill families are measured and assessed.*

The Conundrum of Human Behavior in the Social Environment, edited by Marvin D. Feit, PhD, and John S. Wordarski, PhD (Vol. 10, No. 3, 2004). *A text for graduates, undergraduates, and human services professionals focusing on revising the current HBSE content with a micro and macro evidence-based curriculum.*

Diversity and Aging in the Social Environment, edited by Sherry M. Cummings, PhD, and Colleen Galambos, DSW (Vol. 9, No. 4, 2004, and Vol. 10, No.1, 2004). *Explores the impact of race/ethnicity, gender, sexual orientation, and geographic location on elders' strengths, challenges, needs, and resources.*

How Institutions Are Shaping the Future of Our Children: For Better or for Worse?, edited by Catherine N. Dulmus, PhD, and Karen M. Sowers, PhD (Vol. 9, No. 1/2, 2004). *"A great resource for child welfare professionals working in institutional settings, providing guidance regarding the practices found in one's own agency. The chapter authors are notable experts, and their writing reflects this experience. A highly recommended volume!" (Bruce A. Thayer, PhD, LCSW, Dean & Professor, School of Social Work, Florida State University, Tallahassee)*

Women and Girls in the Social Environment: Behavioral Perspectives, edited by Nancy J. Smyth, PhD, CSW, CASAC (Vol. 7, No. 3/4, 2003). *"At last, a human behavior text in which the unit of analysis is not boys and men, but girls and women. Thoroughly researched. . . . This collection would make an excellent addition to the standard HBSE course." (Katherine Van Wormer, PhD, MSSW, Professor of Social Work, University of Northern Iowa; Author of* Addiction Treatment: A Strengths Perspective*)*

Charting the Impacts of University-Child Welfare Collaboration, edited by Katharine Briar-Lawson, PhD, and Joan Levy Zlotnik, PhD, ACSW (Vol. 7, No. 1/2, 2003). *"An excellent comprehensive compilation of Title-IVE collaborations between public child welfare agencies and university settings at both BSW and MSW levels . . . " (Rowena Fong, MSW, EdD, Professor of Social Work, The University of Texas at Austin)*

Latino/Hispanic Liaisons and Visions for Human Behavior in the Social Environment, edited by José B. Torres, PhD, MSW, and Felix G. Rivera, PhD (Vol. 5, No. 3/4, 2002). *"An excellent example of scholarship by Latinos, for Latinos. . . . Quite useful for graduate social work courses in human behavior or social research." (Carmen Ortiz Hendricks, DSW, Associate Professsor, Hunter College School of Social Work, New York City)*

Violence as Seen Through a Prism of Color, edited by Letha A. (Lee) See, PhD (Vol. 4, No. 2/3, 4, 2001). *"Incisive and important. . . . A comprehensive analysis of the way violence affects people of color. Offers important insights. . . . Should be consulted by academics, students, policymakers, and members of the public." (Dr. James Midgley, Harry and Riva Specht, Professor and Dean, School of Social Welfare, University of California at Berkeley)*

Psychosocial Aspects of the Asian-American Experience: Diversity Within Diversity, edited by Namkee G. Choi, PhD (Vol. 3, No. 3/4, 2000). *Examines the childhood, adolescence, young adult, and aging stages of Asian Americans to help researchers and practitioners offer better services to this ethnic group. Representing Chinese, Japanese, Filipinos, Koreans, Asian Indians, Vietnamese, Hmong, Cambodians, and native-born Hawaiians, this helpful book will enable you to offer clients relevant services that are appropriate for your clients' ethnic backgrounds, beliefs, and experiences.*

Voices of First Nations People: Human Services Considerations, edited by Hilary N. Weaver, DSW (Vol. 2, No. 1/2, 1999). *"A must read for anyone interested in gaining an insight into the world of Native Americans. . . . I highly recommend it!" (James Knapp, BS, Executive Director, Native American Community Services of Erie and Niagara Counties, Inc., Buffalo, New York)*

Human Behavior in the Social Environment from an African American Perspective, edited by Letha A. (Lee) See, PhD (Vol. 1, No. 2/3, 1998). *"A book of scholarly, convincing, and relevant chapters that provide an African-American perspective on human behavior and the social environment . . . offer[s] new insights about the impact of race on psychosocial development in American society." (Alphonso W. Haynes, EdD, Professor, School of Social Work, Grand Valley State University, Grand Rapids, Michigan)*

Contemporary Issues of Care

Roberta R. Greene, PhD

Editor

Contemporary Issues of Care has been co-published simultaneously as *Journal of Human Behavior in the Social Environment*, Volume 14, Numbers 1/2 2006.

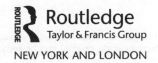
Routledge
Taylor & Francis Group

NEW YORK AND LONDON

First Published by
The Haworth Press, Inc., 10 Alice Street, Binghamton, NY 13904-1580 USA.

This edition published 2011 by Routledge
711 Third Avenue, New York, NY 10017
2 Park Square, Milton Park, Abingdon, Oxon, OX14 4RN

Contemporary Issues of Care has been co-published simultaneously as *Journal of Human Behavior in the Social Environment*™, Volume 14, Numbers 1/2 2006.

Library of Congress Cataloging-in-Publication Data

Contemporary issues of care / Roberta R. Greene, editor.
    p. cm.
    "Contemporary Issues of Care has been co-published simultaneously as Journal of Human Behavior in the Social Environment, Volume 14, Numbers 1/2 2006."
    Includes bibliographical references and index.
    ISBN-13: 978-0-7890-3241-6 (hard cover : alk. paper)
    ISBN-10: 0-7890-3241-4 (hard cover : alk. paper)
    ISBN-13: 978-0-7890-3242-3 (soft cover : alk. paper)
    ISBN-10: 0-7890-3242-2 (soft cover : alk. paper)
    1. Social case work. 2. Caregivers. I. Greene, Roberta R. (Roberta Rubin), 1940- II. Journal of human behavior in the social environment.
HV43.C584 2006
361.3'2–dc22   2006020030

Contemporary Issues of Care

CONTENTS

ABOUT THE EDITOR

Roberta R. Greene, PhD, is the Louis and Ann Wolens Centennial Chair in Gerontology and Social Welfare at the School of Social Work, University of Texas-Austin. Her career activities include clinical social work practice, curriculum construction, policy advocacy, and social work education. She has worked at schools of social work at George Mason University, the University of Georgia, the University of Maryland, and Indiana University. Dr. Greene has numerous publications including *Human Behavior Theory and Social Work Practice* and *Social Work with the Aged and Their Families*. Her most recent text is *Resiliency Theory: An Integrated Framework for Practice, Research, and Policy.*

About the Contributors

Harriet L. Cohen, PhD, LCSW, has served since August 2001 as assistant professor and director of the social work program in the Department of Rehabilitation, Social Work and Addictions at the University of North Texas in Denton. She teaches courses in social justice, community practice and aging. Her areas of research and training include spirituality, midlife and older women, lesbian and gay issues, and intergenerational service learning.

Harriet brings professional and personal experience to her research and writing on caregiving. As the former executive director of the Atlanta Area Chapter of the Alzheimer's Association (1989-1996) and assistant director for Aging, Volunteers, and Special Populations at Jewish Family and Career Services of Atlanta, Georgia (1985-1989), Harriet developed numerous caregiver training and support services for informal and formal caregivers of people with dementia. Also, she has had extensive personal experience caring for family members with chronic and acute disabilities. In addition to her professional responsibilities, Harriet works as a diversity trainer with the National Coalition Building Institute and the Ally training program on campus. She serves on the Steering Committee of the National Association of Social Workers North Texas Chapter and a member of the Texas Department on Aging Policy Resource Group. She is a member of the Council on Social Work Education, AGE-SW, and the Social Work Baccalaureate Program Directors (BPD) Association where she is actively involved with the BDP Educators and Friends of Lesbian and Gays (EFLAG) Committee and the Gerontology Committee.

Harriet received a doctorate in Adult Education (2001) and an MSW (1975) from The University of Georgia. She holds certificates in Women's Studies and Qualitative Research from The University of Georgia.

Tara R. Earl, PhD, MSW, is the recipient of the Margaret Cole Davis Scholarship, and a Houston Endowed Fellow. She is an African American woman who was raised in the multicultural setting of Williamsburg, Virginia. Tara earned her BSW from Virginia Commonwealth University in 1998 and her MSW from the University of Pennsylvania in 2000. Tara regards social work as being an avenue that will equip her with a solid research and theoretical foundation to be able to advance the field's current knowledge of sibling caregiving practices and mental health policy. Her previous work experience includes Philadelphia Elywn, the Pennsylvania Health Law Project, the Center for Mental Health Policy and Services Research at the University of Pennsylvania, and the Philadelphia Behavioral Health System. In addition to sibling caregiving research, other interests for Tara include, the linkages between primary and behavioral health care service delivery; outcomes research and public versus private managed care systems; issues of stigma and minority populations; and disparities in mental health treatment. Upon graduation, Tara hopes to utilize her training to serve the world of minority behavioral health. Outside school, Tara loves to explore local restaurants and to travel.

Kimberly D. Farris, PhD, MSW, received her doctorate at The University of Texas at Austin. She is originally from Atlanta, Georgia. Kimberly received her undergraduate degree BA in psychology from the University of Georgia, located in Athens in 1996. Before returning to school, she worked for one year as a residential treatment counselor at Three Springs Therapeutic Outdoor Treatment Center, located in Trenton, Alabama and one year as a residential treatment counselor, followed by the position of admissions coordinator for The Village of St. Joseph, located in Atlanta, Georgia. In 1998, Kimberly began attending Clark Atlanta University School of Social Work (now formally known as the Whitney M. Young, Jr., School of Social Work) and graduated in 2000 with an MSW degree with a specialization in Health/Mental Health concentration.

John M. Gonzalez, MSW, is currently a third-year doctoral student at the University of Texas at Austin School of Social Work. He is a CSWE Minority Research Fellow. He received his BA in Psychology and Sociology from the University of Texas at Austin and received his MSW from Texas State University at San Marcos, formerly Southwest Texas State University in San Marcos. Mr. Gonzalez is a Licensed Master Social Worker in the state of Texas. He has worked in the area of gerontology, specifically in mental health with older minority adults. He has also worked in the area of chemical dependency with involuntary clients. He has presented at national and state conferences on humor intervention strategies and stress management. He is interested in older Latinos and the delivery of mental health services. He loves competing in sprint triathlon and is a member of USA Triathlon.

Sandra A. Graham, PhD, received her doctorate and has a degree in health education and kinesiology from the University of Texas-Austin. She has a special interest in physical activity among older adults. She formerly worked for FEMA where she assisted older adults following traumatic events.

Laura M. Hopson, PhD, received her doctorate at the University of Texas at Austin School of Social Work. She received her MSW in 1998 from the Columbia University School of Social Work and practiced as a social worker in New York City for four years before beginning work on her doctoral degree in 2002. Laura's research interests include school-based intervention with adolescents to decrease risk behavior, HIV prevention, and improving the quality of life for those living with HIV/AIDS.

Barbara L. Jones, PhD, MSW, is Assistant Professor in the School of Social Work at the University of Texas at Austin. She received her doctorate in 2004 from the University at Albany School of Social Welfare. Dr. Jones is a Project on Death in America Social Work Leader and the principal investigator on a study of the role of social work in pediatric palliative care. Dr. Jones is president-elect of the National Board of the Association of Pediatric Oncology Social Workers and a steering committee member of the National Alliance for Children with Life Threatening Conditions. Dr. Jones is also a member of the Children's Oncology Group End-Of-Life Committee. Dr. Jones's clinical experience has been primarily in the field of pediatric oncology, palliative and end-of-life care, grief, bereavement and trauma.

Sally Hill Jones, PhD, LCSW, received her MSW from the University of Chicago School of Social Service Administration, and her PhD from the Institute for Clinical Social Work in Chicago, Illinois. She has 25 years of social work experience, working in a variety of settings with a wide range of client populations, including family service, private practice and hospice. She has been teaching at Texas State University San Marcos for three years. To request a copy of her vita or more information, contact her at <sh29@txstate.edu>.

Mary Margaret Just, PhD, MSW, teaches Human Behavior and the Social Environment and Policy at Morehead State University. Before she started teaching full-time, she worked for the Oklahoma Department of Human Services as an eligibility worker, service worker, service supervisor, and adult protective service worker. She served as social work consultant for the Oklahoma State Department of Health Eldercare program from its beginning until 1991 when she entered the PhD program at the University of Texas at Austin. While in the doctoral program, she served as the nursing home social worker for several rural nursing homes in central and east central Texas, and as assistant instructor for the Dynamics of Chemical Dependency, and Social Welfare Policy courses. Her dissertation topic was social support for nursing home residents.

Eunkyung Kim, PhD, was a visiting scholar at the University of Texas-Austin School of Social Work's Life Care Institute when she wrote her article for this volume. Her research was financially supported by Changwon National University in 2005.

Nancy Kropf, PhD, MSW, is Director and Professor in the School of Social Work at Georgia State University. She has numerous publications in gerontology and social work, with specific emphasis on older adults in caregiving roles. In addition, she has held national leadership roles in social work and aging, such as a Past President of the Association for Gerontology Education in Social Work (AGE SW), and a John A. Hartford Geriatric Social Work Scholar.

Youjung Lee, MSSW, is a doctoral student at the University of Texas Austin School of Social Work. She received the Helen Farabee Memorial Endowed Presidential Scholarship in 2003 and the Robert Lee Sutherland Scholarship in 2004. Youjung completed her BSW from Sung-Kyun-Kwan in Seoul, Korea in 2000. While working on her bachelor's, she volunteered at Sung-Shim General Hospital and led groups with dementia patients. She received her MSSW from the University of Texas-Austin School of Social Work in 2002. Youjung has worked with Dr. Roberta Greene on the Risk and Resilience Perspective and has presented at the 2002 Gerontological Society of America Conference at Boston. She has also worked with Dr. Gayle Acton on a meta-analysis of interventions for dementia caregivers. She is currently a third-year doctoral student concentrating on aging and resilience of Asian-American dementia caregivers research. Youjung loves to cook Korean dishes and share them with her friends.

Olivia Lopez, PhD, MSW, is completing the second year of her doctoral studies in social work at the University of Texas at Austin. It is her goal to complete and defend her dissertation by August 2005. She holds a bachelors degree in Psychology and Criminal Justice from the Texas A & M University, Corpus Christi, and a MSW from California State University–Fresno. Olivia was selected, by her peers, as the keynote speaker representing her graduating class. She has been the recipient of the South Texas Graduate Fellowship; a research internship with Dr. Yollanda Padilla, and of the Robert Carl Nesbitt Memorial Endowed Presidential Scholarship. She has recently been selected as a winner of the Dean Jack Otis Social Policy Award for a policy paper she authored entitled "Farmworkers and Social Work: The Unanswered Call."

Olivia has a longstanding interest in the living conditions and health status of migrant and seasonal farmworkers. Most recently she has focused her research area on seasonal female farmworkers and health. This population of farmworkers has virtually been ignored by pundits and researchers alike, and particularly by the social work profession. The purpose of her qualitative dissertation research is twofold. To establish baseline demographics about this population and to highlight the serious and potentially debilitating and fatal nature and risk factors related to type II Diabetes Mellitus, which befalls this population at much higher rates than those found within other groups in the general population. Given the substantial, and often insurmountable barriers facing seasonal farmworkers, they may be forced to use traditional self-care practices rather than Western medicine to manage their diabetes. It is essential that we understand the self-care practices themselves and their origins and include these practices in combination with Western medicine to provide the best care available to this extremely ignored and poor segment of the population.

Yvette Murray, PhD, is a consultant with the Texas Long Term Care Institute. She received her doctorate in social work from the University of Texas at Austin in 1987. Her practice credentials include board-certified diplomat and licensure in clinical social work. She has taught social work at the Texas State University and the University of Texas at Austin. Her practice experience spans over twenty-five years in mental health and gerontology.

Michael Uebel, PhD, LMSW, is a former professor of English and is now in practice as a psychotherapist with Sol Associates, Austin, Texas. Also in Austin he volunteers as a psychotherapist at Capitol Area Mental Health Center and as a crisis counselor with Victim Services, APD. He is currently a Fellow at the Houston-Galveston Psychoanalytic Institute. He is at work on a book, *Masochism in America*, which examines the formation of moral consciousness in post-war America.

Michael A. Wright, PhD, MSW, is Assistant Professor of Social Work at Andrews University where he facilitates learning in organizational development, social welfare policy, and diversity. He has 11 years of experience with Internet and related technologies. Michael has 7+ years in post-masters macro level practice building the capacity of organizations to meet their missions as owner/President of MAWMedia Consulting & Development, Inc. MAWMedia has consulted with not-for-profits, membership organizations, and educational units to which it brings research-based practice in organizational development utilizing technology to maximize capacity.

Michael's formal training is in Social Work focusing in administration and other macro issues including organizational and community development, and innovation. His dissertation research focused on the process of innovation in social work schools and educational institutions overall. In addition to research in educational practice, he examines adult development, prevention education, resilience, and many facets of not-for-profit organizational process including fundraising, evaluation, and technology integration. Michael is a member of many broader-based associations that fit his interest areas including the Association of Fundraising Professionals, Association for Supervision and Curriculum Development, Association for Metro/Urban Ministry, and Computer Professionals for Social Responsibility.

Preface:
Contemporary Issues of Care

The Life Care Institute of the University of Texas-Austin School of Social Work is proud to contribute this volume on contemporary issues in giving care. Focusing on caregiving situations across the life span, the purpose of the Institute is to use research findings to shape curriculum and to improve social work practice and services. The intergenerational Life Care Institute is based on a wellness philosophy congruent with a strengths-based approach to social work practice. Recognizing diversity among families in a variety of caregiving situations, the Institute strives to overcome racial, ethnic, and cultural disparities in care.

The volume offers articles that encompass research findings on human behavior and the social environment necessary to inform social work practice at the individual, family, and community level. The role of the social worker in processing and integrating assessment information to arrive at family-centered and community-based interventions is explored.

Roberta R. Greene, Editor

[Haworth co-indexing entry note]: "Preface" Greene, Roberta R. Co-published simultaneously in *Journal of Human Behavior in the Social Environment* (The Haworth Press, Inc.) Vol. 14, No. 1/2, 2006, p. xxvii; and: *Contemporary Issues of Care* (ed: Roberta R. Greene) The Haworth Press, Inc., 2006, p. xxiii. Single or multiple copies of this article are available for a fee from The Haworth Document Delivery Service [1-800-HAWORTH, 9:00 a.m. - 5:00 p.m. (EST). E-mail address: docdelivery@haworthpress.com].

Available online at http://jhbse.haworthpress.com

Chapter 1

Introduction:
The Functional-Age Model
of Intergenerational Treatment

Roberta R. Greene
Sally Hill Jones

SUMMARY. This chapter introduces the Functional-Age Model and its recent modifications. It describes how FAM is used to assess and intervene with families of later years who are experiencing potentially stressful caregiving situations. The chapter also presents research on interventions designed for caregivers. doi:10.1300/J137v14n01_01 *[Article copies available for a fee from The Haworth Document Delivery Service: 1-800-HAWORTH. E-mail address: <docdelivery@haworthpress.com> Website: <http://www.HaworthPress.com> © 2006 by The Haworth Press, Inc. All rights reserved.]*

KEYWORDS. Family of later years, family therapy, caregiving, caregiver support

This volume explores human behavior and research content pertinent to various caregiving situations across the life course. Authors apply the

---

[Haworth co-indexing entry note]: "Introduction: The Functional-Age Model of Intergenerational Treatment." Greene, Roberta R., and Sally Hill Jones. Co-published simultaneously in *Journal of Human Behavior in the Social Environment* (The Haworth Press, Inc.) Vol. 14, No. 1/2, 2006, pp. 1-30; and: *Contemporary Issues of Care* (ed: Roberta R. Greene)The Haworth Press, Inc., 2006, pp. 1-30. Single or multiple copies of this article are available for a fee from The Haworth Document Delivery Service [1-800-HAWORTH, 9:00 a.m. - 5:00 p.m. (EST). E-mail address: docdelivery@haworthpress.com].

Available online at http://jhbse.haworthpress.com
© 2006 by The Haworth Press, Inc. All rights reserved.
doi:10.1300/J137v14n01_01

1

functional-age model of intergenerational therapy (FAM) to address the interplay between the care recipient's biopsychosocial and spiritual functioning and the adaptive capacity of the family/caregiver. The mutual interdependence among family members and the dynamic development of family structure and organization are examined. The function of various social systems as caregiving entities is also considered. The role of the social worker in processing and integrating assessment information to arrive at family-centered and community-based interventions is explored.

This chapter re-introduces FAM (Greene, [1986] 2000) and its recent modifications. It describes how FAM is used to assess and intervene with families of later years who are experiencing potentially stressful caregiving situations. The chapter also presents research on interventions designed for caregivers. The illustration of the model in various situations and contexts is provided throughout the volume.

THE SCOPE OF FAMILY CAREGIVING

The family remains the primary caregiving institution in the United States. These unpaid caregivers are an estimated 44.4 million Americans, representing 21 percent of the U.S. population eighteen years or older (U.S. Census, 2002). In recent studies of those forty-five and older, almost one in five surveyed indicated they were involved in providing personal care such as bathing and dressing to a family member or friend with a disability (AARP, 2003). Unpaid care of family and friends is valued at an estimated 257 billion dollars a year (Arno, 2002).

About 70 percent of caregivers help only one person (NAC, 2003). However, the larger and modified extended families of African-American and Latino families may exhibit cultural differences in family reciprocity important to social work practice (Tennstedt & Chang, 1998). For example, they are more likely than the general population to live with the care recipient and to provide care for more than one person (NAC/AARP, 1997; NAC/AA, 1999). In general, African-American caregivers are more likely to say they spend nine to twenty hours a week providing care than white non-Hispanic caregivers. They also are more likely to remain working than are white caregivers, finding care a financial burden. Latina caregivers are more likely to live with the person they care for than white caregivers, continuing to give care for relatives in serious conditions. Asian caregivers are generally well-educated, with 61 percent having college degrees. Their reported higher household incomes present less of an economic burden than other ethnic groups.

Nearly half (48 percent) of all caregivers provide eight hours or less of care per week but one in five provide more than forty hours of care per week. The average length of caregiving is 4.3 years (NAC & AARP, 2004). Research has made profiles of care providers and care recipients available: Many caregivers who are helping relatives have multiple roles managing work and caregiving responsibilities. Although the typical caregiver is a forty-year-old woman who provides more than twenty hours of care each week to her mother, a sizable number of caregivers are men: nearly four in ten. Care recipients are often female (65 percent) with eight in ten care recipients age fifty years or older.

More than a third (37 percent) of caregivers have no one else helping them give care. Only four in ten (41 percent) of caregivers use paid services from an aide or nurse, hired housekeeper, or others during a twelve-month period. Formal services are more common in urban areas where it is more readily available. Finally, people may need care for various reasons including help with physical or mental illness, developmental disabilities, or at end-of-life. However, it is important to realize that most people who require caregiving are among the frail elderly. In 2002, there were 69.6 million U. S. citizens over fifty-five years of age. Advances in medical care will contribute to their longevity and a sharp increase in the older population. As the family has become reduced in size, the responsibility for looking after older family members will fall on fewer adult children for longer periods of time (Rapp & Chao, 2000). Attention to this cohort as they age will test the viability and high solidarity of intergenerational family supports (Greene, 2005).

FUNCTIONAL-AGE MODEL
OF INTERGENERATIONAL TREATMENT:
THEORETICAL BACKGROUND

From the very inception of the profession, social workers have viewed the family as the major unit of their attention and sought avenues of intervention to enhance family life (Hartman, 1978). In the 1940s, as psychodynamic theory came to the fore, caseworkers increasingly emphasized individual treatment. It was not until well after World War II that practitioners once again realized that to effectively enhance client functioning, it is necessary to consider his or her role within the family system.

By the 1960s, family interventions once again were taking hold. Theorists such as Nathan Ackerman (1972) argued that the family needed to be understood as an emotional system. From this perspective, family treatment centered on helping members develop insight and gain a positive emotional therapeutic experience. At the same time, another group of family theorists became interested in systems thinking, emphasizing the structural and behavioral nature of family relationships (Bowen, 1971; Minuchin, 1974). Therapeutic interventions involved changes in the family as a group and the role of individuals within that group context (Greene, [1986] 2000).

Ironically, general systems theory is actually not a theory at all, but "a working hypothesis, the main function of which is to provide a theoretical model for explaining, predicting, and controlling phenomena" (Bertalanffy, 1962, p. 17). Models may be described as a way of looking at and thinking about selected aspects of reality that are at a higher level of abstraction than a theory (Anderson & Carter, [1984] 1990). Because of this level of abstraction, systems theory provided social workers with a means of simultaneously understanding the interrelatedness of several complex variables including physical/biological, social, and psychological functioning. Thus general systems theory became a conceptual tool used in FAM to help study and explain such complex phenomena as role behavior and gender identity, by considering a number of contributing variables.

Although the family therapy movement was an important feature of child guidance work, it was not until the 1980s that models were developed to work with the family of later years (Greene, first edition, 1986; 2000; Silverstone & Burack-Weiss, 1983). FAM (Figure 1) adopted both the insight-oriented and structural change thinking of the family therapy movement. As an intergenerational model, it assumes that families are characterized by connecting ties based on loyalty and reciprocal indebtedness. *Indebtedness* or obligations that come out of commitment to one another might be expressed through visiting or physical caregiving (Boszormenyi-Nagy & Spark, 1973). Indebtedness varies from one family to another and in some instances may be denied or expressed by feelings of anger about past "wrongs." In other families, loyalty may be fostered by the cultural norms involving familism.

FIGURE 1

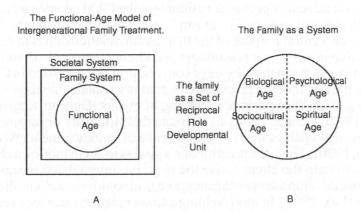

The Functional-Age Model of
Intergenerational Family Treatment.

The Family as a System

A

B

SHIFTS IN HUMAN BEHAVIOR PARADIGMS: AUGMENTING FAM

Ecological-Systems Beginnings

Since its inception in 1986, shifts in emphasis in human behavior theory have brought about modifications to FAM. For example, when FAM was originated, systems theory was prevalent and played an important role in defining caregiving situations. It has been used as an integrating tool in assessing an older adult's biopsychosocial functional capacity within a family and community context (Greene, 2000; Greene, Kropf, & MacNair, 1994; Martin & O'Connor, 1989). Combined with the ecological perspective, it has drawn attention to the need for the social worker to examine the multiple systems in which caregiving occurs.

In addition, FAM addresses the role of various social systems and the part they play in supporting the care recipient and caregiver. For example, the African-American pastor may be the primary caregiver for parishioners with mental illness (see Farris article). Or students from grand-parent-headed families–at any one time, 10 percent of U.S. grandparents (Fuller-Thomson, Minkler, and Driver, 1997)–constitute an increasing proportion of students in schools (Rothenberg, 1996). FAM suggests that the extent to which these various systems collaborate with formal social services is critical to successful caregiving.

Postmodern Influence

With the advent of postmodern thinking, the FAM adopted additional theoretical points of view. For example, postmodern practitioners maintain that the central purpose of the therapeutic relationship is to create a partnership in which the practitioner and client create new meanings of adverse events through dialogue or conversation. As discussed in Greene (1999), the postmodern practitioner's goal is to obtain client-generated meaning to enable a positive reframing of events (Duncan, Solovey, & Rusk, 1992). Clients' ability to re-create their life story or rename their problem also enables them to gain a sense of empowerment (White & Epston, 1990). Thus, the practitioner's goal is to set in motion a change process to help the client revise the negative internalized meaning of problems, develop a sense of agency, and find solutions–a client-directed therapy (Lax, 1992). In short, helping a client make sense of the events on his or her own terms allows the client to integrate the critical event into his or her life story (Hallberg, 2001). Restorying can lead people to have confidence that their environment is somewhat predictable and explicable (Antonovsky & Sourani, 1988).

This knowledge has resulted in important changes in the model involving the use of interventions derived from postmodern approaches, such as narrative and solution-focused therapies. These additions give further emphasis to listening to a particular client story, understanding his or her local, culturally specific experiences, and providing more opportunities following adverse events (Greene, 1999; Greene & Blundo, 1999). Research on risk and resilience suggest that clients better resolve negative events when they are able to derive some positive meaning for themselves or others (Thoits, 1995). Thus, FAM currently offers a wider range of intervention strategies, which will be discussed throughout the volume.

Stress Theory and Caregivers' Burden

During the 1980s and 1990s, the work of Elaine Brody (1985) put forth the idea that family care for older relatives was a normative family life transition. Studies conducted from this perspective revealed that having a dependent elderly relative had an impact on all family members. Researchers began to examine the social and emotional cost of care to family caregivers, prompting an interest in attitudes towards caregiving and caregiver burden (Tables 1, 2).

Caregiver burden is associated with the financial, physical, psychological, and social demands of caregiving (George & Gwyther, 1986). Caregiver burden may be *objective burden,* events and activities associated with negative caregiving experience; or *subjective burden*, emotional re-

TABLE 1. The Burden Interview

1. I feel resentful of other relatives who could but who do not do things for my spouse.
2. I feel that my spouse makes request which I perceive to be over and above what she/he needs.
3. Because of my involvement with my spouse, I don't have enough time for myself.
4. I feel stressed between trying to give to my spouse as well as to other family responsibilities, job, etc.
5. I feel embarrassed over my spouse's behavior.
6. I feel guilty about my interactions with my spouse.
7. I feel that I don't do as much for my spouse as I could or should.
8. I feel angry about my interactions with my spouse.
9. I feel that in the past I haven't done as much for my spouse as I could have or should have.
10. I feel nervous or depressed about my interactions with my spouse.
11. I feel that my spouse currently affects my relationships with other family members and friends in a negative way.
12. I feel resentful about my interactions with my spouse.
13. I am afraid of what the future holds for my spouse.
14. I feel pleased about my interactions with my spouse.
15. It's painful to watch my spouse age.
16. I feel useful in my interactions with my spouse.
17. I feel my spouse is dependent.
18. I feel strained in my interactions with my spouse.
19. I feel that my health has suffered because of my involvement with my spouse.
20. I feel that I am contributing to the well-being of my spouse.
21. I feel that the present situation with my spouse doesn't allow me as much privacy as I'd like.
22. I feel that my social life has suffered because of my involvement with my spouse.
23. I wish that my spouse and I had a better relationship.
24. I feel that my spouse doesn't appreciate what I do for him/her as much as I would like.
25. I feel uncomfortable when I have friends over.
26. I feel that my spouse tries to manipulate me.
27. I feel that my spouse seems to expect me to take care of him/her as if I were the only one she/he could depend on.
28. I feel that I don't have enough money to support my spouse in addition to the rest of our expenses.
29. I feel that I would like to be able to provide more money to support my spouse than I am now.

Source: Zarit, S.H., Reever, K.E. and Bach-Peterson, J.(1980). Relatives of the impaired elderly: Correlates of feelings of burden. *Gerontologist, 20*(6), 649-655. Reprinted with permission.

actions of the caregiver including worry, anxiety, frustration and fatigue (Pinquart & Sorensen, 2003). The phenomenon of caregiver burden is often understood using stress theory. Such theory suggests caregiving responsibilities have the potential to negatively affect the mental and physical well-being of the caregiver, be disruptive to marital or family relationships, or cause problems in meeting work and other social responsibilities (Pearlin, Aneshensel, & Leblanc, 1997).

Research models from the stress perspective make the distinction between primary and secondary stressors. *Primary stressors* are those asso-

TABLE 2. Revised Perceived Caregiver Burden Scale, PCB-13: Items and Subscales

Variable	Factor Loading	Error Term
Subscale 1: Impact on Finances (Mean = 9.00, SD = 3.09)		
30. My financial resources are adequate to pay for things that are required for caregiving	.579	.802
31. It is difficult to pay for the elder's health needs and services	.941	.339
32. Caring for the elder has put a financial strain on the family	.951	.308
33. If I could afford it, I would find some other way to care for the elder	.798	.603
Subscale 2: Impact on Work Schedule (Mean = 6.95, SD = 2.32)		
11. My activities are centered around the care for the elder	.756	.654
12. I have to stop in the middle of my work or activities to provide care	.904	.428
13. I have eliminated things from my schedule since caring for the elder	.961	.276
Subscale 3: Sense of Entrapment (Mean = 11.5, SD = 4.08)		
26. Since caring for the elder, sometimes I hate the way life has turned out	.845	.536
27. I feel I was forced into caring for the elder	.844	.537
28. I feel trapped by my caring role	.947	.322
29. At this time in my life, I don't think I should be caring for the elder	.905	.426
30. Caring for the elder has made me miserable.	.966	.259
31. Just when I thought times were going to be easier for me, I have to be a caregiver	.961	.277

Note: PCB-13 Subscale Item means and standard deviations are for N = 150 participants. EQS standardization factor loadings and error terms are shown for the sample of caregivers.
Adapted from: Gupta (1999). The Revised Caregiver Burden Scale: A preliminary evaluation. *Research on Social Work Practice*, 4, 483-507.

ciated with the necessities of the caregiving role, such as coping with the behaviors associated with dementia. *Secondary stressors* are more peripheral to or outside the caregiving role and may involve social or workplace issues. The practitioner's purpose in using stress models is to better understand a person's reactions when exposed to serious life problems. Understanding may also be gained about *stress proliferation*– the additive or cumulative experience of more stress when caregiving demands increase. (Figure 2).

In addition, further information about the impact of caregiving and the increased recognition that informal caregiving is a typical family experience have moved both practitioners and theorists to seek interventions that might alleviate caregiver stress (Toseland & Rossiter, 1996). Such

FIGURE 2. Stress Proliferation

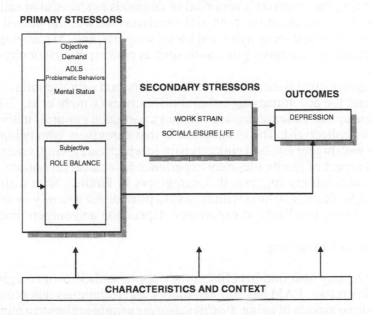

Adapted from: Pearlin, Aneshensel, and Leblanc (1997).

interventions attempt to improve the adjustment of caregivers to increased role demands, using appraisal as a means of reducing negative affect (Rapp & Chau, 2000).

As the client's story unfolds, the practitioner listens to how the client appraises a stressful event: *Appraisal* involves determining whether a client perceives a demand as a threat, loss or challenge; and whether a demand is perceived as controllable or not (Lazarus & Folkman, 1984). How an event is appraised varies with a client's social group status, role demands or conflicts, and belief systems or personal values. The appraisal process may have several outcomes such as having a greater appreciation of life, taking little for granted, or being motivated to live life differently (Janoff-Bulman & Berger, 2000).

Another stress and coping model was developed by Lazarus and Folkman (1984). The model included (1) examining how contextual variables such as gender, age, caregiver's health and relationship of the caregiver to care recipient affect care; (2) exploring the demands on the caregiver, including the extent of disability of the care recipient; (3) understanding the caregiver's appraisal of demands as stressful or satisfying; (4) learning about the potential mediators between appraisal and outcomes such as coping styles and social supports; and (5) realizing the consequences of caregiving demands such as poor emotional or physical health.

Caregiver stress is increasingly being understood with attention to ethnicity and the accompanying cultural differences (Knight et al., 2002). This conceptualization addresses whether a particular culture is individualistic or collectivist. The assumption is that caregivers who belong to groups with higher levels of collectivism–in which caregiving is seen as a natural aspect of family life–may experience less caregiver burden. Research increasingly suggests that caregivers in families with a strong sense of *familism*, a natural willingness to provide for a family member, caregivers are less likely to experience depression and burden (ibid.).

Benefits in Caregiving

People may also find benefits as they appraise their own caregiving story. Therefore, FAM has adopted theory and techniques that promote the positive aspects of aging. *Positive aspects of aging* refers to a number of concepts dealing with individual and family strengths. For example, Walsh (1998; 1999) has pointed out that families have a variety of adaptive mechanisms to help them successfully meet the challenges of later life. Antonovsky (1998) used the phrase *salutogenesis orientation* to describe his philosophy of how people naturally use their resources to strive for health. Similarly, gerontologists, such as Atchley (1999), used the term *continuity strategies* to refer to the means that older adults take to maintain life satisfaction despite disability.

In addition, Greene (2001) has advanced a resilience-based orientation, a theory that builds on social work's strengths perspective and examines what factors contribute to successful outcomes in the face of a crisis. In support of a positive resilience approach, Riley (2007) has contended that it is best for practitioners to explore client attitudes for information about psychological well-being, benefit, or resiliency of the caregiving experience. She went on to state that "the idea that caregiving is *only* a burden does not give credence to how people benefit from adversity, thus skewing perceptions of the caregiving experience and limiting the selection of strengths-based interventions" (p. 252).

Other positive aging concepts that are increasingly being applied to older adults include successful aging and resilience (Rowe & Kahn,

1998). *Successful aging* consists of three major factors: (1) Avoiding disease by adopting a prevention orientation; (2) engaging in life by continuing social involvement; and (3) maintaining high cognitive and physical functioning through ongoing activity. Crowther et al. (2002) have expanded the conceptualization of successful aging expanded to include positive spirituality.

According to Hodge (2005), the recognition of spirituality as important in helping some people to deal with life challenges allows practitioners to integrate spirituality into clinical dialogue for those clients. Greene and Conrad (2002) make a distinction between spirituality, referring to an existential relationship with a higher being; and religion encompassing more formal rituals, beliefs, and practices of a religious community. Spiritual and/or religious experiences when combined with caregiving relationships have been found to sustain families in difficult caregiving situations (Pierce, Lydon, & Yang, 2001).

ASSESSMENT AND THE INTERGENERATIONAL FUNCTIONAL-AGE MODEL

Biopsychosocial-Spiritual Assessment

The functional age model was originally intended to be used to guide a biopsychosocial spiritual assessment of the older adult. Because the older adult often has a complex, chronic illness such as dementia, practitioners want to design a system of care with goals delineated by family caregivers, recipients, and clinicians (Bradley et al., 2000). This allows for clients' input regarding what is appropriate to their own well-being. As discussed (p.15), FAM may be used as a guide to accomplish this task with older adults and their families and is applied with other populations throughout the volume.

Functional age assessment involves an understanding of the biopsychosocial-spiritual behaviors that affect a person's ability/competence to perform behaviors central to everyday life. *Biological factors* are related to functional capacity and include health, physical capacity, or vital life-limiting organ systems; *psychological factors* encompass an individual's affect state or mood, cognitive or mental status, and their behavioral dimensions; *sociocultural aspects* to consider involve the cultural, political, and economic aspects of life events (Greene, 2000). *Spiritual factors* may include a person's relationship with his or her faith/religious community and or an inner system of beliefs, discovering what contributes to a person's ability to transcend the immediate situation and find meaning in seemingly meaningless events.

Biological facts to remember are that older adults are less likely to have an acute sense of smell, touch, vision, and hearing. Psychological facts to remember when conducting assessment involve prior mental health conditions. Older adults may have a history of tiredness, loss of interest and appetite, weight loss, or inability to sleep. They may be disoriented to time and place or not be able to take stock of their situation. Social functioning following an adverse event is related to how a person has made role transitions across his or her lifetime. Social events across the life course may be *normative*, referring to events that most people experience over their lifetime or *nonnormative*, encompassing situations that are not expected to occur and are experienced by an entire cohort such as the Great Depression, the Holocaust, or September 11. Spiritual assessment factors may involve gathering a history of religious traditions, spiritual beliefs, and public rituals such as baptism or bar mitzvah (Hodge, 2001). Spiritual assessment information also reveals possible community support networks.

Family Assessment

The functional-age model of intergenerational family treatment can be used to examine caregiving risk and well-being from a systems perspective. FAM is an approach used to assess and intervene when promoting a family's caregiving capacity. The model suggests that the social worker understand that

> A family is far more than a collection of individuals occupying a specific physical and psychological space together. Rather, it is a natural social system, with properties of its own, one that has evolved a set of rules, roles, a power structure, form of communication, and ways of negotiation and problem solving that allow various tasks to be performed effectively. (Goldenberg & Goldenberg, 2003, p. 3)

In family crisis situations, such as caregiving may be, the practitioner uses assessment and treatment strategies that take into account the developmental issues and the changing biopsychosocial needs of a family member (Figure 1). The practitioner must realize that, throughout the life cycle, family members attempt to negotiate the changes in a member's functioning, shifting and altering their relationships to meet the needs of all. That is, a family is a mutually dependent unit with interdependent pasts and futures. This movement through the life cycle is called *family development*. To accomplish caregiving tasks, a *differentiation* of family roles within a family occurs (Greene, 2000). The extent to which a family is experiencing burden and reward can be assessed using the Caregiver Burden Scale and Farran's Attitude Scales (see Table 3).

To make this assessment, the social worker explores the functional capacity of the person needing care: What are the factors affecting his or her biological, psychological, and sociocultural capacity? How is he or she able to perform activities of daily living? The model also suggests that family be understood as a *social system*, referring to how a group of people interact and influence each other; a *set of reciprocal roles*, involving the behavioral expectations members have for each other; and as a *developmental unit*, encompassing how the family faces life transitions. In essence, systems thinking allows the practitioner to understand that as individual family members interact, patterns such as the division of labor, authority structure, and rules for behavior emerge and evolve over time (Greene, 1999).

Family assessment may also involve an assessment of the family members' resilience, or the fit between family strengths and their specific circumstances, the path a family follows as it adapts and prospers in the face of stress (Hawley & DeHaan, 1996, p. 293).

According to Walsh (1998, 1999), a family's ability to withstand and rebound from disruptive life challenges can be assessed by examining its functioning in three domains: (1) belief systems, including values and attitudes about how they should act [in caregiving situations]; (2) organizational patterns, referring to expectations for behavior and structures to carry out stressful [caregiving] tasks; and (3) communication patterns, encompassing the exchange of information in the family (Table 4).

Similarly, McCubbin et al. (1994) developed a model of family adaptation that can be used to assess how a family is appraising a crisis situation (see Figure 3). The practitioner explores five levels of family functioning: (1) the *family schema*, referring to the general shared values, beliefs, goals, expectations, and priorities, shaped and adopted by the family unit, thus formulating a generalized informational structure against and through which information and experiences are compared, sifted, and processed; (2) *family coherence*, encompassing the motivational and cognitive bases for transforming the family's potential resources into actual resources; (3) *family paradigms*, including shared beliefs and expectations that guide *specific* patterns of functioning around *specific* aspects

FIGURE 3. Focus on Appraisal Processes in the Resiliency Model of Family Adjustment and Adaptation

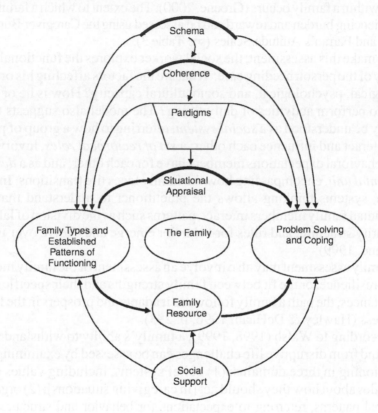

From "Ethnicity, Schema, and Coherence: Appraisal Processes for Families in Crisis," by H.I. McCubbin, E.A. Thompson, A.I. Thompson, K.M. Elver, and M.A. McCubbin, (1994). In *Stress, Coping and Health in Families: Sense of Coherency and Resiliency* (p. 44). Thousand Oaks, CA: Sage Publications. Reprinted by permission of Sage Publications, Inc.

of family life such as work and family, spiritual/ religious orientation, or caregiving; (4) *situational appraisal*, involving the family's shared assessment of their ability to manage a stressor, the hardship created by the stressor, and the demand upon the family system to change some established patterns of functioning; and (5) *Stressor appraisal*, referring to the family's definition of the stressor and its severity, which is the initial level of family assessment (pp. 43-46).

TABLE 3. Attitudes Toward Caregiving

This questionnaire contains a number of statements related to opinions and feelings about yourself, your impaired relative, and your caregiving experience. Read each statement carefully, then indicate the extent to which you agree or disagree with the statement. Circle one of the alternative categories.

	SA STRONGLY AGREE	A AGREE	U UNDECIDED	D DISAGREE	SD STRONGLY DISAGREE
Loss/Powerless Subscale (LP)					
1. I miss the communication and companionship that my family member and I had in the past.	SA	A	U	D	SD
2. I miss my family member's ability to love me as he/she did in the past.	SA	A	U	D	SD
3. I am sad about the mental and physical changes I see in my relative.	SA	A	U	D	SD
4. I miss the little things my relative and I did together in the past.	SA	A	U	D	SD
5. I am sad about losing the person I once knew.	SA	A	U	D	SD
6. I miss not being able to be spontaneous in my life because of caring for my relative.	SA	A	U	D	SD
12. I miss not having more time for other family members and/or friends.	SA	A	U	D	SD
13. I have no hope; I am clutching at straws.	SA	A	U	D	SD
18. I miss our previous social life.	SA	A	U	D	SD
19. I have no sense of joy.	SA	A	U	D	SD
24. I miss not being able to travel.	SA	A	U	D	SD
25. I wish I were free to lead a life of my own.	SA	A	U	D	SD
30. I miss having given up my job or other personal interests to take care of my family member.	SA	A	U	D	SD
31. I feel trapped by my relative's illness.	SA	A	U	D	SD
34. We had goals for the future but they just folded up because of my relative's dementia.	SA	A	U	D	SD
36. I miss my relative's sense of humor.	SA	A	U	D	SD
37. I wish I could 'run away.	SA	A	U	D	SD
41. I feel that the quality of my life has decreased.	SA	A	U	D	SD
7. My situation feels endless.	SA	A	U	D	SD

15

TABLE 3 (continued)

	SA STRONGLY AGREE	A AGREE	U UNDECIDED	D DISAGREE	SD STRONGLY DISAGREE
Provisional Meaning (PM)					
8. I enjoy having my relative with me: I would miss it if he/she were gone.	SA	A	U	D	SD
9. I count my blessings.	SA	A	U	D	SD
10. Caring for my relative gives my life a purpose and a sense of meaning.	SA	A	U	D	SD
14. I cherish the past memories and experiences that my relative and I have had.	SA	A	U	D	SD
15. I am a strong person.	SA	A	U	D	SD
16. Caregiving makes me feel good that I am helping.	SA	A	U	D	SD
20. The hugs and "I love you" from my relative make it worth it all.	SA	A	U	D	SD
21. I'm a fighter.	SA	A	U	D	SD
22. I am glad I am here to care for my relative.	SA	A	U	D	SD
26. Talking with others who are close to me restores my faith in my own abilities.	SA	A	U	D	SD
27. Even though there are difficult things in my life, I look forward to the future.	SA	A	U	D	SD
28. Caregiving has helped me learn new things about myself.	SA	A	U	D	SD
32. Each year, regardless of the quality, is a blessing.	SA	A	U	D	SD
33. I would not have chosen the situation I'm in, but I get satisfaction out of providing care.	SA	A	U	D	SD
38. Every day is a blessing.	SA	A	U	D	SD
39. This is my place: I have to make the best out of it.	SA	A	U	D	SD
40. I am much stronger than I think.	SA	A	U	D	SD
42. I start each day knowing we will have a beautiful day together.	SA	A	U	D	SD
43. Caregiving has made me a stronger and better person.	SA	A	U	D	SD

TABLE 3 (continued)

Ultimate Meaning (UM)					
11. The Lord won't give you more than you can handle.	SA	A	U	D	SD
17. I believe in the power of prayer: without it I couldn't do this.	SA	A	U	D	SD
23. I believe that: the Lord will provide.	SA	A	U	D	SD
29. I have faith that the good Lord has reasons for this.	SA	A	U	D	SD
35. God is good.	SA	A	U	D	SD

Farran, C., Miller, B., Kaufman, J., Donner, D., & Fogg, L. (1999). Finding meaning through caregiving: Development of an instrument for family caregivers of persons with Alzheimer's disease. Journal of Clinical Psychology, 55(9), 1107-1125. Reprinted with permission of John Wiley & Sons, Inc.

TABLE 4. Key Processes in Family Resilience

Belief Systems

Making meaning of adversity
- Affiliative value: resilience as relationally based
- Family life cycle orientation: normalizing, contextualizing adversity and distress
- Sense of coherence: crisis as meaning, comprehensible, manageable challenge
- Appraisal of crisis, distress, and recovery: facilitative versus constraining beliefs

Positive outlook
- Active initiative and perseverance
- Courage and en-courage-ment
- Sustaining hope, optimistic view: confidence in overcoming odds
- Focusing on strengths and potential
- Mastering the possible; accepting what can't be changed

Transcendence and spirituality
- Larger values, purpose
- Spirituality; faith, communion, rituals
- Inspiration: envisioning new possibilities, creativity, heroes
- Transformation: learning and growth from adversity

Organizational Patterns

Flexibility
- Capacity to change: rebounding, reorganizing, adapting to fit challenges over time
- Counterbalancing by stability: continuity, dependability through disruption

Connectedness
- Mutual support, collaboration, and commitment
- Respect for individual needs, differences, and boundaries
- Strong leadership: nurturing, protecting, guiding children and vulnerable members
- Varied family forms: cooperative parenting/caregiving teams
- Couple/coparent relationship: equal partners
- Seeking reconnection, reconciliation of troubled relationships

Social and economic resources
- Mobilizing extended kin and social support; community networks
- Building financial security; balancing work and family strains

Communication Processes

Clarity
- Clear, consistent messages (words and actions)
- Clarification of ambiguous situation; truth-seeking/truth-speaking

Open emotional expression
- Sharing range of feelings (joy and pain; hopes and fears)
- Mutual empathy; tolerance for differences
- Responsibility for own feelings, behavior: avoid blaming
- Pleasurable interactions: humor

Collaborative problem solving
- Creative brainstorming; resourcefulness
- Shared decision making: negotiation, fairness, reciprocity
- Conflict resolution
- Focusing on goals: taking concrete steps, building on success, learning from failure
- Proactive stance: reinventing problems, crises; preparing for future challenges

---

Ecological Assessment

Ecological assessments involve understanding the role that various social systems play in caregiving situations. This multisystemic approach allows practitioners to work with small-scale *microsystems*, such as families and peer groups; the connection between systems, known as *mesosystems*, such as the family and health care systems; *exosystems*, the connections between systems that do not directly involve the person, such as Social Security and Medicare; and *macrosystems*, or overarching large-scale systems, such as legal, political, and value systems about the role of informal versus formal caregiving.

According to Greene (1999), the following principles can be used to develop an ecological perspective on assessment:

- View the person and environment as inseparable.
- Be an equal partner in the helping process.
- Examine transactions between the person and environment by assessing all levels of systems affecting a client's adaptiveness. Assess life situations and transactions that induce high stress levels.
- Attempt to enhance a client's personal competence through positive relationships and life experiences.
- Seek interventions that affect the goodness-of-fit among a client and his or her environment at all systems levels.
- Focus on mutually sought solutions and client empowerment.

INTERVENTIONS AND THE FUNCTIONAL AGE MODEL OF INTERGENERATIONAL TREATMENT

FAM: Family Systems Interventions

The FAM model is in the eclectic tradition involving a wide range of interventions ranging from life review therapy, family counseling, and linkages to provide supplemental family supports (Greene, [1986] 2000). Practitioners are encouraged to:

- Promote the adaptive capacity of the older adult and his or her family;
- Help members adapt to changes in an older adults' biopsychosocial functioning;
- Counteract the effects of depletion and loss;

- Mobilize the family system on behalf of the older adult;
- Deal with the stress and strain in caregiving;
- Seek means to enable the older adult to remain autonomous as possible (or the least restrictive environment);
- Promote positive interdependence among generations;
- Deal with the dynamics of dependency, loyalty, loss, and anger; and
- Use resources from an ecological perspective (p. 138).

These treatment goals were accomplished through six overlapping phases: (1) connecting with the client system; (2) determining the problems and issues; (3) reframing the problem to arrive at solutions; (4) setting mutual goals with the family; (5) evaluating progress and providing feedback, and (6) terminating.

Interventions: A Wellness Perspective

Since its inception, the model has been augmented with a wellness perspective associated with resiliency and the *positive psychology movement*–a science based on the idea that people are and can be taught to be resilient. In addition, the approach assumes that practitioners can instill hope and optimism ultimately promoting health and well-being (Ryff & Singer, 2002; Seligman, 2002). Positive psychologists center their attention on adaptive functioning, particularly taking into account how people maintain well-being despite various stumbling blocks or trauma. Techniques to accomplish well-being following adversity have been outlined in the REM (Resilience Enhancing Model) developed by Greene and Armenta (2007; Table 5).

Research: Special Intervention for Caregivers

Research is increasingly illuminating the efficacy of caregiver interventions. Intervention for caregivers has developed from general education and support programs to more specific skills training, so that the complexity of the caregiver's needs are being recognized (Bourgeois, Schulz, & Burgio, 1996). Current research is focusing on learning what specific interventions meet what specific needs, and tailoring intervention to specific groups of caregivers. Studies also indicate that a long-term, intensive, individually tailored, multicomponent intervention is more effective than brief, single-factor interventions (Clark et al., 2001; Mittelman et al., 1996; Coon, Gallagher-Thompson, & Thompson, 2003; Oswald et al., 1999).

TABLE 5. Intervention Strategies: The REM

Practitioners who use a resilience-based approach to social work practice,

- Acknowledge client loss, vulnerability, and future.
- Identify the client's source of stress.
- Recognize client stress.
- Stabilize or normalize the situation.
- Help clients take control.
- Provide resources for change.
- Promote client self-efficacy.
- Collaborate in client self-change.
- Strengthen a client's problem-solving abilities.
- Address positive emotions.
- Listen to client stories.
- Make meaning of client's critical events.
- Help clients find the benefits of adverse events.
- Assist clients in transcending the immediate situation.

Adapted from: Greene, R. R. & Armenta, K. (2007). The REM Model: Phase II–Practice Strategies. In R. R. Greene, *Social Work Practice: A Risk and Resilience Perspective*. Monterey, CA: Brooks/Cole.

Interventions can include individual and/or family counseling, case management, skills training, support groups, respite and day care services, and different combinations of these factors. Some programs include continuous availability of counselors to help caregivers and families deal with crises. Several examples of comprehensive programs exist in the literature (Reifler & Eisdorfer, 1980; Ferris et al., 1987; Mohide et al., 1990; Seltzer et al., 1987; Mittelman et al., 2003) and have shown significant reductions in caregiver depression, anger, insomnia, and anxiety, as well as increased ability to cope, quality of life, and longer time to institutionalization. Some studies show that more services bring about better results (Montgomery & Borgatta, 1989) while others show this may not be the case (Gray, 1983). Analysis of the effectiveness of different components is needed to determine which services are effective for which caregivers.

Individual and Family Counseling. Bourgeois et al. (1996) found individual and family counseling described only narrowly defined efforts from a variety of theoretical approaches, making it difficult to make generalizations about the efficacy of this approach. However, studies by Toseland and colleagues (1990) revealed greater gains for daughters and daughters-in-law in individual counseling as compared with group counseling.

Role changes are one aspect of the strains of family caregiving. Family interventions can be helpful for the family to manage these strains. Different theoretical approaches can be used. Marriott et al. (2000) had satisfactory results using a cognitive-behavioral family therapy approach with Alzheimer's caregivers.

Support Groups. The caregivers in Berg-Weger, Rubio, and Tebb's (2001) research mentioned caregiver support groups as a helpful but often an unmet need. However, much empirical evidence suggests support groups are not helpful (Lavoie, 1995). Gottlieb and Wolfe (2002) suggest identifying those who already effectively use their social support networks and therefore drop out of support groups, and those who do not have those networks. They also suggest support groups that have different foci for different needs, e.g., educational versus support. Likewise, in a review of caregiver interventions by Bourgeois et al. (1996), it was found that support groups provide information and informal support networking, but that more emphasis is needed on tailoring the support group format to the different needs and developmental timeline of caregivers.

Support groups have not been well-attended by ethnic minority caregivers. Henderson et al. (1993) reported on the successful use of a model for an Alzheimer's disease support group for African-American and Hispanic populations. They spent a great deal of time and effort developing the program, used extensive, active, and culturally sanctioned ways of recruitment for members, trained indigenous support group leaders, chose meeting locations that would be welcoming to the groups involved. The Hispanic group chose to speak in Spanish although almost all of the members were bilingual. Another adaptation of a support group involved a rural Mexican-American population (Gallagher-Thompson et al., 1996), in which a van picked up the support group members and drove them to the meeting site, with much of the support occurring during the transport.

Little research has been done on the effectiveness of support groups for men; however, one study indicates that they are helpful (Kaye & Applegate, 1993). Some authors found that dementia caregiving men did better in small, men-only groups that include discussion of concrete caregiving skills, educational components, and skills to manage emotions (Davies et al., 1986; Moseley, Davies, & Priddy, 1988; McFarland & Sanders, 2000). Lauderdale, D'Andrea and Coon (2003) found success with a cognitive-behavioral psychoeducational group format. Information about caregiving men of color is limited.

Diversity and Family Interventions. Szapocznik et al. (1997) developed a structural ecosystems approach for Hispanic/Latino families caring for someone with dementia. However, little research has been done in this area. Qualls (1997, 1999) reported two broad categories of issues: the impact of the caregiving on the family and the conflicts related to caregiving duties. Family meetings, focused on practical planning and behavior management, were differentiated from family therapy, which focuses on changes in the family patterns and interactions (Zarit & Edwards, 1996). For GLBT caregivers, family work may revolve around tensions between family-of-origin and partners in terms of decision-making.

Diversity and Community-Based Services. An example of an interorganizational community-based collaborative model of intervention for Latino dementia caregivers is "El Portal" (Aranda et al., 2003). A group of public, private and voluntary agencies involving community-based providers, grassroots groups, and elected officials successfully provided an array of culturally and linguistically competent services including outreach and education, a helpline, support groups, day care services, legal services, transportation, counseling, in-home respite, diagnostic consultations, and case management. The authors suggested services aimed specifically at the caregiver including grief work, cognitive-behavioral treatment programs, indigenous mental health interventions, retreats and weekend getaways, and spiritual consultations.

A model suggested by Coon and Zeiss (2003) for GLBT dementia caregivers, the SURE 2 Framework, combined cognitive-behavioral techniques with grassroots support groups. This model includes education, support, and cognitive-behavioral strategies such as reframing.

Respite Services. Respite care research demonstrates only modest benefits, and Bourgeois et al. (1996) suggested that respite needs to be more frequent and for longer periods of time, as well as the need to explore the different levels of caregiver acceptance of respite earlier in the caregiving process. Gottlieb and Johnson (2000) found mixed results for respite services, perhaps because the caregivers did not use their time to get effective relief for themselves.

Skills Training. Skills training has had significant positive results when well defined, practiced, and used to solve real-life difficulties. These skills are sometimes aimed at managing care recipient behaviors, but can also result in caregiver improvements, (Burgio et al., 2002; Teri et al., 1997). These skills can include educational instruction, role-playing, corrective feedback, and data collection in order to manage patient behaviors (Pinkston & Linsk, 1988; Pinkston, Linsk, & Young, 1988). In addition, problem-solving strategies, including an increase in pleasant activities, resulted in less stress and depression and increased morale (Lovett & Gallagher, 1988). Skills in managing anger and hostility about caregiving (Gallagher-Thompson & Devries, 1994) have shown success. Teaching the caregiver skills in managing her thoughts, feelings and behaviors in response to caregiving is helpful (Gallagher-Thompson et al., 2000; Oswalt et al., 1999). Relaxation training resulted in significant decreases in caregiver anxiety and depression (Greene & Monahan, 1989). Making these skills programs culturally relevant is needed and has begun to be addressed (Burgio et al., 2002; Gallagher-Thompson et al., 2001; Gallagher-Thompson et al., 2002). Kaye and Applegate (1993) suggested approaching male dementia caregivers with attempts to combine their "workmanship and nurturant" qualities. Educational approaches are often more acceptable to those who view the illness of their care recipient as a stigma, as well as to those caregivers who equate outside help as a failure on their part.

Empowerment. An empowerment approach assumes individual strengths and capacities, and facilitates the client to use these to bring about change in the environmental resources that will impact upon the client's needs. Clients who are from marginalized and oppressed groups have many internal, family, and community strengths and capacities, along with the vulnerabilities that accompany oppression, powerlessness and lack of access to resources (Chadiha et al., 2004). African-American women are often seen as central in their families and perform several caretaking roles. As Krieger et al. (1993) suggested, "Conspicuously absent is any caring source for black women themselves" (p. 90).

Chadiha et al. (2004) suggest three empowerment strategies for working with African-American female caregivers. One is using group support to raise consciousness through a narrative or storytelling approach, which serves many functions. It helps women know they are not alone, helps them restory their experiences from a strengths perspective and fosters collaboration. The women take turns telling a personal story about a recent caregiving experience, which the other members can then comment or build. This has also worked well with Latino groups (Gutierrez & Ortega, 1991). The second strategy is concrete problem-solving skills, tied to the specific problems identified by the caregivers. Finally, the authors recommend the strategy of teaching advocacy skills and mobilizing resources, assisting the caregivers in techniques of self-advocacy as well as advocacy on a macro level.

Technology Aids. More is being done with the use of advanced technology to complement existing programs for caregivers. These include psychoeducational videotape programs, email support, on-line support and psychoeducational groups, web-based information, and conference calling within a network of informal and formal supports. Extensive telephone-based intervention systems have included check-in calls, automated advice on handling difficult behaviors, an individualized recorded message for the care recipient to disrupt difficult behaviors, voice-mail connections to a support group and geriatric care specialists, as well as automated alerts when call patterns indicate need for intervention. One website has sections on self-care with screenings and tips, and journaling. Initial research shows that these approaches hold promise (Steffen, Mahoney, & Kelley, 2003).

REFERENCES

Ackerman, N. (1972). Family therapy: Theory and practice. In G. D. Erikson & T. P. Hogan (Eds.), *Family therapy: An introduction to theory and technique*. Monterey, CA: Brooks/Cole.

Anderson, R. E., & Carter, L. ([1984] 1990). *Human behavior in the social environment*. Hawthorne, NY: Aldine de Gruyter.

Antonovsky, A. (1998). The sense of coherence: An historical and future perspective. In H. I. McCubbin, E. A. Thompson, A. I. Thompson, & J. E. Fromer (Eds.), *Stress, coping, and health in families* (pp. 3-20). Boston: Allyn & Bacon.

Aranda, M. P., Villa, V. M., Trejo, L., Ramirez, R., & Ranney, M. (2003). El Portal Latino Alzheimer's Project: Model Program for Latino Caregivers of Alzheimer's Disease-Affected People. *Social Work, 48* (2), 259-272.

Atchley, R. C. (1999). *Continuity and adaptation in aging*. Baltimore: Johns Hopkins University Press.

Berg-Weger, M., Rubio, D. M., & Tebb, S. S. (2001). Strengths-based practice with family caregivers of the chronically ill: Qualitative insights. *Families in Society: The Journal of Contemporary Human Services, 82* (3), 263-272.

Bertalanffy, L. (1962). General systems theory: A critical review. *General Systems Yearbook, 7:*1-20.

Boszormenyi-Nagy, I., & Spark, G. (1973). *Invisible loyalties*. New York: Harper & Row.

Bourgeois, M. S., Schulz, R., & Burgio, L. (1996). Interventions for caregivers of patients with Alzheimer's disease: A review and analysis of content, process and outcomes. *International Journal of Aging and Human Development, 43:*35-92.

Burgio, L., Steven, A., Guy, D., Roth, D. L. & Haley, W. F. (2003). Impact of two psychosocial interventions on White and African American family caregivers of individuals with dementia.*The Gerontologist, 43* (4), 568-579.

Bowen, M. (1971). Aging: A symposium. *Georgetown Medical Bulletin, 30:*4-27.

Bradley, E. H., Bogardus, S., van Doorn, C., Williams, C. Cherlin, E., & Inouye, S. (2000). Goals in geriatric assessment: Are we measuring the right outcomes? *Gerontologist, 40*(2):191-96.

Brody, E. (1985). Parent care as normative family stress. *Gerontologist, 25:*19-29.

Chadiha, L. A., Adams, P., Biegel, D. E., Auslander, W., & Gutierrez, L. (2004). Empowering African American women informal caregivers: A literature synthesis and practice strategies. *Social Work, 49* (1):97-109.

Clark, F., Azen, S. P., Zemke, R., Jackson, J. Carlson, M., Mandel, D., Hay, J., Josephson, K., Cherry, B., Hessel, C., Plamer, J., & Lipson, L. (2001). Occupational therapy for independent-living older adults: A randomized controlled trial. *Journal of the American Medical Association, 278:*1321-1326.

Coon, D. W., Gallagher-Thompson, D., & Thompson, L. W. (2003). *Innovative interventions to reduce dementia caregiver distress: A clinical guide.* New York: Springer.

Coon, D. W., & Zeiss, L. M. (2003). The families we choose: Intervention issues with LBGT caregivers. In D. W. Coon, D. Gallagher-Thompson, & L. W. Thompson (Eds.), *Innovative interventions to reduce dementia caregiver distress: A clinical guide.* New York: Springer.

Crowther, M. R., Parker, M. W., Achenbaum, W. A., Larimore, W. L., & Koenig, H. G. (2002). Rowe and Kahn's model of successful aging revisited: Positive spirituality–the forgotten factor. *Gerontologist, 42*(5):613-620).

Davies, H., Priddy, J. M., & Tinklenberg, J. R. (1986). Support groups for male caregivers of Alzheimer's patients. *Clinical Gerontologist, 5:*385-395.

Farran, C. J., Keane-Hagerty, E., Salloway, S., Kupferer, S., & Wilken, C. S. (1991). Finding meaning: An alternative paradigm for Alzheimer's disease caregivers. *Gerontologist, 31:*483-489.

Farran, C. J., Miller, B., Kaufman, J., Donner, D., & Fogg, L. (1999). Finding meaning through caregiving: Development of an instrument for family caregivers of persons with Alzheimer's disease. *Journal of Clinical Psychology, 55*(9):1107-1125.

Fuller-Thomson, E., Minkler, M., & Driver, D. (1997). A profile of grandparents raising grandchildren in the United States. *The Gerontologist, 37,* (3), 406-411.

Gallagher-Thompson, D., & Devries, H. M. (1994). "Coping with frustration" classes: Development and preliminary outcomes with women who care for relatives with dementia. *Gerontologist, 34:*548-552.

Gallagher-Thompson, D., Lovett, S., Rose, J., McKibbin, C., Coon, D., Futtterman, A., & Thompson, L. W. (2000). Impact of psychoeducational interventions on distressed family caregivers. *Journal of Clinical Geropsychology, 6:*91-110.

Gallagher-Thompson, D., Talamantes, M., Ramirez, R. & Valverde, I. (1996). Service delivery issues for working with Mexican American family caregivers. In Yeo, G. & Gallagher-Thompson (Eds.), *Ethnicity and the Dementias.* Washington, D. C.: Taylor & Francis

George, L. K., & Gwyther, L. P. (1986). Caregiver well-being: A multidimensional examination of family caregivers of demented adults. *Gerontologist, 26:*253-259.

Goldenberg, I., & Goldenberg, H. (2003). *Family therapy: An overview* (5th ed.). Monterey, CA: Brooks/Cole.

Gottlieb, B. H., & Johnson, J. (2000). Respite programs for caregivers of persons with dementia: A review with practice implications. *Aging and Mental Health, 4*(2): 119-129.

Gottlieb, B. H., & Wolfe, J. (2002). Coping with family caregiving to persons with dementia: A critical review. *Aging & Mental Health, 6*(4):325-342.

Gray, V. K. (1983). Providing support for home caregivers. In M. Smyer & M. Gatz (Eds.), *Mental Health and Aging,* Beverly Hills, CA: Sage.

Greene, R. R. ([1986] 2000). *Social work with the aged and their families.* Hawthorne, NY: Aldine de Gruyter.

Greene, R. R. (1999). *Human behavior theory and social work practice.* Hawthorne, NY: Aldine de Gruyter.

Greene, R. R. (2000). Serving the aged and their families in the 21st century using a revised practice model. *Journal of Gerontological Social Work, 34*(1):43-62.

Greene, R. R. (2002). *Resiliency Theory: An Integrated Framework for Practice, Research, and Policy.* Washington, DC: NASW Press.

Greene, R. R. (2005). The changing family of later years and social work practice. In L. Kaye (Ed.), *Perspectives on aging.* Washington, DC: NASW Press.

Greene, R. R., & Armenta, K. (2007). The REM Model: Phase II–Practice strategies. In R. R. Greene (Ed.), *Social work practice: A risk and resilience perspective.* Monterey, CA: Brooks/Cole.

Greene, R. R. & Conrad, A. (2002). Basic assumptions and terms. In R. R. Greene, (2002). *Resiliency Theory: An Integrated Framework for Practice, Research, and Policy.* Washington, DC: NASW Press.

Greene, R. R., & Barnes, G. (1998). The ecological perspective, diversity, and culturally competent social work practice. In R. R. Greene & M. Watkins (Eds.), *Serving diverse constituencies: Applying the ecological perspective* (pp. 63-96). Hawthorne, NY: Aldine de Gruyter.

Greene, R. R., & Blundo, R. (1999). Post modern critique of systems theory in social work with the aged and their families. *Journal of Gerontological Social Work, 31:*87-100.

Greene, R. R., Kropf, N., & MacNair, N. (1994). A family therapy model for working with persons with AIDS. *Journal of Family Psychotherapy, 5*(1): 2-19.

Greene, V. L., & Monahan, D. J. (1989). The effect of a support and education program on stress and burden among family caregivers to frail elderly persons. *Gerontologist, 29*(4):472-477.

Gutierrez, L., & Ortega, R. (1991). Developing methods to empower Latinos: The importance of groups. *Social Work with Groups, 14:*23-43.

Hartman, A. (1978). Diagrammatic assessment of family relationships. *Social Casework, 59:*465-476.

Hawley, D., & DeHaan, L. (1996). Towards a definition of family resilience. *Family Process, 35:*283-289.

Henderson, J. N., Gutierrez-Mayka, M., Garcia, J., & Boyd, S. (1993). A model for Alzheimer's disease support group development in African American and Hispanic populations. *Gerontologist, 33:*409-414.

Hodge, D. R. (2001). Spiritual assessment: A review of major qualitative methods and a new framework for assessing spirituality. *Social Work, 46*(3):203-211.

Hodge, D. R. (2005). Spiritual lifemaps: A client-centered pictorial instrument for spiritual assessment, planning, and intervention. *Social Work, 50*(1):77-87.

Kaye, L. W., & Applegate, J. S. (1993). Family support groups for male caregivers: Benefits of participation. *Journal of Gerontological Social Work, 20:*167-185.

Knight, B. G., Robinson, G. S., Longmire, C. Chun, M., Nakao, K., & Kim, J. (2002). Cross cultural issues in caregiving for persons with dementia: Do familism values reduce burden and distress? *Ageing International, 27*(3, Summer):70-94.

Krieger, N., Rowley, D. L., Herman, A. A., Avery, B., & Phillips, M. T. (1993). Racism, sexism, and social class: Implications for studies of health, disease, and well-being. *American Journal of Preventive Medicine, 2:*82-122.

Lauderdale, S. A., D'Andrea, J. A., & Coon, D. W. (2003). Male caregivers: Challenges and opportunities. In Coon, D. W., Gallagher-Thompson, D., & Thompson, L. W. (Eds.), *Innovative interventions to reduce dementia caregiver distress: A clinical guide.* New York: Springer.

Lazarus, R. S., & Folkman, S. (1984). *Stress, appraisal, and coping.* New York: Springer.

Lovett, S., & Gallagher, D. (1988). Psychoeducational interventions for family caregivers: Preliminary efficacy data. *Behavior Therapy, 19:*321-330.

Marriott, A., Donaldson, C., Tarrier, N., & Burns, A. (2000). Effectiveness of cognitive-behavioral family intervention in reducing the burden of care in carers of patients with Alzheimer's disease. *British Journal of Psychiatry, 176:* 557-562.

McCubbin, H. I., Thompson, E. A., Thompson, A. I., Elver, K. M., & McCubbin, M. A. (1994). Ethnicity, schema, and coherence: Appraisal processes for families in crisis. In *Stress, coping and health in families: Sense of coherency and resiliency* (p. 44). Thousand Oaks, CA: Sage.

Minuchin, S. (1974). *Families and family therapy.* Cambridge, MA: Harvard University Press.

Mittelman, M. S., Ferris, S. H., Steinberg, G., Shulman, E., Mackell, J., Aminder, A., & Cohen, J. (1996). A comprehensive support program: Effect on depression in spouse-caregivers. *Gerontologist, 35:*792-802.

Mittelman, M. S., Zeiss, A., Davies, H., & Delois, G. (2003). Specific stressors of spousal caregivers: Difficult behaviors, loss of sexual intimacy, and incontinence. In Coon, D. W., Gallagher-Thompson, D., & Thompson, L. W. (Eds.), *Innovative interventions to reduce dementia caregiver distress: A clinical guide.* New York: Springer.

Mohide, E. A., Pringle, D. M., Streiner, D. L., Gilbert, J. R., Muir, G., & Tew, M. (1990). A randomized trial of family caregiver support in the home management of dementia. *Journal of the American Geriatric Society, 38:*446-454.

Montgomery, R., & Borgatta, E. (1989). The effects of alternative support strategies on family caregiving. *Gerontologist, 29:*457-464.

Moseley, P. W., Davies, H. D., & Priddy, J. M. (1988). Support group for male caregivers of Alzheimer's patients: A follow-up. *Clinical Gerontologist, 7:*127-136.

National Alliance for Caregiving (2003). *Family caregiving and public policy principles for change.*http://www.caregiving.org

National Alliance for Caregiving & AARP (1997). *Family Caregiving in the U.S.: Findings from a National Survey.* Washington, DC: AARP.

Oswald, S. K., Hepburn, K. W., Caron, W., Burns, T., & Mantell, R. (1999). Reducing caregiver burden: A randomized psychoeducational intervention for caregivers of persons with dementia. *Gerontologist, 39:*299-308.

Pearlin, L. I., Aneshensel, C. S., & Leblanc, A. J. (1997). The forms and mechanisms of stress proliferation: The case of AIDS caregivers. *Journal of Health and Social Behavior 38*(3):223-236.

Pierce, T., Lydon, J. E., & Yang, S. (2001). Enthusiasm and moral commitment: What sustains family caregivers of those with dementia. *Basic and Applied Social Psychology, 23*(1):29-41.

Pinkston, E. M., & Linsk, N. L. (1988). Behavioral family interventions with the impaired elderly. *Gerontologist, 24:*576-583.

Pinkston, E. M., Linsk, N. L., & Young, R. N. (1988). Home based behavioral family treatment of the impaired elderly. *Behavior Therapy, 19:*331-344.

Pinquart, M., & Sorensen, S. (2003). Associations of stressors and uplifts of caregiving with caregiver burden and depressive mood: A meta-analysis. *Journal of Gerontology: Psychological Sciences, 58B*(2):112-128.

Qualls, S. H. (1997). Transitions in autonomy: The essential caregiving challenge. An essay for practitioners. *Family Relations, 46:*41-45.

Qualls, S. H. (1999). Realizing power in intergenerational family hierarchies: Family reorganization when older adults decline. In M. Duffy (Ed.), *Handbook of counseling and psychotherapy with older adults.* New York: Wiley & Sons.

Rapp, S. R., & Chao, D. (2000). Appraisals of strain and of gain: Effects on psychological wellbeing of caregivers of dementia patients. *Ageing and Mental Health, 4*(2):142-147.

Reifler, B. V., & Eisdorfer, C. (1980). A clinic for the impaired elderly and their families. *American Journal of Psychiatry, 137:*1399-1403.

Rothenberg, D. (1996). Grandparents as parents: A primer for schools. Kid Source Online. Eric Clearinghouse on Elementary and Early Childhood Education. Urbana, IL. http://www.kidsource.com/kidsource/content2/grandparents.3.html

Rowe, J. W. & Kahn, R. L. (1998). *Successful aging.* New York: Pantheon.

Ryff, C. D., & Singer, B. (2002). From social structure to biology: Integrative science in pursuit of human health and well-being. In C. R. Snyder & S. J. Lopez (Eds.), *Handbook of positive psychology* (pp. 541-555). New York: Oxford University Press.

Seligman, M. E. P. (2002). Positive psychology, positive prevention, and positive therapy. In C. R. Snyder & S. J. Lopez (Eds.), *Handbook of positive psychology* (pp. 3-7). New York: Oxford University Press.

Seltzer, M. M., Ivry, J., & Litchfield, L. C. (1987). Family members as case managers: Partnership between the formal and informal support networks. *Gerontologist, 27:*722-728.

Silverstone, B., & Burack-Weiss, A. (1983). *Social work practice with the frail elderly and their families.* Springfield, IL: Charles C. Thomas.

Steffen, A., Mahoney, D. F., & Kelley, K. (2003). Capitalizing on technological advances. In Coon, D. W., Gallagher-Thompson, D., & Thompson, L. W. (Eds.), *Innovative interventions to reduce dementia caregiver distress: A clinical guide.* New York: Springer.

Szapocznik, J., Kurtines, W. M., Santisteban, D. A., Pantin, H., Scopetta, M., Mancilla, Y., Aisenberg, S., McIntosh, S., Perez-Vidal, A., & Coatsworth, J. D. (1997). The evolution of structural ecosystemic theory for working with Latino families. In J. G. Garcia & M. C. Zea (Eds.), *Psychological interventions and research with Latino populations.* Boston: Allyn & Bacon.

Tennstedt, S. & Chang, B. H. (1998). The relative contribution of ethnicity vs. socio-economic status in explaining differences in disability and receipt of national care. *Journal of Gerontology: Social Sciences, 53B*(2), 861-870.

Teri, L., Logsdon, R. G., Uomoto, J., & McCurry, S. M. (1997). Behavioral treatment of depression in dementia patients: A controlled clinical trial. *Journal of Gerontology B: Psychological Science and Social Science, 52:*159-166.

Toseland, R. W., Rossiter, C. M., Peak, T., & Smith, G. C. (1990). Comparative effectiveness of individual and group interventions to support family caregivers. *Social Work, 35:*209-217.

U.S. Census Bureau (2002). The older population in the United States. *Current Population Reports* (pp. 20-546). Washington, DC: U.S. Department of Commerce.

Walsh, F. (1998). *Strengthening Family Resilience.* New York: Guilford.

Walsh, F. (1999). Families in later life: Challenges and opportunities. In E. A. Carter & M. McGoldrick (Eds.), *The expanded life cycle: Individual, family, and social perspectives* (pp. 307-324). Boston: Allyn & Bacon.

Zarit, S. H., & Edwards, A. (1996). Family caregiving: Research and clinical intervention. In R. T. Woods (Ed.), *Handbook of the clinical psychology of ageing.* New York: Wiley & Sons.

doi:10.1300/J137v14n01_01

Chapter 2

Intervention Continued:
Providing Care Through Case Management

Roberta R. Greene
Michael Uebel

SUMMARY. This chapter describes the case management process–a process for assisting individuals and families with multiple service needs–and its use in various fields of practice including mental health, human immunodeficiency virus and acquired immune deficiency syndrome (HIV/AIDS), and services for older adults. It addresses the role of the case manager as the person responsible for ensuring the timely and adequate delivery of suitable community-based services. The integration of formal services with informal care by family and friends as an intervention strategy is also discussed. doi:10.1300/J137v14n01_02 *[Article copies available for a fee from The Haworth Document Delivery Service: 1-800-HAWORTH. E-mail address: <docdelivery@haworthpress.com> Website: <http://www.HaworthPress.com> © 2006 by The Haworth Press, Inc. All rights reserved.]*

KEYWORDS. Case management, families, community-based services

Because the care an individual may need is often obtained from multiple sources, effective coordination and monitoring of care is essential.

[Haworth co-indexing entry note]: "Intervention Continued: Providing Care Through Case Management." Greene, Roberta R., and Michael Uebel. Co-published simultaneously in *Journal of Human Behavior in the Social Environment* (The Haworth Press, Inc.) Vol. 14, No. 1/2, 2006, pp. 31-50; and: *Contemporary Issues of Care* (ed: Roberta R. Greene) The Haworth Press, Inc., 2006, pp. 31-50. Single or multiple copies of this article are available for a fee from The Haworth Document Delivery Service [1-800-HAWORTH, 9:00 a.m. - 5:00 p.m. (EST). E-mail address: docdelivery@haworthpress.com].

Available online at http://jhbse.haworthpress.com
doi:10.1300/J137v14n01_02

This article describes the case management process–a process for assisting individuals and families with multiple service needs–and its use in various fields of practice including mental health, human immunodeficiency virus and acquired immune deficiency syndrome (HIV/AIDS), and services for older adults. It addresses the role of the case manager as the person responsible for ensuring the timely and adequate delivery of suitable community-based services (Rose & Moore, 1995). The integration of formal services with informal care by family and friends as an intervention strategy is also discussed.

Case management is a process that assists people traverse the long-term care system. Ideally, community resources form a long-term care service continuum, including a range of services that address the health, psychosocial, and personal care needs of individuals who are lacking some capacity for self-care (Daatland, 1983). Long-term care encompasses resident facilities as well as social service and health programs designed to provide supportive care for an individual over a prolonged period of time at home or in a variety of protective and semi-protective settings (Figure 1 and Table 1). Services may be a combination of formal ones delivered by health and social service agencies and informal ones provided by significant others and people in a person's social support network. Furthermore, informal helping is dependent on people's natural tendency to care for others (Hooyman, 1983).

The focus of a long-term care system is the person (and his or her family) whose decreased functional capacity places him or her in a position to need assistance with activities of daily living, such as housekeeping, finances, transportation, meal preparations, or administering medication. As discussed in Chapter One, the delivery of appropriate long-term care services involves an assessment of the biopsychosocial aspects of functional capacity and an understanding of the specific conditions that can interfere with autonomous functioning. Case management also involves social work skills at the macro systems level including system design and analysis.

SOCIAL WORK CASE MANAGEMENT

Social work case management dates back to the Charity Organization Societies of the 1880s when case workers were faced with limited resources and numerous families in need of financial resources and other tangible assistance (Vourlekis & Greene, 1992). The Charity Organization Societies' friendly visitors "had to be trained in investigation, diag-

FIGURE 1. Five Continua for the Elderly

1. Continuum of Need					
Independent (Little or no need)			Moderately dependent		Dependent (Multiple Need)
2. Continuum of Services					
Health promotion/ disease prevention	Screening and early detection	Diagnosis and pre-treatment evaluation	Treatment	Rehabilitation: skilled nursing services	Continuing care and hospice
3. Continuum of Service Settings					
Own home, apartment, etc.	Friend or relative's home apartment, etc.	Congregate living situation	Sub-acute care facility (e.g., day hospital)	Acute care facility (e.g., hospital)	Skilled long-term care facility (e.g., nursing home) · Continuing care and hospice
4. Continuum of Service Providers					
Self-care	Family friends (support network)		Para-professionals		Professionals
5. Continuum of Professional Collaboration					
Single discipline		Multidisciplinary			Interdisciplinary

Hooyman, N., Hooyman, G., & Kethley, A. (1981). The role of gerontological social work in interdisciplinary care. Paper presented at Council on Social Work Education Annual Program Meeting, Louisville, Kentucky, March. Used with permission.

33

TABLE 1. Long-Term Continuum of Care

Access to Service	Array of Service	Setting
		FAMILY
	Least restrictive	
• Outreach	Monitoring services	
	Homemaker	In Home
	Home health care	
• Informational/referral	Nutrition programs	
	Legal protective services	
	Senior centers	
• Assessment	Community medical services	
	Dental services	Community
• Case management	Community mental health	
	Adult day care	
• Linkages	Respite care	
	Hospice care	
	Retirement villages	
• Evaluation quality	• life care	
	• service	
	Domiciliary care	
	Foster home	
	Personal care home	
Special housing	Group home	Institutional
	Congregate care	
	• meals	
	• social services	
	• medical services	
	• housekeeping	
	Intermediate care	
	Skilled nursing care	
	Mental hospitals	
	Acute care hospitals	
	Most restrictive	

Adapted from: Brody, E. (1979). Planning for the Long-Term Support/Care System: The Array of Services to Be Considered. Philadelphia: Region III Center for Health Planning.

nosis, preparations of case records, and treatment, all of which required guidance, counsel, supervision, and the knowledge of scientific philanthropy" (Trattner, 1994, p. 238). During the 1970s, the deinstitutionalization of the mental health community, whereby large numbers of people were moved from self-contained institutions to community-based settings such as halfway houses, group homes, family homes, and single residential dwellings, resulted in a shifted perspective on case management. As Lourie (1978), a member of the American Psychiatric Association's Ad Hoc Committee on the Chronic Mental Patient, noted, case management had become "a vital, perhaps the most primary, device in management for any individual with a disability where the requirements demand differential access to and use of various resources" (p. 159). In the 1980s, further shifts in state policies and funding priorities once again drew attention to the need for case management services to address uncoordinated or fragmented services for vulnerable clients (Rose, 1992).

Social work case management shares particular features that are congruent with our professional mission and responsibility to client and societal well-being. The purpose of social work case management at the client level is to achieve quality and continuity of care by:

- Working within a mutual relationship;
- Setting mutual goals for the service plan;
- Focusing on client strengths and capabilities;
- Blending therapeutic help with advocacy and resource allocation;
- Striving for the highest level of client functionality and competence;
- Using the least restrictive services;
- Reaching out to natural support systems; and
- Mutually evaluating service implementation and outcomes.

Goals at the systems level include:

- Developing resource systems;
- Linking people to resource systems; and
- Making systems more accessible and responsive.

Case Management Functions

There are several models of case management, each characterized by the specific target population to be served, staff capabilities, and the financial resources and organizational structure of the agency (Greene & Kropf, 2003). For example, broker models of case management, such as that in the generalist approach discussed below, involve the social worker's attention to referrals and linkages in the effort to achieve intersystem or interagency cooperation between and among agencies. Assertive outreach workers focus on the attainment of the treatment plan (Austin, 1992). In the advocacy empowerment case management approach, as discussed below in the client-driven approach, the case manager has a dual commitment to meeting vulnerable clients' needs and challenging dysfunctional service delivery systems (Rose, 1992).

According to Rose and Moore (1995), when case management systems began to focus on the process used in setting client goals, the case managers' tasks were "rearranged" (p. 337). The authors indicate that goal setting may begin with the preset services of the provider or the unique interests of the client. In an individualized service plan, goals may be measured by how the client believes the quality of his or her life has improved. In the broker model, more attention is given to the measurement of the client's pattern of service usage. However, in reality there does appear to be general agreement and overlap about basic social work case management functions. A comprehensive list is outlined by Weil and Karls (1985):

1. client identification and outreach, determining the target population and eligibility;
2. client assessment and diagnosis, evaluating a client's level of functioning and service needs;
3. service planning and resource identification with clients and members of service networks, describing the steps and issues in service delivery, monitoring, and evaluation;
4. linking clients to needed services, connecting or securing client services;
5. service implementation and coordination, service assessment and trouble shooting, getting the work done or putting all the plan's pieces in place;
6. monitoring service delivery, overseeing and supervising client services;
7. advocacy for and with client in service network, pressing for client needs; and
8. evaluation of service delivery and case management, determining the progress of the service plan that may result in continued service with same or revised service plan, termination, or basic follow up.

Three key elements for success in the case management process, compatible with the description provided by Weil and Karls (1985), have been identified by Ozarin (1978): responsibility, continuity, and accountability. *Responsibility* depends upon a network model of service agencies that, when called upon, provide specific resources without assuming total responsibility for the client, "unless responsibility for carrying out the total plan is also transferred and accepted" (p. 167). There must be, in other words, a clear and well-articulated line of responsibility for the case and the client. The second crucial element of sound case management is *continuity*. Continuity depends upon planning, which is important during both the intensive treatment phase and aftercare. *Accountability* methods must also be in place, as they "assure the patient is not lost" (p. 168), wherein, through the case management process, the client is helped to increase his or her own ability to function independently and to assume self-responsibility. The social work ethical value of self-determinacy is paramount here as the goal is to involve the client in all aspects of decision making.

A GENERALIST APPROACH TO CASE MANAGEMENT

In the generalist approach to case management, the case manager follows a method that closely resembles traditional casework (Levine & Fleming, 1984), carrying out a variety of roles that assist a client's access to the service delivery system (Rothman, 1992). According to Rubin (1987), in this instance, case management is a boundary-spanning strategy used by the case manager to link the multiple services that an individual client may need. Holding one person accountable for all services a client may need requires the case manager to carry out several roles and functions compatible with a generalist social work approach.

Generalist social work practice–taught in some form in most every social work program–is considered "a form of professional practice competently conducted in a variety of settings with client systems of varying size at several levels of prevention, using a transferable body of knowledge, values, and skills" (Norlin & Chess, 1997, p. 10). In addition, Miley, O'Melia, and DuBois (2001) contend that a generalist approach is "an integrated and multilevel approach for meeting the purpose of social work" (p. 9). Therefore, the case manager must assess the situation and decide which system will be the unit of attention (Johnson, 1992; see Chapter 1).

A generalist view of case management is rooted in ecological and systems theory. A systems-derived ecological model is particularly appropriate for social work intervention and case management since the ways in which persons interact with their family environments, non-kin environments (e. g., neighbors), and community, regional, national, and international environments are the very keys to their functioning and thus to the ways they can be helped to function better. Individual persons (as systems), in relation to the complex external world (comprised of multiple systems or ecology), are not viewed only as products of their environment but are seen as capable of influencing or changing their ecological setting. Early social work ecological and systems theory (Coulton, 1981; Engel,

1980; Germain, 1973) emphasized that the object of intervention can be a single person, a social collectivity such as a non-profit organization, or a culturally and geographically spanning system such as a metropolis or a rain forest. In short, from a case management perspective, the systems ecological model can incorporate thinking about the interactions and interconnections among the smallest micro and the broadest macro social systems.

In an increasingly complex technological society, the ecological scope of systems analysis becomes more and more relevant (Hawley, 1979). Germain's (1973; 1978; 1987) pioneering work on redefining casework from ecological perspectives in the systems model, with its emphasis on the interface between person and environment, amounted to a challenge to caseworkers to promote change in the client as well as in his or her environment, the site from which many difficulties issue (e. g., inadequate housing, education, medical care, or the power differentials that favor those already in power). The challenge, then, for ecologically-oriented case management is to develop treatment plans that incorporate new service-delivery arrangements, tap volunteer and paraprofessional resources, and employ interdisciplinary consultations. For Germain (1978), the very health of the ego depends upon case management strategies that allow for active and even creative responses of the ego to environmental changes. As the pace of contemporary life continues to speed up, the quick adaptations facilitated by ecologically-based case management are vital.

A Client-Driven Approach to Case Management

A client-driven approach to case management was fueled by case managers who were faced with the conflict of restrictive funding and large case loads. These social workers hoped to "implement a client-driven, systems-impact paradigm" (ibid, p. v) in which the values of self-determination and human dignity were upheld. The importance of monitoring, linkage, and advocacy activities also were viewed as a means of systems reform as were the need to have goals and outcome measures. In the client-driven approach, a client's goals or desired outcomes are the basis for evaluating the adequacy and appropriateness of services rather than the provider system's imposition of identified targets. Thus, social work case management processes were intended to combat the ill effects of poor resource allocation (Table 2).

A strengths-perspective on case management came to the fore in the late 1980s following the deinstitutionalization movement. As the population in state mental hospitals from 1955 to 1980 was reduced from

TABLE 2. Client-Driven versus Provider-Driven Case Management Models

Case Management Characteristics	Client-Driven Models	Provider-Driven Models
Fundamental perception of Client	Clients as subjects who know and act	Clients as objects who are known and acted on
Case manager sees client's	Strengths to identify and Develop	Problems to identify and Pathology to manage
Case manager seeks	Active participation, Reframing deficits, Producing direction	Compliance, adaptation to service plans
Case management goals	Positive direction, Implementation steps, and self-confidence	Improved patterns of service consumption and patient-role behavior
Case management needs Assessment	Derived directly from the Client's direction plan and goals	Derived directly from the Service provider's Definitions and outputs
Linking	Resources seen as total Community, with emphasis on informal social networks	Referrals to existing service providers and use of the formal system
Monitoring	Mutual evaluation of process In relation to direction of Plan	Assures compliance With treatment plan
Evaluation	Increasing autonomy, critical assessment of social context, growing self-confidence. Involvement with informal networks	Increased units of service consumed, use of fewer inpatient days, improved compliance
Focus	Identify strengths and obstacles to the attainment of goals, develop social networks, free the client from clinical judgment and contempt, assess the role of each service system as a support or obstacle	Identify problems, make referrals, and assure the client's compliance with the treatment plan. Keep attention on the client's behavior and functioning, family interaction, keeping appointments

Adapted from: Rose, S. M. & Moore, V. L. (1995). Case Management. In R. L. Edwards (Ed.-in-Chief), *Encyclopedia of social work* (19th edition, p. 338). Washington, DC: NASW Press.

558,992 to 175,000 (Rapp, 1992), many became homeless without access to suitable housing and services. Studies conducted during that time documented six basic principles as the core of a strengths-based model:

1. The focus is on individual strengths not pathology.
2. The case manager-client relationship is primary and essential.
3. Interventions are based on client self-determination.

4. The community is viewed as an oasis of resources, not as an obstacle.
5. Aggressive outreach is the preferred mode of intervention.
6. People suffering from severe mental illness can continue to learn, grow, and change (ibid., p. 46).

This strengths-based perspective involves a view of human behavior that focuses on people's inherent capacity to respond to and confront daily challenges (Kisthardt, 1992) as well as adverse events (Masten & Coatsworth, 1998). Concepts such as maintaining self-efficacy (Bandura, 1994) or resilience (Greene, 2002) address how people cope with stress successfully.

Client-driven or -focused case management derives from the strengths-perspective the essential belief that a person's quality of life, achievement, and life satisfaction are attributable to the type and quality of niches (or systems) that the person inhabits. Niches can be understood as imbricated life domains: living arrangements, work, education, recreation, social relationships, and so on. The quality of niches for any one is a function of that person's:

- Aspirations,
- Competencies,
- Confidence,
- Environmental resources,
- Opportunities, and
- People available to that person.

By tapping into and drawing upon a client's resiliency, this set of personality characteristics, dispositions, and resources comprises the biopsychosocial elements that enable stressed persons to maintain a sense of competence and control in their lives. Additional factors contributing to a successful individual's enhanced resiliency include the family interaction system and the work and community milieu (Norman, 2000). The strengths approach favors the establishment of niches or environmental conditions, such as those in family and community, which enable rather than stigmatize individuals. Once again, the focus is on seeing possibilities rather than problems, options rather than restrictions, and well-being rather than pathology (Rapp, 1998).

FAMILY-CENTERED CASE MANAGEMENT

Family case management is based on family systems thinking that examines the behavior of the inner workings of the family unit–its roles, rules, power relationships, and sharing of responsibilities. The family is the "basic social unit on society in which relations are culturally and socially defined either by law, tradition, religion, and/or some combination of these" (Goode, 1964, p. 2). As such, its recognition by social workers as a system depends upon one of two perspectives: (1) the family viewed as *inclusive*, and (2) the family viewed as *included*. The view of the family by the case manager as an inclusive system focuses on how the family shapes or influences the behaviors and perceptions of its members. The emphasis is thus upon the form and quality of intrafamilial relationships and the impact these have on involved family members. The family is itself among the most interdependent of all social systems, where "the essence of a social system is interdependence and the essence of interdependence is people's investment of themselves in other people and in collectivities. . . . It is these investments that tie the system together and give it strength" (Coleman, 1963, p. 3). Family therapists have long viewed the family as an interpersonal or group phenomenon (Minuchin, 1974; Satir, 1967). Treating the family as an included system focuses not on its interpersonal systemic nature but rather on its institutional dimensions and functions. The central point of interest here is how the family fits with other social institutions (e.g., the educational system, the health sector, and social and governmental institutions such as the church or the military). Within the frame of case management, an analysis of the family as an included system directs concern toward identifying the consequences for the family of its multiple linkages with the broader ecological system (Verzaro-Lawrence, 1981). The following linkages are among the most important:

- Kin networks
- Social or friendship networks
- Occupational or labor market ties
- Education system ties
- Memberships/activities of family members in voluntary organizations
- Religious activities (Martin & O'Connor, 1989, p. 127).

The key question concerns whether or not the family is integrated in the broader social system, and to what degree. Family-centered case management, from the perspective of its status as an included system, is thus primarily concerned with linking families with other institutional dimensions of the social system (see Table 3).

The necessity of forging linkages between families and the broader social system is dramatized, for example, by some of the major changes that have led to the partial isolation of older persons in Western society. Changes in family structure or residential arrangements have been typically offered as explanations for this isolation, while the more compelling explanation may have to do with the transformation and redefinition of family functions and values (Hareven, 2001). The interdependence between members of the nuclear family and extended kin, for instance, has been weakened by an erosion of the instrumental view of family relations and the resulting shift toward sentimentality and intimacy as the significant cohesive forces in the family (ibid.). Add to this the family's retreat from the community–a feature of the erosion of social capital–and the increasing privatization of the modern middle-class family, all of which results in sharper boundaries between family and community and more intense segregation of different age groups within the family. When ger-

TABLE 3. Key Features of Family-Focused Social Work Case Management

---

Family-focused social work requires that the case manager
- identify the family as the unit of attention
- access the frail or impaired person's biopsychosocial functioning and needs within a culturally sound family context
- write a mutually agreed on family care plan
- refer client systems to services and entitlements not available within the natural support system
- implement and coordinate the work that is done with the family
- determine what services need to be coordinated on behalf of the family
- intervene clinically to ameliorate family emotional problems and stress accompanying illness or loss of functioning
- determine how the impaired person and family will interact with formal care providers
- integrate formal and informal services provided by the family and other primary groups
- offer or advocate for particular services that the informal support network is not able to offer
- contact client networks and service providers to determine the quality of service provision
- mediate conflicts between the family and service providers to empower the family when they are not successful
- collect information and data to augment the advocacy and evaluation efforts to ensure quality of care

---

Adapted from: Vourlekis, B., & Greene, R. R. (1992). *Social work case management*. New York: Aldine de Gruyter.

ontologists write about the elimination of older persons from viable family roles, they often have these social changes in mind.

The needs and situations of parents and children (in the nuclear family) or grandparents, parents, and children (in the extended family) shift over the life course, and do so perhaps no more dramatically than when an aging parent's health declines or when children become sick with a life-threatening illness such as AIDS. Informal kinds of support, help ranging from emotional support to hands-on nursing care and received from someone more intimate such as a family member, friend, or neighbor, constitute the vast majority of help provided to vulnerable populations such as the frail elderly. Because families and friends are the major care providers for person's needing care, they are often in the "interstitial" position of case manager (Sussman, 1976). That is, they are in the role coordinating plan services on behalf of relatives (Greene, 1992; Seltzer, Ivry, & Litchfield, 1992). According to Greene and Kropf (2003), "this perspective generally views the family as promoting positive interdependence and problem resolution, and uses intervention strategies aimed at developing the family as a system of mutual aid" (p. 93).

The family conceived of as a mutual aid system is the ideal of "interstitial" case management. While older persons often give and receive assistance, the imbalanced focus on help provided by children often adds to the more general societal impression that all older people need help and downplays their role as helpers in old age. Dowd (1980) showed that support between parent and child is more accurately viewed as an exchange relationship, including assumptions of reciprocity (Gouldner, 1967), the presence of which affects the perceived quality of the relationship. Among older persons, for example, emotional functioning is better if exchanges are characterized by reciprocity (Black, 1985). Indeed, reciprocal relationships enhance life satisfaction for adults of all ages. It is not surprising, then, that reciprocity, the root of filial responsibility, is reflected in the fact that one of the chief reasons children take care of their parents is because their parents took care of them when they were young (Dwyer, Lee, & Jankowski, 1994). An important aspect of family-centered case management will be recognizing (and working to enhance) the extent to which support between family members flows in more than one direction. Despite real limits to which parties may feel that the intergenerational bond is a balanced one, the optimal condition is one of reciprocity. Recent studies (Rossi, 2001) have suggested that close kin relationships in the U.S. are marked by a high degree of reciprocity, supporting the image of families as interdependent and multigenerational, with "considerable social interaction and helping behavior between the generations," both contributing to social cohesion (ibid., p. 344).

NORMATIVE FAMILY CAREGIVING

Commitments and obligations, crisscrossing generational lines, are taken to be elemental components of family organization, evidence of family solidarity (Bengtson, Burgess, & Parrott, 1997). Indeed, Brody (1985) has proposed that caregiving is a normative family task. Yet its normativity should not mask the diverse ways in which intergenerational ties are negotiated in the family. Structured social relations, such as those based on gender, class, ethnicity, and race, play a key role in how support exchanges will play out within families. Socially sanctioned reasons for avoiding obligations to provide care in particular situations (Finch, 1989) may include gendered family roles as, for example, when a married father in the labor force declines caring for his mother, arguing that his prior claims as father, husband, and worker excuse him, especially since there is a sister (a married homemaker with no children) who is more available. From the perspective of case management, it will be crucial to know the history of relationships within a family so that it can be better determined who will assume what obligation to give care.

As illness, disability, and death are universal family occurrences, family theorists have addressed the normative context in which these events take place. For example, Rolland (2003) has contended that practitioners use the concept of goodness-of-fit as a standard of how families are mastering the challenge of serious illness and disability. That is, what is the fit between the psychosocial demands of the disorder and the family style of functioning and the resources available? He suggests that assessment address the family and individual life cycles at the time of the disorder, the multigenerational legacies related to illness and loss, and the family belief system (see Chapter one, Table 4). He goes on to propose that practitioners examine the onset of the disorder, whether it is gradual or sudden and acute, requiring families to rapidly mobilize their crisis management skills. The course of the illness is another matter for practitioners to consider. Is it a progressive disease in which the family is faced with continued decline and loss? Is it a constant-course disease in which the relative experiences a relatively stable biological course? Or is it a relapsing or episodic illness in which families are strained by inconsistencies of symptoms?

In addition, practitioners will want to be aware of the initial expectation the family has for the disease. The outcome is usually equated with whether or not the disease will shorten the relative's lifespan. Finally, whether or nor a disease is incapacitating is often a worry for the family and can be addressed by the social worker. Rolland developed schema to describe the timeline and phases of illness that families may go through (see Figure 2). The phases and their critical tasks include:

- The *crisis phase* encompasses the time period before there are symptoms and the initial diagnosis has been made. It also includes the period after diagnosis has been made and initial adjustment starts to occur. Families learn to cope with symptoms; adapt to health care settings and treatment(s); and establish and maintain working relationships with health care professionals (Moos, 1984). They also create meaning of the illness that maximizes mastery; grieve for the loss of life before the illness; gradually accept the illness as permanent; pull together to cope with the immediate crisis; and face the uncertainty of the future. Practitioners when involved have the tasks framing events so that families may stay as competent as possible.
- The *chronic phase* is the time between the initial phase and the third phase when issue of death and terminal illness predominate. The ability of the family to maintain the day-to-day semblance of "normal" life is the key task. Emotions of blame, shame, and guilt are not uncommon and can be helped by psychoeducational groups.
- The *terminal phase* emerges when the family realizes that their family member's death is inevitable. The primary tasks often are coping

FIGURE 2. Timeline and Phases of Illness

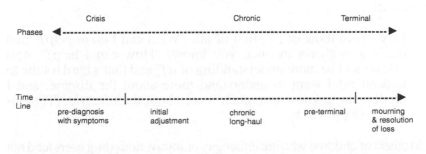

Adapted from: Rolland (1984)

with issues of separation, death, mourning, and the resumption of family life beyond the loss (Rolland, 2003, pp. 469-470).

NON-NORMATIVE FAMILY CARE

Not all family caregiving follows universal patterns. For example, according to Greene, Kropf, and MacNair (1994), an HIV positive diagnosis and the need to provide care is not considered a predictable part of family development. The spread of AIDS among young and middle-aged adults has produced a challenging and often overwhelming situation for many older adults who must face their child's illness and, often, death, during the prime of life (Mullan, 1998). Partners, parents, and grandparents–to take the three most common caregiving groups–who confront this now chronic disease, must deal with grief, loss, and death long before the "normal time." In many HIV-affected families, the burden of caregiving falls on older extended family members, usually grandmothers, who must not only cope with the loss of their adult child but must assume the responsibilities of caring for the surviving grandchildren (Itin, McFeaters, & Taylor-Brown, 2004). Often the grief of these older caregivers can be complicated by feelings of anger and resentment toward their own children for leaving them with the burden of providing childcare "at an unanticipated time in their own life cycle" (ibid., p. 646; Boyd-Franklin, Drelich, & Schwolsky-Fitch, 1995). The settling of old scores with families of origin may also be an issue. In addition, negative social attitudes and stigmatization may mean diminished social support systems.

Despite some discomfort with the link between AIDS and being gay, among older mothers of children with HIV/AIDS, there is a marked tendency to focus on their child's illness rather than the issue of sexual orientation (Brennan & Moore, 1994; Thompson, 2000). One mother puts it very clearly:

> I try . . . to think of . . . first of all, "What can I do to help?" and that's a mother's instinct, you know, "How can I help?" And "How can I be more understanding of it?" and that's hard for me to understand–I want to understand more about the disease, and I don't want to know too much more about the lifestyle. (Thompson, 2000, p. 161)

Mothers of children who are either gay or intravenous drug users tend not to blame their children, although some blame for their child's situation will be self-directed (ibid.). For practitioners, the challenge is to set parental boundaries that amount to limits to their responsibility for their children, thereby permitting and encouraging them to focus on the present and the caregiving and support of their child.

In addition to personal beliefs, beliefs inflected by race, culture, or religion, for example, are also a major influence on how families perceive health and illness. Cultural differences thus have an influence on how caregiving is administered. While, for many persons with AIDS, an older mother serves as a crucial source of care and support, this is especially true among gay men and bisexual African American men who are less likely to be part of a gay support network than their white counterparts (Brown & Sankar, 1998). For families affected by HIV/AIDS, another important social difference from the perspective of case management is the extent to which the family may be experiencing social isolation issuing from a fear of stigma. Families may isolate themselves, drawing a boundary between the immediate family and those outside of it by choosing not to disclose the diagnosis to those in the wider social network (Bor, Miller, & Goldman, 1993).

Alternatively, families, especially low-income ones, may not have the privacy necessary to draw such a protective boundary. Their close physical proximity to neighbors and institutions may make it exceedingly difficult to conceal personal information or behaviors. If an individual's diagnosis of HIV/AIDS becomes public knowledge, this can have significant negative impact on the family, marking family relations with shame and stigma, and negatively affecting self-esteem and identity (Dane & Miller, 1992). The fear of stigma can lead to the isolation of HIV/AIDS-impacted families, removing them from the potential support networks of family, friends, community, and professionals. Therefore, case management with families must realize a culturally appropriate plan of care.

REFERENCES

Austin, C. (1992). Case management in long-term care: Options and opportunities. In S. M. Rose (Ed.), *Case management and social work practice.* (pp.199-218). New York: Longman.

Bandura, A. (1994). Self-efficacy. In V. S. Ramachaudran (Ed.), *Encyclopedia of human behavior* (Vol. 4, pp. 71-81). New York: Academic Press.

Bengtson, V. L., Burgess, E. O., & Parrott, T. M. (1997). Theory, explanation, and a third generation of theoretical development in social gerontology. *Journals of Gerontology: Social Sciences, 52B,* S72-S88.

Black, M. (1985). Health and social support of older adults in the community. *Canadian Journal on Aging*, 4(4), 213-226.

Bor, R., Miller, R., & Goldman, E. E. (1993). HIV/AIDS and the family: A review of research in the first decade. *Journal of Family Therapy, 15*, 187-204.

Boyd-Franklin, N., Drelich, E. W., & Schwolsky-Fitch, E. (1995). Death and dying: Bereavement and mourning. In N. Boyd-Franklin, G. Steiner, & M. Boland (Eds.), *Children, families, and HIV/AIDS: Psychosocial and therapeutic issues* (pp. 167-178). New York: Guilford.

Brennan, P. F., & Moore, S. M. (1994). Caregivers of persons with AIDS. In E. Kahana, D. E. Biegel, & M. L. Wykle (Eds.), *Family caregiving across the lifespan* (pp. 159-177). Thousand Oaks, CA: Sage.

Brody, E. M. (1985). Parent care as a normative family stress. *The Gerontologist, 25(1)*, 19-29.

Brown, D. R., & Sankar, A. (1998). HIV/AIDS and aging minority populations. *Research on Aging 20(6)*, 865-884.

Canda, E. (2002). The significance of spirituality for resilient response to chronic illness: A qualitative study of adults with cystic fibrosis. In D. Saleebey (Ed.), *The strengths perspective* (3rd edition, pp. 63-79). Boston: Allyn & Bacon.

Coleman, J. (1963). Comments "On the concept of influence." *Public Opinion Quarterly, 27*, 63-82.

Coulton, C. J. (1981). Person-environment fit as the focus in health care. *Social Work, 26*, 26-35.

Daatland, S. O. (1983). Care systems. *Aging and Society, 3*, 1-21.

Dane, B., & Miller, S. (1992). *AIDS: Intervening with hidden grievers*. Westport, CT: Auburn House.

Dowd, J. J. (1980). *Stratification among the aged*. Monterey, CA: Brooks/Cole.

Dwyer, J. W., Lee, G. R., & Jankowski, T. B. (1994). Reciprocity, elder satisfaction, and caregiver stress and burden: The exchange of aid in the family caregiving relationship. *Journal of Marriage and the Family, 56(1)*, 35-43.

Engel, G. L. (1980). The clinical application of the biopsychosocial model. *American Journal of Psychiatry, 137*, 535-544.

Germain, C. B. (1973). An ecological perspective in casework practice. *Social Casework*, 54, 323-330.

Germain, C. B. (1978). General systems theory and ego psychology. *Social Service Review, 52*, 535-550.

Germain, C. B. (1987). Human development in contemporary environments. *Social Service Review, 61*, 565-580.

Goode, W. J. (1964). *The family*. Englewood Cliffs, NJ: Prentice-Hall.

Gouldner, A. J. (1967). Reciprocity and autonomy in functional theory. In N. J. Demerath III, & R. A. Peterson (Eds.), *System, change, and conflict* (pp. 141-169). New York: Free Press.

Greene, R. R. (1992). Case management: An arena for social work practice. In B. S. Vourlekis & R. R. Greene (Eds.), *Social work case management* (pp. 11-25). New York: Aldine de Gruyter.

Greene, R. R. (2000). Social work with the aged and their family. New York: Aldine de Gruyter.

Greene, R. R. & Kropf, N. P. (2003). A family case management approach for level I needs. In A. C. Kilpatrick & T. P. Holland (Eds.), *Working with families: An integrative model by level of care* (pp. 85-103). Boston: Allyn & Bacon.

Greene, R. R., Kropf, N. P., & MacNair, N. (1994). A family therapy model for working with persons with AIDS. *Journal of Family Therapy, 5*(1), 1-20.

Hareven, T. K. (2001). Historical perspectives on aging and family relations. In R. H. Binstock & L. K. George (Eds.), *Handbook of aging and the social sciences* (pp. 141-159). New York: Academic Press.

Hawley, A. H. (1979). *Societal growth: Processes and implications.* New York: Free Press.

Hooyman, N. R., Hooyman, G., & Kethly, A. (1981). The role of gerontological social work in interdisciplinary care. Paper presented at the Council on Social Work Education Annual Program Meeting, Louisville, Kentucky, March.

Itin, C., McFeaters, S., & Taylor-Brown, S. (2004). The family unity program for HIV-affected families: Creating a family-centered and community-building context for interventions. In J. Berzoff & P. R. Silverman (Eds.), *Living with dying: A handbook for end-of-life health care practitioners* (pp. 642-660). New York: Columbia University Press.

Johnson, L. C. (1992). *Social work practice: A generalist approach.* Boston: Allyn & Bacon.

Kirst-Ashman, K. K., & Hull, G. H. (2002). *Understanding generalist practice.* Chicago: Nelson-Hall.

Kisthardt, W. E. (1992). A strengths model of case management. In D. Saleebey (Ed.), *The strengths perspective in social work* (pp. 59-83)). New York: Longman.

Lourie, N. (1978). Case management. In J. Talbott (Ed.), *The chronic mental patient* (pp. 159-164). Washington, DC: American Psychiatric Association.

Martin, P. Y., & O'Connor, G. G. (1989). *The social environment: Open systems applications.* New York: Longman.

Miley, K. K., O'Melia, M., & DuBois, B. (2001). *Generalist social work practice: An empowerment approach.* Boston: Allyn & Bacon.

Minuchin, S. (1974). *Families and family therapy.* Cambridge, MA: Harvard University Press.

Mullan, J. T. (1998). Aging and informal caregiving to people with HIV/AIDS. *Research on Aging, 20(6)*, 712-738.

Norman, E. (Ed.) (2000). *Resiliency enhancement: Putting the strengths perspective into social work practice.* New York: Columbia University Press.

Ozarin, L. (1978). The pros and cons of case management. In J. Talbott (Ed.), *The chronic mental patient* (pp. 165-170). Washington, DC: American Psychiatric Association.

Rapp, C. A. (1992). The strengths perspective of case management with persons suffering from severe mental illness. In D. Saleebey (Ed.), *The strengths perspective* (pp. 45-58). New York: Longman.

Rapp, C. A. (1998). *The strengths model: Case management with people suffering from severe and persistent mental illness.* New York: Oxford University Press.

Rolland, J. S. (1984). Toward a psychosocial typology of chronic and life-threatening illness. *Family Systems Medicine, 2*(3), 245-263.

Rolland, J. S. (2003). Mastering family challenges in serious illness and disability. In F. Walsh (Ed.), *Normal family processes: Growing diversity and complexity* (3rd edition, pp. 460-492). New York: Guilford Press.

Rose, S. M. (1992). *Case management and social work practice.* New York: Longman.

Rose, S. M. & Moore, V. L. (1995). Case Management. In R. L. Edwards (Ed.-in-Chief), *Encyclopedia of social work* (19th edition, pp. 335-340). Washington, DC: NASW Press.

Rossi, A. S. (2001). The impact of family problems on social responsibility. In A. S. Rossi (Ed.), *Caring and doing for others: Social responsibility in the domains of family, work, and community* (pp. 321-347). Chicago: University of Chicago Press.

Rubin, A. (1987). Case management. In A. Minahan (Editor-in-Chief), *Encyclopedia of social work* (18th edition, pp. 212-222). Silver Spring, MD: NASW Press.

Satir, V. (1967). *Conjoint family therapy* (2nd ed.). Palo Alto, CA: Science and Behavior Books.

Seltzer, M. M., Ivry, J., & Litchfield, L. C. (1992). Family members as case managers: Partnership between the formal and the informal support networks. In S. M. Rose (Ed.), *Case management and social work practice* (pp. 229-242). New York: Longman.

Sussman, M. B. (1976). The family life of older people. In R. H. Binstock & E. Shanas (Eds.), *Handbook of aging and the social sciences* (pp. 415-449). New York: Van Nostrand Reinhold.

Thompson, E. (2000). Mothers' experiences of an adult child's HIV/AIDS diagnosis: Maternal responses to and resolution of accountability for AIDS. *Family Relations, 49(2),* 155-164.

Trattner, W. I. (1994). *From poor law to welfare state: A history of social welfare in America.* New York: Free Press.

Verzaro-Lawrence, M. (1981). Shared childbearing: A challenging alternative lifestyle. *Alternative Lifestyles, 4(2),* 205-217.

Vourlekis, B. & Greene, R. R. (1992). *Social work case management.* New York: Aldine de Gruyter.

Weil, M., & Karls, J. (1985). *Case management in human service practice.* San Francisco: Jossey-Bass.

doi:10.1300/J137v14n01_02

Chapter 3

Mental Health Care Policy: Recognizing the Needs of Minority Siblings as Caregivers

Tara R. Earl

SUMMARY. This chapter presents a review of the research on sibling related caregiving issues and their implications for social work practice and mental health policy. Specifically, it discusses the concerns of ethnic minority siblings as caregivers for their mentally ill family member. doi:10.1300/J137v14n01_03 *[Article copies available for a fee from The Haworth Document Delivery Service: 1-800-HAWORTH. E-mail address: <docdelivery@haworthpress.com> Website: <http://www.HaworthPress.com> © 2006 by The Haworth Press, Inc. All rights reserved.]*

KEYWORDS. Mental illness, caregiving, minority siblings

SEVERE MENTAL ILLNESS IN SOCIETY

Severe mental illness (SMI) or severe and persistent mental illness (SPMI) affects a significant proportion of those diagnosed with mental disorders, and it is considered a more debilitating class of disorders than

[Haworth co-indexing entry note]: "Mental Health Care Policy: Recognizing the Needs of Minority Siblings as Caregivers." Earl, Tara R. Co-published simultaneously in *Journal of Human Behavior in the Social Environment* (The Haworth Press, Inc.) Vol. 14, No. 1/2, 2006, pp. 51-72; and: *Contemporary Issues of Care* (ed: Roberta R. Greene) The Haworth Press, Inc., 2006, pp. 51-72. Single or multiple copies of this article are available for a fee from The Haworth Document Delivery Service [1-800-HAWORTH, 9:00 a.m. - 5:00 p.m. (EST). E-mail address: docdelivery@haworthpress.com].

other forms of mental illness (U.S. DHHS, 1999; Table 1). The 1999 U.S. Surgeon General's Report on Mental Illness estimated that, in any given year, between ten to eleven million people are diagnosed with a mental illness and five to six million people meet the criteria for SMI (U.S. Surgeon General, 1999). This means approximately five to six percent of the adult population in the U.S. is diagnosed with a mental illness and three percent of the adult population in the United States meets the criteria for SMI (Biegel & Shulz, 1999; Kessler, Abelson, & Zhao, 1998; Kessler et al., 1996; U.S. DHHS, 1999).

Defining Severe Mental Illness

There does not seem to be a consensus on the clinical delineation of the classification of mental illness and severe mental illness (SMI) (Biegel & Shulz, 1999; Kuntz, 1995). However, the United States Senate National Advisory Mental Health Council (1993) describes severe mental illness as being

> defined through diagnosis, disability, and duration, and includes disorders with psychotic symptoms such as schizophrenia, schizoaffective disorder, manic depressive disorder, autism, as well as severe forms of other disorders such as major depression, panic disorder, and obsessive compulsive disorder.

This definition is consistent with other descriptions and definitions of severe mental illness. For instance, the National Alliance for the Mentally Ill reported that an individual experiencing a severe mental illness is someone who has mental conditions that are characterized by alterations in thinking, mood, or behavior (or some combination thereof) associated with distress and/or impaired functioning.

Schizophrenia

Schizophrenia, the most common diagnostic category associated with SMI, is a chronic, severe, and disabling brain disease (NIMH, 2001). Schizophrenia ranks among the top ten causes of disability in developed countries, including the United States (Murray & Lopez, 2004). Schizophrenia and other severe mental illnesses—schizoaffective disorder, major depressive disorder (clinical depression), and manic depressive disorder/bipolar disorder—are commonly diagnosed during early or later

TABLE 1. Percentage of People Experiencing Psychiatric Disorders During Their Lifetime**

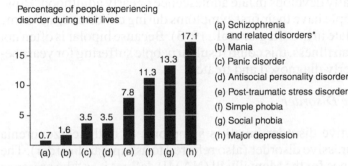

Percentage of people experiencing disorder during their lives

(a) Schizophrenia and related disorders*
(b) Mania
(c) Panic disorder
(d) Antisocial personality disorder
(e) Post-traumatic stress disorder
(f) Simple phobia
(g) Social phobia
(h) Major depression

*Related disorders include schizophreniform disorder, schizoaffective disorder, delusional disorder, and atypical psychosis.
**The percentages are lower than in other reported documents because homeless people and those living in prisons, nursing homes, or other institutions, were not included in the survey.
Adapted from: National Comorbidity Survey, *Archives of General Psychiatry*, (Kessler et al., 1994). Researchers interviewed more than 8000 people aged 15 to 54 years.

adulthood when most individuals are linked to varying family systems (Greenberg, Seltzer, Orsmond, & Krauss, 1999).

The onset of schizophrenia is commonly referred to as an acute phase, characterized by a state of mental impairment, hallucinations, delusions, and disorganized speech and behavior, all of which may cause the person to become fearful and withdrawn from family and friends (NIMH, 2001). The National Alliance of Research on Schizophrenia and Depression (NARSAD) reported that in any given year there are more than two million people affected by schizophrenia in the United States. It is further estimated that approximately one percent of the world population will develop schizophrenia.

Bipolar Disorder

Bipolar disorder, also known as manic-depressive disorder, is a brain disorder that causes unusual shifts in a person's mood, energy, and ability to function (Baldessarini et al., 2003). The disorder is generally considered to be a biochemical disorder of the brain and its associated hormonal systems. Different from the normal ups and downs that everyone goes through, the symptoms of bipolar disorder are severe.

More than two million American adults, or about 1 percent of the population age 18 and older in any given year, have bipolar disorder. Bipolar disorder typically develops in late adolescence or early adulthood. However, some people have their first symptoms during childhood, and some develop them late in life (Regier et al., 1993). Because bipolar is often not recognized as an illness, this could result in people suffering for years before it is properly diagnosed and treated.

Schizoaffective Disorder

Schizoaffective disorder involves symptoms of both schizophrenia and manic depressive disorder (also referred to as bipolar disorder). The National Alliance for the Mentally Ill (NAMI) defines it as "the presence of psychotic symptoms in the absence of mood changes for at least two weeks in a patient who has a mood disorder." The diagnosis is used when an individual does not fit diagnostic standards for either schizophrenia or "affective" (mood) disorders such as depression and bipolar disorder (manic depression). The onset of the illness usually begins in early adulthood and is more commonly diagnosed in women.

Major Depressive Disorder

Major depression disorder is also referred to as clinical depression. It is characterized by a severely depressed mood that persists for at least two weeks (DSM-IV, 2000). Episodes of major depressive disorder may start suddenly or slowly and can occur several times through a person's life. This disorder may occur or coexist as a result of another serious illness such as diabetes or HIV/AIDS (www.nimh.gov).

THE BIOLOGICAL, PSYCHOLOGICAL, AND SOCIAL COMPONENTS OF MENTAL ILLNESS

Mental health (not to be confused with mental illness) is as important as physical health to daily living. In fact, the two are intertwined. Individuals with physical health problems often experience anxiety or depression that affects their response to the physical illness. Individuals with mental illnesses can develop physical symptoms and illnesses, such as weight loss and blood biochemical imbalances associated with eating disorders. Feelings, attitudes and patterns of thought strongly influence people's experience of physical health or illness, and may affect the course of illness and the effectiveness of treatment.

Addressing the biological, psychological and social components of mental illness can promote mental health and perhaps prevent some mental illnesses. For the individual, factors such as proper medication treatment and compliance, appropriate diet and lifestyle, social supports, meaningful employment or social roles, physical activity, and an internal locus of control will strengthen mental health and, indirectly, reduce the impact or incidence of some mental illness episodes.

Biological Components

Research suggests that mental illness is the result of a complex interaction of genetic, biological, personality, and environmental factors; however, the brain is the final common pathway for the control of behavior, cognition, mood, and anxiety. At this time, the links between specific brain dysfunction and specific mental illnesses are not fully understood (Schwartz, 1999). It is important not to over-interpret the available evidence about the role of either genetic or environmental factors in causing mental illnesses as much more research is needed to fully understand the cause of mental illness.

Most mental illnesses are found to be more common in close family members of a person with a mental illness, suggesting a genetic basis to the disorders (Schwartz, 1999). In some instances there is research evidence suggesting that particular genetic factors affecting brain chemistry contribute to the onset and progression of mental illness. However, there is also increasing evidence that long-term changes in brain function can occur in response to factors in the environment such as stimulation, experiences of traumatic or chronic stress, or various kinds of deprivation (Schwartz, 1999). In other words, the interaction between brain biology and lived experience appears to work both ways.

For reasons that may be biological, psychosocial, or both, age and sex affect rates of mental illness. Environmental factors such as family situation, workplace pressures, and the socio-economic status of the individual can precipitate the onset or recurrence of a mental illness. Lifestyle choices (e.g., substance abuse) and learned patterns of thought and behavior can influence the onset, course, and outcome of mental illness (Schwartz, 1999).

Psychological Components

The serious stigma and discrimination attached to mental illnesses are among the most tragic realities facing ethnic minorities with mental illness in our society. Arising from racism, superstition, lack of knowledge and empathy, old belief systems, and a tendency to fear and exclude people who are perceived as different, stigma and discrimination have existed throughout history (Whaley, 1997). Such perceptions or feelings force people to remain quiet about their mental illness, often causing them to delay seeking health care, to avoid following through with recommended treatment, and to evade sharing their concerns with family, friends, co-workers, employers, health service providers, and others in the community (Snowden, 2001).

Ironically, most mental illnesses can be treated. Treatment must reflect the complex origins of mental illnesses. A variety of interventions, such as psychotherapy, cognitive behavioral therapy, medication, occupational therapy, and social work, can improve an individual's functioning and quality of life. Since mental illnesses involve disorders of brain functioning, medication often forms an important part of treatment.

Making the correct diagnosis and tailoring effective treatment to the individual's needs are essential components of an overall management plan, especially with persons of ethnic/minority backgrounds. The active involvement of the individual in the choice of therapy and his/her adherence to the chosen therapy are critical to successful treatment.

Treatment requires a variety of health and social service providers and volunteers organized into a comprehensive system of services. Service providers need to work as a team to ensure continuity of care. For maximal effectiveness, a treatment system should provide all individuals with access to services where needed.

Social Components

At the public mental health system level, strategies that create supportive environments, strengthen community action, and put the proper resources in the community, can help to ensure that individuals living in the community have some control over the psychological and social determinants of their illness.

FAMILIES AND MENTAL ILLNESS

Parents to Siblings

The literature on the ways in which families provide care to a relative has offered many contributions to the study and treatment of severe mental illness (Goldman, 1982; Goldstein & Canton, 1983, Lefley, 1987; NIMH, 1994; NAMI, 2004; Steinwachs, Kasper, & Skinner, 1992a). Despite the fact that parents initially assume responsibility for their severely mentally ill children, there is a growing recognition that the ability of parents to provide care for their child eventually diminishes and ultimately ends (Lefley, 1987). Research to date has focused either globally on the family or specifically on the mother. As a result, there is a major gap about the specific role of the sibling as caregiver. As parents begin to "age out," the responsibility of providing care increasingly shifts to the adult sibling (Greenberg et al., 1999; Horwitz, 1993a, 1993b, 1994; Horwitz, Tessler, Fisher, & Gamache, 1992).

Sibling Relationships and Bonds

Sibling relationships are the least studied relationships in the family system, yet they are one of the longest-lasting relationships in people's lives (Shortt & Gottman, 1997). Moreover, siblings share a common social, cultural, and genetic heritage, making the sibling bond an unique factor within the family network (Nechmad et al., 2000). Sibling support is intense during childhood and adolescence (Shortt & Gottman, 1997; Jenkins, 1992), weakens in adulthood (Bank & Kahn, 1982), and strengthens again in old age (Cicirelli, 1989; Connidis, 1989).

The relationship between siblings may vary through the years, but many people find that it helps to keep them rooted to their past, to cope with the present, and be willing to hope for the future (Bank & Kahn, 1982; Cicirelli, 1995). For instance, when parents were neglectful or abusive, Jenkins (1992) found that siblings leaned on one another for support, a finding that further confirms the notion about the strong bond between siblings. That is, "when other relationships cannot be relied upon, intense sibling relationships are activated" (Bank & Kahn, 1982, p. 19). Moreover, research shows that after the death of a parent, the relationship between siblings becomes more powerful (Greenberg, Seltzer, Orsmond, & Krauss, 1999; Horwitz, 1994; Horwitz, Tessler, Fisher, & Gamache, 1992).

Bank and Kahn (1982) attempted to develop a unified and comprehensive theory that would integrate various perspectives and provide a better understanding of the nature of the bond between siblings. The authors suggested that there were three recurring, predictable conditions that allowed a strong bond to develop: (1) high access or frequent contact between siblings; (2) the need for meaningful personal identity; and (3) sufficient influence. They observed that

> sibling bonds will become intense and exert a formative influence upon personality when, as children or adolescents, the siblings have had plentiful access and contact *and* have been deprived of reliable parental care. In this situation, siblings will use one another as major influences, or touchstones, in a search for personal identity. When other relationships–with parents, children, or spouses– are emotionally fulfilling, the sibling bond will be weaker and less important. (p. 19)

Recognizing the Role of the Sibling as a Caregiver

Over the past ten to fifteen years there has been an increased recognition of the role of adult siblings as caregivers for relatives with severe mental illness. In the United States, siblings represent more than 80% of the population (Marsh, 1998). Despite these numbers, with respect to their role as potential primary caregivers of their relatives with mental illness, siblings are often ignored by practitioners who fail to consider and understand their experiences, needs, or concerns (Greenberg et al., 1999). The major reason is that, historically, the caregiver role has primarily focused on the parent, specifically, the mother who has received the label of "primary caregiver" (Lefley, 1987; Maltiades & Pruncho, 2002).

Despite common beliefs, as parents grow older either they become too tired to continue to care for their mentally ill child or they die. This is commonly known as "aging out." The aging out phenomenon is particularly germane because it highlights the fact that siblings are often overlooked when practitioners and clinicians develop treatment plans or utilize the person in environment treatment model (Cook et al., 1997; Marsh et al., 1993a; Marsh et al., 1993b; Thompson & Doll, 1982). Nonetheless, the literature consistently informs us that the sibling is the family member who is most likely to end up taking on the caregiving responsibility(Greenberg et al., 1999; Hatfield & Lefley, 1993; Horwitz, 1993a; Horwitz, 1993b; Seltzer, Greenberg, Krauss, Gordon, & Judge, 1997). For example, the following is a narrative of a sibling recalling her mother's burden and how her mother became too tired to continue providing care for her child:

Well, my mom predominantly, has dealt with, I hate to call it a burden, but it has been for her. From the time of my sister being diagnosed with a developmental disability, let alone a mental illness, which my parents sorta understood but not really, she was the one who looked at the programs and was there when Evelyn had issues or was "not behaving well, was not feeling well, or something's going wrong," but literally she was decompensating, that's what it was. My mom had to deal with it and just dealt with it. She didn't communicate to any body until she realized, about 15 years ago, she could clearly communicate to me about it. She didn't communicate much with my oldest sister, she would tell my dad, but wouldn't tell anyone at church . . . wouldn't tell her good friends. It was "her burden" that she kept and wore and ironically when my dad retired, even more so since they've been in Austin, which has been about 7 years now, she told my dad, "it's your turn now to do the ripping and running to do the meds and do the doctors exams and so forth." (Earl, T.R., unpublished data, 2003)

Siblings and Social Support

The literature has increasingly presented research in which caregiving is understood as a form of social support. For example, Horwitz and colleagues (1992) examined the role of adult siblings in providing social support to their severely mentally ill relatives. The researchers interviewed a sample of 283 patients from state hospitals in Ohio and 24-hour crisis care facilities shortly after they were discharged. The researchers asked for permission to interview close family members, such as parents, siblings, or extended family. The study was based on personal interviews from a sub-sample of 109 sibling respondents, out of a list of 146 respondents.

The study categorized the responses to the interviews with siblings into two dimensions of support: (1) subjective feelings, and (2) provision of concrete forms of material, financial, or other kinds of assistance. They compared predictors of sibling caregiving versus parental caregiving according to six main areas: (1) need, (2) personal relationships, (3) caregiver involvement, (4) social networks, (5) gender of caregiver, and (6) race. Findings indicated that greater patient need, positive attitudes towards the mentally ill sibling (personal relationships), and other role involvement (caregiver involvement) were the major factors influencing sibling caregiving. Comparative analyses showed that personal relationships and alternative role involvements (caregiver involvement) were better predictors of sibling caregiving rather than parental caregiving.

Horwitz (1993) tested the hypothesis, derived from the serial model of social support, that adult siblings will provide more support to their seriously mentally ill relative when parents are not available. He interviewed 108 siblings. Results supported the serial model, and indicated that, over the life course, siblings could in part replace parental caretakers as providers of social support to their seriously mentally ill relative.

Specifically, siblings with one or no living parents provided more help than siblings with two living parents. Siblings with only one brother or sister provided more help than siblings with multiple brothers or sisters. Finally, siblings who provided more assistance were more likely to be African American or Puerto Rican, to live at a closer distance, and to regard their siblings as having a very serious illness.

Horwitz (1994) also conducted an exploratory study to examine how obligation, reciprocity, and the quality of personal relationships affected whether siblings provided social support to their relative diagnosed with a mental illness. The primary question in this study was whether or not "kinship responsibilities extend beyond spousal and parental/child bonds so that relationships between adult siblings can become sources of long-term social support?" (p. 274). In order to answer this, Horwitz interviewed 108 siblings who had a brother or sister diagnosed with schizophrenia (80%) and manic-depression (15%). The diagnoses for the remaining 5% were unknown.

Reciprocity or mutual caregiving stood out as the best predictor of sibling social support. In other words, reciprocity was important in creating bonds when one sibling was mentally ill. Siblings reported more help and more willingness to provide help to mentally ill relatives who reciprocated through affection, gifts, chores, and so on. When siblings did not perceive reciprocity, they tended to withhold support without guilt or worry about how they would be perceived by others.

Horwitz's studies were the first to systematically examine the possibility of viewing the sibling as one who could provide support to a sibling diagnosed with a mental illness. This research study, however, explored the siblings as being potential supports for their brother or sisters diagnosed with a severe mental illness, and not as being the primary caregiver, thus offering little insight into the experiences of individuals actively serving as primary caregivers.

Qualitative Research on Sibling Caregiving

Qualitative research studies have also informed sibling caregiving, raising questions, providing narratives, and giving voice to the personal experiences of siblings who had a brother or sister diagnosed with a severe mental illness (Landeen et al. 1992; Marsh, Dickens, Koeske, Yackovich, Wilson, & McQuillis, 1993a; Marsh, Appleby, Dickens, Owens, & Young, 1993b). For example, Landeen et al. (1992) examined the practical concerns of well siblings of persons with schizophrenia. A descriptive study was conducted that included a needs assessment survey and a workshop designed to increase well siblings' knowledge about schizophrenia. The results of their study indicated that well siblings wanted more information about schizophrenia. The 88 sibling respondents expressed a desire to learn more about the prognosis of mental illness and ways in which they could improve how they communicated and problem solved with their mentally ill siblings. Overall, the study's findings highlighted that well siblings of persons with schizophrenia had specific needs that varied from other family members, such as parents.

Another study by Marsh et al. (1993a; 1993b) examined the experiences of both siblings and children of people with serious mental illnesses over three phases of the life span: (1) childhood, (2) adolescence, and (3) adulthood. The researchers pointed out that the response patterns varied over the life span. For example, siblings reported that they did not really deal with the mental illness of a family member until adolescence or adulthood.

The results from the 1993 study *Troubled journey: Siblings and children of people with mental illness* pointed to the impact that severe mental illness had on the lives of the respondents. Some respondents reported major transformations in their lives, such as having to deal with an illness that was not familiar and having to figure a way to respond to the needs of their sibling, while taking care of their personal responsibilities. Others shared stories about how they were afraid to have a family of their own because they feared that the mental illness would affect their children. Overall, the respondents expressed a need for more support and information about their relative's illness. On average, sibling respondents ranked needs for personal support, for skills to cope with the illness, and for working through their reactions to the illness as being "very important."

The findings from the subsequent study, *Anguished voices: Impact of mental illness on siblings and children* (1993b), were consistent with the first study. In this study, respondents participated in interviews and two national surveys. The respondents presented at a workshop before a group of psychologists who were attending an annual meeting of their state psychological association. The respondents first shared their experiences and then made recommendations to the audience. This study took excerpts from the detailed discussions and utilized the narratives to explain how mental illness impacts both siblings and children of relatives diagnosed with a mental illness.

FAMILY CAREGIVING BURDEN

Earlier research defined family as one unit, and tended to compare the amount of support provided by parents or spouses, rather than by siblings (Horwitz et al., 1992; Horwitz, 1993; Horwitz, 1994). Investigations during the 1950s and 1970s were based on the theory of familial transmission of schizophrenia and focused on siblings from the aspect of their susceptibility to the disease (Lidz, 1963, 1973, 1976; Lidz, Fleck, Alanen, Cornilson, 1963; Lidz, Fleck, & Cornilson, 1966). Case studies were often used to explain how some well siblings escaped the pathological family network (Adams, 1968; Glick et al., 1967).

With the introduction of the concept of family burden in the 1960s, research shifted to the emotional impact of growing up with a brother or sister with schizophrenia. This was accompanied by the emergence of self-help groups and published case histories of siblings themselves. In the 1980s, research was mostly descriptive. Researchers studied sibling shame, poor self-esteem, and feelings of stigmatization. Different patterns of subjective burden were distinguished. Recently, greater efforts have been made to systematically define the variables associated with the burden experienced by siblings (Greenberg, Kim, & Greenley, 1997; Greenberg, Seltzer, Orsmond, & Krauss, 1999; Horwitz & Reinhard, 1995; Landeen et al., 1992; Marsh, Dickens, Koeske, Yackovich, Wilson, & McQuillis, 1993a; Marsh, Appleby, Dickens, Owens, & Young, 1993b).

Researchers have explored and investigated family burden as it relates to caregivers of mentally ill relatives (Cook, Cohler, Pickett, & Beeler, 1997; Greenberg et al., 1997; Karp, 2003; Kung, 2001; Lefley, 1998; Lefley, 2003; Marsh et al., 1993a; Tessler & Gamache, 2000). For example, Muhlbauer (2002) used qualitative methods to examine different phases in the journey or experiences of family members as caregivers. The findings indicated that family members (parents, siblings, and significant others) of a relative diagnosed with a mental illness experience substantial difficulty with memory and concentration, and problems with hallucinations, delusions, violent behavior, substance abuse, social skills, money, and coping with stress and change.

Much of the literature has described families as being highly burdened by their relative's mental illness, revealing two primary domains: (1) objective burden, and (2) subjective burden. *Objective burden* involves environmental constraints including loss of financial income and *subjective burden* pertains to personal affective states such as emotional distress (Cook et al., 1997). However, the literature on family burden included only a brief description of the sibling experience.

SIBLING CAREGIVING PRACTICES

Using a sample of 164 siblings, Greenberg, Kim, and Greenley (1997) examined the relationship between various factors associated with the subjective caregiving burden experienced by siblings of adults with severe mental illness. Subjective burden, the variable of interest, was measured using four scales: a global measure of subjective burden and three measures of specific types of subjective burden, stigma, fears, and worries about the future. They also examined objective burden, family attributions, caregiving context, health, gender differences, and the nature of the disabled sibling's illness. Findings suggested that:

- Older siblings tended to worry less about their ill sibling's future care than did younger siblings.
- The well sibling's gender and education were positively related to global feelings of burden. Sisters and those siblings with higher education reported significantly greater subjective burden.
- Younger siblings taking care of an older sibling reported higher levels of subjective burden and stigma than those taking care of a younger sibling.
- There was a trend in which siblings worried more about the future care of a sister than of a brother with mental illness.
- Siblings who provided more care tended to report more feelings of subjective burden than did less involved siblings.
- Well siblings who thought their ill sibling had control over their symptoms experienced higher levels of subjective burden, stigma, fears, and worries about the future.
- Psychiatric symptoms were significantly related to higher levels of stigma.

Greenberg and colleagues (1999) completed another study in which they investigated the current involvement and expectations of future caregivng roles for siblings of adults with mental illness or mental retardation. The study highlighted a set of *push* and *pull* factors that influenced the extent to which a person was or became a caregiver. The researchers defined *push* factors as those that propelled siblings towards greater involvement with caring for their brother or sister and *pull* factors as those that drove them away. Some of the factors that would push a sibling into an increased caregiving role included childhood socialization experiences and feelings of closeness within the family. Some examples of factors that would pull a sibling away from providing care to their brother or sister diagnosed with a severe mental illness involved midlife roles such as marriage, parenthood, and a career. The severity of the brother or sister's behavior problems was also identified as a pull factor.

Ethnic Minority Siblings as Caregivers

> . . . I'm the oldest of nine children and in our culture, the oldest always takes over after mom and dad decides that they can't handle it . . . I'm very much involved in taking my brother to the doctors, being a part of his treatment. . . . By helping my brother, I feel very strongly that I help my mom and I help myself and I help others.

Research that focuses on Asians, Hispanic/Latinos, Pacific Islanders, and Native Americans is needed. Additionally, the research on African Americans is by no means comprehensive and is in need of enhancement. Ethnicity is a critical factor affecting levels of informal caretaking for persons with serious mental illness. The role of a person's ethnic background should be given substantial consideration as it will influence the manner in which care is provided.

Very little attention has been given to minority siblings as caregivers for relatives diagnosed with mental illness, contributing to the failure of the mental health system in reaching this population. The need for more research and information is further illustrated in the following narrative from a forty-four year old African American sibling who refers back to the time when her sister was diagnosed with schizophrenia in middle adulthood:

> Yeah, my parents would always say, "oh she's shy." I think that even to tell family members that there was something wrong was not right and my parents just never had that comfort level. And I don't think really they had that comfort level until about 10 years ago when I "came out of the closet" and publicly acknowledged that I had a sister with a mental illness and a sister with developmental disabilities. It was so freeing for me and I think it helped

them know that it was "okay." Whether it be family members or even friends.

They were aware of the mental retardation but I think embarrassed or not really knowing how to explain it to folks. But when the schizophrenia developed, quite candidly, I don't think they understood or knew what schizophrenia was. It wasn't until about 15 years ago when I "came out of the closet" and started pursuing and really trying to understand the medications she was on, she had a couple of in patient episodes and I would say even one commitment or two other inpatient incidents and it was then that I said, "you know this is what's going on" and actually I explained it to them [her parents] because the doctors really never did. She was about 32 or 33 at the time. (Earl, 2003)

Horwitz and Reinhard (1995) reported that ethnicity had a significant impact on the caregiving duties family members perform and the burden that results from such duties. The researchers examined questions about the sibling caregiving process related to the extended kinship network more common in the Black community versus the more individualistic networks among white siblings. They anticipated that study participants who were Black had a sense of family obligation that extended beyond parent-child ties, suggesting that sibling caregiving would be a more normative event in these communities. If this expectation was accurate, then the researchers posited that comparable levels of caregiving would seem less burdensome for Blacks than for whites. The findings from the study with a sample of 70 siblings and 78 parents reported that Black siblings reported having more caregiving duties, but experienced less caregiver burden, than the white siblings.

IMPLICATIONS FOR SOCIAL WORK PRACTICE

As it is important not to stereotype, social workers need to remember that different individuals from the same cultural background may have very different views, especially those that are the second or third generation Americans. The policy, research, and especially practice communities must continue to become familiar with cultural differences and the diversity within cultures. The key is to treat each client as an individual with particular needs and values.

There are many perspectives on what would constitute a comprehensive, effective mental health care system. The following model is derived from the Public Health Agency of Canada-PHAC's *A Report on Mental Illnesses in Canada* (2001). This report details a number of elements that could be regarded as essential to such a system.

Education for Users of Services and Their Families

Individuals and families directly affected by mental illness need information about the signs and symptoms of these illnesses, sources of help, medications, therapy, and early warning signs of relapse. Booklets, videotapes, and family consultations can help to raise awareness. Outcomes may be improved by educating people in order to enhance their abilities to identify episodes in the earlier stages and to respond with appropriate actions.

Community Education

Dispelling the myths surrounding mental illness requires community education programs, including programs in schools. Such programs could help to reduce the stigma associated with mental illness and improve the early recognition of a problem. They may be instrumental not only in encouraging people to seek care but also in creating a supportive environment for the individual.

Case Management/Community Outreach Programs

Case management programs (sometimes referred to as community outreach) come in many forms, but generally consist of multidisciplinary teams that share the clinical responsibility for each individual receiving care in the community. A team aims to help individuals with mental illness to achieve the highest level of functioning possible in the least restrictive setting. To this end, the team works to ensure compliance with treatment (particularly for those with schizophrenia and other psychotic illnesses) and, consequently, improve functioning in order to reduce the need for hospital readmission.

The program also focuses on obtaining and coordinating needed services from a variety of health and social agencies; resolving problems with housing, employment, leisure, relationships and activities of daily living; and providing social skills training to improve social functioning. Two key features of case management include: (1) providing a caring, supportive relationship between the team and the individual and (2) emphasizing flexibility and continuity of care–that is, supports provided as long as needed, across service and program settings, even when the person's needs changes over time.

Self-Help/Mutual Aid Network

Self-help (advocacy) organizations and programs connect individuals to others facing similar challenges and provide support to both individuals and family members. Mutual aid groups have been found to empower individuals, in particular by providing information, reducing isolation and teaching coping skills. They can work in effective partnerships with professional services if their strengths are recognized and the boundaries between formal health care and mutual aid are acknowledged.

Primary and Specialty Care

For most, the primary care physician is the first and often only contact with the health care system. Under-diagnosis, misdiagnosis, and under-treatment of mental illness can result in poor outcomes. As a result, educating primary care physicians to properly recognize, diagnose, treat most mental illnesses, and to know when to refer the affected individuals to others, has a crucial role in maximizing the care that they provide. Training of family medicine residents in these topics is also essential. Creating and distributing consensus treatment guidelines that are relevant to persons of various cultural and ethnic backgrounds is a first step to increase knowledge about mental illnesses, their diagnosis and treatment. Encouraging the use of these guidelines requires attention to the predisposing, enabling, and reinforcing factors that exist in the clinical setting. Health professions, such as psychology and social work, also provide essential services to those with mental illness. An ideal primary care model would involve psychologists, social workers, family physicians, psychiatrists, nurses, pharmacists, and others working in a collaborative and integrated system.

ADDRESSING POLICY NEEDS OF MINORITY SIBLING CAREGIVERS

The community mental health revolution dates back many years. In 1961, President John F. Kennedy proposed a new national mental health program and appropriated fund for planning grants. After the death of

President Kennedy, Public Law 88-164, the Community Mental Health Centers Act of 1963, was passed by the U.S. Congress. Several characteristics of the community mental health movement were embedded in community mental health centers (CMHS), which have direct relevance to ethnic minority groups (Bloom, 1984). These include an emphasis on (1) delivering services or practices in the community, (2) providing comprehensive and continuity of services, (3) offering disease-prevention and health-promotion services, (4) designing innovative clinical strategies to meet the needs of community residents, (5) tapping new sources of personnel, including paraprofessionals and indigenous mental health workers, (6) providing opportunities for community control, and (7) identifying and eliminating sources of stress within the community.

Forty years after the Act, and despite several failed attempts at new designs, ethnic minority communities continue to have unmet needs. One solution would be to design practice around identified cultural and ethnic sibling caregiving practices. But the system must first prioritize and educate itself about diversity within minority groups, and then, and only then, will it be able to respond to their needs and attain effectiveness. By making this a mental health policy priority, the field will be able to better understand *who* will need what type of services.

It is recommended that the next steps involve:

1. Supporting systematic research geared specifically to the sibling caregiving population and their needs.
2. Developing a forum for siblings of various backgrounds to express their needs, raise concerns, support one another, and share information that will enable them to better manage and prepare for their responsibilities.
3. Making sibling caregiving practices a policy priority area for social work and other social service professions.
4. Expanding efforts to collaborate with consumer advocacy groups around the needs of minority sibling caregivers.

REFERENCES

Adams, B. (1968). *Kinship in an urban setting.* Chicago, IL: Markham.
Baldessarini, R. J. et al. (2003). Lithium treatment and suicide risk in major affective disorders: Update and new findings. *Journal of Clinical Psychiatry, 64* (Suppl 5), 44-52.
Bank, S. P., & Kahn, M. D. (1982). *The sibling bond.* NY: Basic Books.

Biegel, D., & Shultz, R. (1999). Caregiving and caregiver interventions in aging and mental illness. *Family Relations, 48 (4)*, 345-353.

Bloom, B. L. (1984). *Community mental health: A general introduction* (2nd ed.). Monterey, CA: Brooks/Cole.

Cicirelli, V. G. (1989). Feelings of attachment to siblings and well-being in later life. *Psychology and Aging, 4*, 211-216.

_____. (1995). *Sibling relationship across the life span*. New York: Plenum.

Connidis, I. A. (1989). Siblings as friends in later life. *American Behavioral Scientist, 33*, 81-93.

Cook, J. A., Pickett, S. A., & Cohler, B. J. (1997). Families of Adults with Severe Mental Illness–The Next Generation of Research: Introduction. *American Journal of Orthopsychiatry, 67*, 172-176.

Diagnostic and Statistical Manual of Mental Disorders, Fourth Edition, Text Revision (2000). Washington, DC, American Psychiatric Association, 2000.

Earl, T. R. (2003). Identifying the impact of knowledge development about schizophrenia among African American Caregiver siblings. Unpublished.

Goldman, H. (1982). Mental illness and family burden: A public health perspective. *Hospital and Community Psychiatry, 33*, 557-560.

Greenberg, J. S., Seltzer, M. M., & Greenley, J. R. (1993). Aging parents of adults with disabilities: The gratifications and frustrations of later-life caregiving. *Gerontologist, 33*, 542-550.

Greenberg, J. S., Kim, H. W., & Greenley, J. R. (1997). Factors associated with subjective burden in siblings of adults with severe mental illness. *American Journal of Orthopsychiatry, 67*, 231-241.

Greenberg, J. S., Seltzer, M. M., Orsmond, G. I., & Krauss, M. W. (1999). Siblings of adults with mental illness or mental retardation: Current involvement and expectation of future caregiving. *Psychiatric Services, 50*, 1214-1219.

Horwitz, A. V. (1993a). Adult siblings as sources of social support for the seriously mentally ill: A test of the Serial Model. *Journal of Marriage and the Family, 55*, 623-632.

_____. (1993b). Siblings as caregivers for the seriously mentally ill. *Milbank Quarterly, 71*, 323-339.

_____. (1994). Predictors of adult sibling social support for the seriously mentally ill: An exploratory study. *Journal of Family Issues, 15(2)*, 272-289.

Horwitz, A. V., & Reinhard, S. C. (1992). Family management of labeled mental illness in a deinstitutionalized era. *Perspectives on Social Problems, 4*, 111-127.

_____. (1995). Ethnic differences in caregiving duties and burdens among parents and siblings of persons with severe mental illnesses. *Journal of Health and Social Behavior, 36*, 138-150.

Horwitz, A. V., Tessler, R., Fisher, G., & Gamache, G. (1992). The role of adult siblings in providing social support to the severely mentally ill. *Journal of Marriage and the Family, 54*, 233-241.

Jenkins, J. (1992). Sibling relationship in disharmonious homes: Potential difficulties and protective effects. In F. Boer & J. Dunn (Eds.), *Children's siblings relationships: Developmental and clinical issues*. Hillside, NJ: Erlbaum.

Karp, D. A. (2003). The burden of sympathy: How families cope with mental illness. *Australian & New Zealand Journal of Psychiatry, 37*, 253-254.

Kessler, R., Abelson, J., & Zhao, S. (1998). The epidemiology of mental disorders. In J. Williams & K. Ell (Eds.), *Advances in mental health research: Implications for practice*. Washington, D.C.: NASW Press.

Kessler, R., Berglund, P., Zhao, S., Leaf, P., Kouzis, A., Bruce, M., Friendman, R., Grossier, R., Kennedy, C., Narrow, W., Kuehnel, T., Laska, E., Manderscheid, R., Rosenheck, R., Santoni, T., & Schneier, M. (1996). The 12-month prevalence and correlates of serious mental illness. In R. W. Manderscheid & M. A. Sonnenschein (Eds.), *Mental Health, United States, 1996*. DHHS Publication No. (SMA) 96-3098. Washington, D.C.: U.S. Government Printing Office.

Kessler, R., McGonagle, K., Zhao, S., Nelson, C., Hughes, M., Eshleman, S., Wittchen, H., & Kendler, K. (1994). Lifetime and 12-month prevalence of DSM-III-R psychiatric disorders in the United States: Results from the National Comorbidity Survey. *Archives of General Psychiatry, 51*, 8-19.

Landeen, J., Whelton, C., Dermer, S., Cardamone, J., Munroe-Blum, H., & Thornton, J. (1992). Needs of well siblings of persons with schizophrenia. *Hospital and Community Psychiatry, 43*, 266-269.

Lefley, H. P. (1987). Aging parents as caregivers of mentally ill adult children: An emerging social problem. *Hospital and Community Psychiatry, 38*, 1063-1070.

_____. (2003). Changing caregiving needs as persons with schizophrenia grow older. In C. I. Cohen (Ed.), *Schizophrenia into later life: Treatment, research, and policy*. (pp. 251-268). Washington, D.C.: American Psychiatric Publishing, Inc.

Lefley, H., & Hatfield, A. (1999). Helping parental caregivers and mental health consumers cope with parental aging and loss. *Psychiatric Services, 50*, 369-375.

Lidz, T. (1963). Parents whose children become schizophrenic. *Journal of Nervous and Mental Disease, 172 (7)*, 408-411.

_____. (1973). *The origin and treatment of schizophrenic disorders*. New York: Basic.

Lidz, T. (1976). Commentary on 'a critical review of recent adoption, twin, and family studies of schizophrenia: Behavioral genetics perspectives'. *Schizophrenia Bulletin, 2 (3)*, 402-412.

Lidz, T., Fleck, S., Alanen, Y., & Cornilson, A. (1963). Schizophrenic patients and their siblings. *Psychiatry, 26(1)*, 1-18.

Lidz, T., Fleck, S., Cornilson, A. (1966). *Schizophrenia and the family*. New York: International University.

Maltiades, H. B. & Pruncho, R. (2002). The effect of religious coping on caregiving appraisals of mothers of adults with developmental disabilities. *The Gerontologist, 42 (1)*, 82-91.

Marsh, D. T. (1992). *Families and mental illness: New directions in professional practice*. New York: Praeger.

_____. (1998). *Serious mental illness and the family: The practitioner's guide*. New York: John Wiley & Sons.

Marsh, D. T., Appleby, N. F., Dickens, R. M., Owens, M., & Young, N. O. (1993a). Anguished voices: Impact of mental illness on siblings and children. *Innovations & Research, 2*, 25-34.

Marsh, D. T., Dickens, R. M., Koeske, R. D., Yackovich, N. S., Wilson, J. M., Leichliter, J. S. et al. (1993b). Troubled journey: Siblings and children of people with mental illness. *Innovations & Research, 2,* 13-23.

Muhlbauer, S.A. (2002). Navigating the storm of mental illness: Phases in the family's journey. *Qualitative Health Research, 12 (8),* 1076-1092.

Murray C. J. L., Lopez A. D. (Eds.) (1996). *The Global Burden of Disease: A Comprehensive Assessment of Mortality and Disability from Diseases, Injuries, and Risk Factors in 1990 and Projected to 2020.* Cambridge, MA: Harvard University Press.

National Advisory Mental Health Council. (1993). The report of the National Advisory Mental Health Council. *American Journal of Psychiatry, 150 (10),* 1445-1465.

National Institute of Mental Health (2001). *When someone has schizophrenia.* Retrieved October 16, 2004 from the World Wide Web: http://www.nimh.nih.gov/publicat/schizsoms.cfm

Nechmad, A., Fennig, S., Ternochiano, P., Treves, I., Fennig-Naisberg, S., & Levkovich, Y. (2000). Siblings of schizophrenic patients–A review. *Israel Journal of Psychiatry and Relational Science, 37,* 3-11.

Neighbors, H. W., Bashshur, R., Price, R., Selig, S., Donabedian, A., & Shannon, G. (1992). Ethnic minority mental health service delivery: A review of the literature. *Research in Community and Mental Health, 7,* 55-71.

Neighbors, H. W., Musick, M. A., & Williams, D. R. (1998). The African American minister as a source of help for serious personal crises: Bridge or barrier to mental health care? *Health Education & Behavior, 25,* 759-777.

Narrow W.E. (1998). One-year prevalence of depressive disorders among adults 18 and over in the U.S.: NIMH ECA prospective data. Population estimates based on U.S. Census estimated residential population age 18 and over on July 1, 1998. Unpublished.

Public Health Agency of Canada (2001). *A Report on Mental Illnesses in Canada.* Canada. http://www.phac-aspc.gc.ca

Regier D. A., Narrow W. E., Rae D. S. et al. (1993). The de facto mental and addictive disorders service system: Epidemiologic Catchment Area prospective 1-year prevalence rates of disorders and services. *Archives of General Psychiatry,* 50(2), 85-94.

Schwartz S. (1999). Biological approaches to psychological disorders. In A. V. Horwitz & T. L. Shcid (Eds.), *A Handbook for the Study of Mental Health–Social Context, Theories and Systems* (Ch. 4). Cambridge: Cambridge University Press.

Shortt, J. W., & Gottman, J. M. (1997). Closeness in young adult sibling relationships: Affective and physiological processes. *Social Development, 6 (2),* 142-164.

Snowden, L. R. (2001). Barriers to effective mental health services for African Americans. *Mental Health Services Research, 3*(4), 181-187.

Steinwachs, D., Kasper, J., & Skinner, E. (1992a). *Family perspectives on meeting the needs for care of severely mentally ill relatives: A national survey.* Baltimore, MD: Johns Hopkins University Press.

Tessler, R., & Gamache, G. (2000). *Family experiences with mental illness.* Westport, CT: Auburn Press.

Thompson Jr., E. H., & Doll, W. (1982). The burden of families coping with the mentally ill: An invisible crisis. *Family Relations: Journal of Applied Family & Child Studies, 31,* 379-388.

U.S. Department of Health and Human Services (1999). *Mental Health: A Report of the Surgeon General*. Rockville, MD: U.S. Department of Health and Human Services, Substance Abuse and Mental Health Services Administration, Center for Mental Health Services, National Institutes of Health, National Institute of Mental Health.

Whaley, A. L. (1997). Ethnic and racial differences in perceptions of dangerousness of persons with mental illness. *Psychiatric Services, 48*(10), 1328-30.

_____ . (1998). Racism in the provision of mental health services: A social-cognitive analysis. *American Journal of Orthopsychiatry 68(1)*, 47-57.

doi:10.1300/J137v14n01_03

Chapter 4

Older Latinos and Mental Health Services: Understanding Access Barriers

John M. Gonzalez

SUMMARY. This article discusses the biopsychosocial and spiritual aspects related to older Latinos' use of mental health care. It also addresses the environment that older Latinos have to navigate to access mental health services. Structural barriers to mental health services are emphasized as critical to a holistic assessment of the client's situation. doi:10.1300/J137v14n01_04 *[Article copies available for a fee from The Haworth Document Delivery Service: 1-800-HAWORTH. E-mail address: <docdelivery@haworthpress.com> Website: <http://www.HaworthPress.com> © 2006 by The Haworth Press, Inc. All rights reserved.]*

KEYWORDS. Mental health services, barriers, Latino elders

INTRODUCTION

The United States Surgeon General's Report on Mental Health (1999) underscored the idea that culture has an impact on mental illness and mental health, contributing to how patients communicate and exhibit symptoms, cope with mental illness, and the way families and communities cope with

[Haworth co-indexing entry note]: "Older Latinos and Mental Health Services: Understanding Access Barriers." Gonzalez, John M. Co-published simultaneously in *Journal of Human Behavior in the Social Environment* (The Haworth Press, Inc.) Vol. 14, No. 1/2, 2006, pp. 73-93; and: *Contemporary Issues of Care* (ed: Roberta R. Greene) The Haworth Press, Inc., 2006, pp. 73-93. Single or multiple copies of this article are available for a fee from The Haworth Document Delivery Service [1-800-HAWORTH, 9:00 a.m. - 5:00 p.m. (EST). E-mail address: docdelivery@haworthpress.com].

mental illness. The Report goes on to identify several methods to improve the nation's mental health services including tailoring mental health treatments to diverse, age, gender, racial, and cultural needs.

This article discusses the biopsychosocial and spiritual aspects related to older Latinos' use of mental health care. It also addresses the environment that older Latinos have to navigate to access mental health services. Structural barriers to mental health services are emphasized as critical to a holistic assessment of the client's situation. The author makes the assumption that it is not enough to provide a Latino client with a Latino professional. Rather, it is necessary to understand the client's culture. Culture is discussed as more than language and shared ethnicity; it is treated as shared values, expressions, thoughts, and traditions that may or may not bring a Latino who is mentally ill into treatment. Practice and policy implications are also provided.

POPULATION GROWTH

In 2002, most older Latinos resided in four states: California (27 percent), Florida (16 percent), New York (9 percent), and Texas (20 percent) (USDHHS, 2003). Older Latinos are concentrated in these areas because they originally immigrated there. Mexican Americans are the largest groups in California and Texas because of the close proximity. Cubans are concentrated in Florida, and Puerto Ricans are concentrated in New York. Latinos are now the nation's largest minority group (U. S. Census, 2002). Minority Americans make up 14% of the country's elderly population and 16% of the Medicare population (Henry J. Kaiser Family Foundation, 1999). Estimates have Latino Americans making up six percent of the older population. By the year 2050, reports estimate that Latino Americans will make up 16 percent of the older population (Federal Interagency Forum on Aging Related Statistics, 2000).

There is much diversity among the Latino population. Mexican-Americans, Puerto Rican Americans, and Cuban Americans are just a few cultures within the Latino culture including many immigrants from South America. The distribution of the Hispanic population in the 2000 census was 58.5 percent Mexican, 9.6 percent Puerto Rican, 3.5 percent Cuban, and 28.4 percent "other" Hispanic, a catergory that includes Dominicans, Central Americans, South Americans, Spaniards, and all other Hispanic peoples (Bureau of the Census, 2000).

BIOPSYCHOSOCIAL AND SPIRITUAL FACTORS AFFECTING HEALTH CARE AMONG LATINOS

Biological Issues of Care

Older Latinos experience several chronic medical conditions that contribute to mental distress. Black, Goodwin, and Markides (1998) examined the association between specific chronic conditions, individual functional disabilities, and depressive symptoms in older Mexican Americans. Using data from the Hispanic Epidemiologic Study for the Elderly (HEPESE) that consisted of 2823 Mexican Americans aged 65 and older, they found that diabetes, arthritis, urinary incontinence, bowel incontinence, kidney disease, and ulcers were predictive of high levels of depressive symptoms.

Some other major medical problems older Latinos report include arthritis, diabetes, cardiovascular disease, depression, and hypertension (Espino, 1990). Older Latinos have higher rates of diabetes and hypertension than white counterparts, and older Latinos are at greater risk for stroke, obesity, and some heart disease (Markides & Black, 1996; Mutchler & Burr, 1991). Within the ethnic group, older Mexican Americans have high prevalence rates of diabetes (Hazuda & Espino, 1997).

One or more functional limitations often accompany some of the medical conditions affecting the older Latino. Functional limitations are activities of daily living (ADLs) such as needing assistance bathing or walking. Johnson and Wolinsky (1994) found that older Latinos also report more difficulty with functioning and limitations in activity than whites. Espino (1993) estimated that 45 percent of older Latinos had some limitation in ADLs. These biological/medical conditions of older Latinos mean living with chronic and disabling conditions, which may lead to a low quality of life (Crimmins, Hayward, & Saito, 1994; Angel & Angel, 1997).

Psychological Issues of Care

According to the U.S. Surgeon General's report, 8%-20% of community dwelling older adults have symptoms of depression (USDHHS, 1999). Assessed mental health status served as one indicator of the "The State of Aging and Health in America." Researchers asked respondents to report number of days out of the past 30 days they had experienced stress, depression, or problems with emotions for 14 days or more, indicating poor mental health. Latino Americans reported the highest level of mental distress compared to other racial and ethnic groups (CDC 2004).

The recognition of mental distress in older Latinos is sometimes a problem for professionals as well as the individual and their family. Malgady et al. (1997) studied diagnoses and found that Latino clinicians consistently rated symptoms as more severe than non-Hispanic white clinicians. They also found the symptom severity rating and diagnostic sensitivity highest in bilingual interviews. In addition, Latino clinicians were more consistent in rating symptomology and in recognizing severity of symptoms.

Older minorities access mental health services for several reasons. Most often, the reasons center on loss and adjustment to life changes due to aging. In a pilot study, Choi and Gonzalez (2005a), examined the experiences and perceptions of geriatric mental health clinicians of the circumstances in which older minorities access outpatient mental health treatment. Clinicians reported that the common circumstances for accessing mental health services included:

1. lack of social support in times of loss and life changes such as loss of job or career or loss of spouse;
2. difficulty adjusting to physical illness and related mood disorders, and the loss of independence due to deteriorating health;
3. family conflict and relationship issues like role reversal, or children's continued dependency needs;
4. depletion of family caregiving resources and possible placement in a nursing home; and
5. caregiver stress and guilt issues.

Social Issues of Care

Guarnaccia and Rodriguez (1996) view culture as including ethnic identity, language, material signs and symbols, events and celebrations, shared views, and views of mental illness. Because culture molds a person's conceptions and responses to mental illness, cultural beliefs can sometimes be a barrier to accessing mental health services. Assessment and treatment techniques need to be sensitive to the effect of culture on mental illness and take into account the expressions of culture of mental illness. For example, shame and stigma of mental illness along with self-reliance of family tend to be stronger among Hispanics, sometimes presenting barriers to mental health treatment services (Guarnaccia & Rodriguez, 1996).

One of the social issues related to mental health care usage is educational attainment. Despite the overall increase in educational attainment among older Americans, there are still substantial educational differences among racial and ethnic groups. Older Latinos lag behind in educational attainment, with about 35 percent of the population having finished high school compared to 70 percent of the general older population. In addition, 5.5 percent of older Latinos had a bachelor's degree or higher compared to 16.7 percent of all older persons (USDHHS, 2003).

Another social factor affecting care is whether an elder lives with a family member or lives alone. The number of older Latinos living alone is lower than that of the general population. The number of older Latinos living with other relatives is about twice that of the total population. In 2000, 68 percent of old Latino males lived with their spouses, 16 percent lived with other relatives, and 14 percent lived alone. For older Latino females, 38 percent lived with their spouses, 34 percent lived with other relatives, and 25 percent lived alone (USDHHS, 2003). The poverty rate for older Latinos–another factor influencing access to care– was twice that of the total older population, with 22 percent for older Latinos compared to 10.1 (USDHHS, 2003).

Religious and Spiritual Issues of Care

Hispanics are mostly Christians, the majority being either Roman Catholic or Protestant. Other religious/spiritual practices, region specific in Latin America and among Hispanics, include *Santeria* and *Espiritismo*. *Espiritismo*, part of the Puerto Rican culture, is the belief that a spiritual world exists parallel to our world, and linked to the actual world. The Afro-Cuban belief *Santeria* is a religion that combines African deities and Roman Catholic saints. While these are the more common religions among Hispanics, several other faiths can be found within the population (Vasquez & Clavijo, 1995).

For many Latinos, the church is a primary source of support. Latinos can be described as fatalistic, because they believe their destiny is in the hands of God. When Latinos are in psychiatric distress, they often interpret their symptoms as a deserved punishment for theirs sins. The belief is often "*si Dios quiere*," if God so wishes. Some believe that all they can do is pray (Carrillo, 2001).

FAMILY AND MENTAL HEALTH CARE

In the Latino culture, the family meets several emotional and psychological needs of their elderly. The family network consists of generations that include the nuclear family, extended family, the *compadrazo* system (i.e., godparents), the *barrios* (friends and neighbors), and the larger community. The immediate family usually takes care of older Latinos with help from the extended family in their community. There is a strong connection for Latino elders between mental health, well being, and their health status (Harris, 1998.)

Older Latinos are at the center of the family. When they experience mental distress and aging, the family is strained. Family roles and responsibilities are changed and at times exchanged or reversed. The older Latino gives up the responsibility of being the caregiver to become being cared for. The adult children take on the responsibility of caring for their aging parent. This exchange of responsibilities sometimes leads to stress and distress for the family and the family members involved.

Angel, J. L., Angel, R. J., McClellan, and Markides (1996) studied Latino elders and found they preferred to live with their spouse, live alone, or live with family, instead of in nursing homes or institutions. Rural elders are resistant to outside help and have a strong sense of independence. They often are self-reliant, desirous of aging in place (their home), and dependent on family support and friends to meet health care needs. Keeping medical, mental health, and other problems in the family is a norm that contributes to the reluctance of taking advantage of available health care services (Magilvy, Congdon, Martinez, Davis, & Averill, 2000).

INSTITUTIONAL BARRIERS: CHALLENGES POSED BY DIVERSITY

Historical Background

To understand issues related to older Latinos accessing mental health services, it is important to appreciate their historical background. Three major historical events specifically related to Mexican Americans are the "Battle of the Alamo," the Treaty of Guadalupe Hidalgo, and the Bracero Program during World War II. For Texans, the battle cry "Remember the Alamo" provided inspiration during the Texas Revolution. The Mexican Army defeated the Texans in this battle and set up angry feelings towards Mexicans. For Mexican Americans, however, "Remember the Alamo" has connotations of racism and discrimination (Garcia, 1977). These events set the foundation for the Mexican American experience in the United States.

The second event comes at the end of the U.S.-Mexican War in 1848 with the signing of the treaty of Guadalupe Hidalgo. In this agreement, the U.S. purchased Colorado, Arizona, New Mexico, Texas, California, and parts of Utah and Nevada in return for 15 millions dollars. The treaty guaranteed Mexican landowners their right to land in Arizona, New Mexico, Texas, and California. However, most Mexican Americans lost their land between 1850 and 1870 (Garcia, 1977). During this time, hostility characterized the relationship between Mexican Americans and Anglo Americans.

The third event, the Bracero Program, started in 1942 because of a need for farm labor when many men and women from the U.S. were away fighting in World War II. The governments of the United States and Mexico agreed on a cooperative that allowed Mexican farmhands to work in the United States for a specified time and then return to Mexico. U.S. employers found ways around the Bracero program and hired illegal aliens to do their work. Thus, Braceros found it easier to be illegal. Both the illegal and the Bracero were treated as "foreigners." The program ended in 1964, although the labor practice did not (McLemore, Romo & Gonzalez-Baker, 2001).

Institutional Barriers

From the beginning, the United States has had a population of diverse backgrounds. The multi-ethnic/racial population brings several challenges to health and mental health care. Differences exist in health beliefs and practices and in health care needs including differences in genetic make-up, occupational exposure, resources and nutrition (Trevino, 1999). Several structural barriers at the societal level keep older Latinos from accessing health care, including economic, administrative, cultural, and linguistic barriers. Since these barriers influence older Latinos' decisions to seek help for mental health treatment, understanding them will help social workers foster the access and retention of older Latinos seeking healthcare services. Other barriers include language, lack of appropriate information, a distrust of the delivery system, low income, and low education levels (Administration on Aging, 2001). Older Latinos experience a case of double jeopardy, being aged and ethnic minority, and triple jeopardy for those who experience any access barrier (Kart, 1985). Structural barriers must be evaluated and part of the biopsychosocial assessment for social workers to understand how best to work with older Latinos. Understanding these barriers will also help social workers empower older Latinos to have an advantage when making health decisions.

Acculturation

Mexican Americans have had and continue to have a difficult, sometimes stressful acculturation experience. Acculturative stress is influenced by several factors such as a preference for one's language, family cohesiveness, tenure in residency, and coping resources (Miranda & Matheny, 2000). Smart and Smart (1995) concluded that acculturative stress has a pervasive, life-long influence on Latinos' psychological adjustment, decision-making abilities, occupational functioning, and physical health. Older Mexicans have experienced acculturative stress because of the stigma of their history, often leading to fear and distrust of the mainstream system along with feeling less than or second class.

McLemore, Romo, and Baker (2001) state that colonized minorities remain in their homeland and are committed to the preservation of their culture, while the dominant group prevents them from competing freely for employment and other resources. Mexican American entry into U.S. society was by conquest, and they also experienced dislike by Irish and Germans Americans who immigrated during the same time period. This history of mistreatment and discrimination has caused a distrust and fear that bleed into labor practices, which have not allowed older Latinos to work in jobs that came with good retirement benefits (Villa & Aranda, 2000).

Power

Because of their history and acculturation patterns, older Latinos have experienced power differentials that impact their help-seeking behaviors. Goldenberg (1978) describes power as "the ability to control or influence, directly or indirectly, the conditions under which one lives" (p. 59). Powerlessness, on the other hand, is an inability to exercise this control (Pinderhughes, 1989). In their book *The Gender of Power*, Davis, Leijenar, and Oldersma (1991) discuss several common features used to understand client circumstances in relation power in their society. They suggest that powerlessness can be experienced when there is:

1. inequality in social resources, social position, political, and cultural influences;
2. inequality in opportunities to make use of existing resources;
3. inequality in the division of rights and duties;
4. inequality in implicit or explicit standards of judgement, often leading to differential treatment (in laws, the labor market, educational practices, and so forth);
5. inequality in cultural representations: devaluation of the powerless group, stereotyping, references to the "nature" or (biological) "essence" of the less powerful;
6. inequality in psychological consequences: a "psychology of inferiority" (insecurity, "double-blind" experiences, and symptoms of identification with the dominant group) versus a "psychology of superiority" (arrogance, inability to abandon the dominant perspective); and
7. a social and cultural tendency to minimize or deny power inequality: (potential) conflict often represented as consensus, power inequality as "normal" (p. 52).

In the mental health treatment setting, a power differential is already said to exist in the client-social worker relationship (Saleebey, 1997). Add to this being minority, aged, and feeling powerless and this power differential widens.

Communication/Linguistic

Communication with the mental health care system is another barrier for older Mexican Americans. As generation after generation pass on culture, language, at the core of this communication process, is the very creator of culture. Therefore, speaking the client's language is a key to providing mental health treatment. However, "speaking the client's language" is not always so easy. Staff may be bicultural and bilingual and miscommunication might still happen. Region, socioeconomic status, and acculturation influence linguistic minorities' language (Guarnaccia & Rodriguez, 1996).

In the past, the literature has treated language as a problem rather than seeing language as an expression of one's culture (O'Hagan, 2001). Providers placed an onus on the patient for not communicating in a language that the provider could understand. Currently, it is more accepted that understanding the client's language is a necessary factor in treating mentally ill.

Limited English proficiency applies to persons who cannot speak, read, write, or understand English at a level that yields effective communication (Health Care Financing Administration, 2000). The 2000 U. S. Census reports 17.9 percent of the population five years and older speak a language other than English, and 8.1 percent speak English less than "very well." The United States is home to millions of national origin minority individuals who are limited English proficient (LEP). Due to these limitations, linguistic minorities may experience denial, delays with service delivery, and inaccurate assessment.

Latinos are now the nation's largest minority group (U.S. Census, 2002). One in three Latinos have problems with communicating with their doctor (Collins et al., 2002). Timmins (2002) reported that Latinos with limited English proficiency are at risk for low access to care and low access to quality of care. Powerlessness and lack of ability to gain knowledge that would enable Latinos to make informed choices regarding health care are direct results of language barriers (Juarbe, 1995).

Professionals who are unable to communicate with minority groups cannot provide the same diagnostic expertise, cannot establish the necessary empathy and rapport, and cannot provide the necessary support, comfort, and care (O'Hagan, 2001). Lago and Thompson (1996) believe that the professional's task is always to aspire to communication and understanding that evokes trust. "Culturally skilled counselors take responsibility for interaction in the language requested by the client" (ibid., p. 61). O'Hagan (2001) discussed two main factors in working with linguistic minorities: first, linguistic minorities clients regard their language as significant and important in their daily lives; second, there is enormous potential for discriminatory practice in the professional's attitude and approach to languages other than their own.

Insurance

Many Latinos are uninsured. A study by the Tulane Hispanic Health Initiative (2002) reported almost 60% of Latinos in the U.S. are uninsured. Other significant issues in the assessment of older Latinos are their knowledge level of their insurance benefits (i.e., Medicare, Medicaid, dual-eligibility) and knowledge level and experience with the healthcare system. Latino Medicare beneficiaries are more likely to live in poverty, and one-third of the Latino Medicare beneficiaries have incomes below the poverty level. Twenty-five percent of older Latinos only have

Medicare for insurance and more than a quarter of Latinos receive some level of Medicaid assistance (Henry J. Kaiser Family Foundation, 1999). Collins et al. (2002) reported 46 percent of Hispanic adults lacked health insurance in the past year and forty-one percent of Hispanics reported that following doctor's recommendations would have cost too much.

Medicare comes with many out-of-pocket costs. Many older adults decide against using health care services because of these costs. Angel, Angel, and Markides (2002) analyzed data from the Hispanic Established Populations for Epidemiological Study of the Elderly and found that uninsured Mexicans reported fewer health care visits and were less likely to have a standard source of care. They also went to Mexico more often for health care. Many of the sample relied on Medicare only, which incurs out-of-pocket costs, often resulting in not accessing health care services.

Service Utilization

Older minorities are less likely than non-Hispanic whites to see a mental health specialist for their mental health problems. They turn to traditional self-care and informal support networks, clergy and primary care physicians. Structural barriers contribute to the disparities in mental health service utilization. Using data from the 1990-1992 National Comorbidity Survey, Alegria and colleagues (2002), examined disparities in the rates of specialty mental health care for Latinos and African Americans compared to non-Latino whites in the United States. The sample consisted of 8,098 English-speaking respondents aged 15 to 54 years. They found a significantly higher proportion of non-Latino whites (11.8 percent) received specialty care than African Americans (7.2 percent) or Latinos (5.9 percent). The researchers concluded that to understand ethnic disparities in specialty care, ethnicity needs to be analyzed with variables related to poverty and other environmental contexts.

Sarrett et al. (1989) studied the formal mental health utilization patterns of elderly Hispanics. They analyzed data provided by the National Association for Hispanic Elderly, a sample of 1,805 non institutionalized Hispanic individuals age 55 and over. They found that older Hispanics rely on themselves to solve their mental health issues more often than using the church, a physician, or a professional. The characteristics associated with being more likely to use formal networks included having more psychosocial problems, experiencing bad health, being disabled, Cuban, or female. Other factors contributing to the greater access of services for Hispanic elderly include attending church more frequently, being female, and having a Mexican American heritage (Sarrett et al., 1989).

Using data from the Household Survey of the 1987 National Medical Expenditure Survey, Freimen and Cunningham (1997) analyzed the interactions between race/ethnicity and other characteristics of a person and their local area that are important in determining the probability of mental health care use. (Blacks and Latinos were over sampled.) The researchers found Mexican/Chicanos were less likely to use mental health services when compared to other Hispanics and Blacks. Living in an urban area and the availability of psychiatrists were among the factors that decreased the probability of use for Latinos.

Padgett, Burns, and Schlesinger (1994) conducted an analysis of enrollment data of federal employees to examine factors influencing the use of outpatient mental health services among ethnic groups. They found Hispanics averaged the fewest number of visits, followed by blacks and then whites. Whites were 1.7 times more likely to make a visit compared to Blacks and Hispanics. In addition, they found that whites were estimated to make 2.64 more mental health visits during the year than Hispanics and Blacks. This study demonstrated that ethnic differences in the use of outpatient mental health services persist even in an insured population and showed a clear pattern of lower use by Blacks and Hispanics compared to whites.

Torrez (1998) conducted a qualitative study that examined the service utilization patterns of a group of older Mexican Americans and the barriers encountered when they attempt to access formal services. A purposeful sample of clients was drawn from a social service program in North Texas and forty-six interviews were conducted. They found that deteriorating health exacerbated the need for services. But when adult children had time constraints or there was a need for transportation participants were less likely to access services. This study revealed that older adults not only need health and social service information, they also need assistance to access services.

Another study by Vega, Kolody and Aguilar-Gaxiola (2001) sheds light on some of the factors that contribute to a person accessing mental health services. This study used data from the Mexican American Prevalence and Services Study (MAPPS) to assess utilization patterns of Mexican Americans recently diagnosed with a psychiatric disorder. The MAPPS interviewed 3000 respondents in Fresno, California. Interviews were conducted in the language the respondent preferred, English or Spanish. The researchers found that U.S.-born Mexican Americans had higher utilization of primary care physicians and counselors than immigrants. They also found that neither group relied heavily on informal network providers to treat psychiatric disorders. In addition, they discovered that knowing where to find a specialty mental health provider increased the likelihood of service use as did having private insurance.

HELP-SEEKING BEHAVIOR

Preferences of Latinos

Several studies discuss language and ethnic matching as ways to help the Latino population to access mental health services. Zuniga (1987) notes the Spanish-speaking client can benefit from catharsis, when speaking his or her native language. At the same time, the Spanish-speaking worker can interject *dichos*, cultural anecdotes, to enlighten and maintain the flow of therapy. These familiar phrases enhance the idea that the client's feelings are understood.

In a qualitative study, Lantican (1998) found those who expressed a preference for bilingual bicultural professional staff alluded to the benefits of being better understood in the therapy process. That is, language barriers were overcome. Warda (2000), in a study of professionals and clients, found communication repeatedly identified as a key component of culturally competent care. Adjectives used to describe harmonious verbal and nonverbal communication included "human," "respectful," "professional," and "sensitive." Another finding of the study was that the use of the Spanish language by health care professionals was a component of system support. These findings also reveal that the providers' bilingual abilities affect the content of the interaction and the patient's recall of the information.

Models of Behavior

Kleinman's Explanatory Model (1980) is frequently used to examine help seeking behaviors. According to Kleinman, *explanatory models* are the notions a person has about an episode of illness and its treatment delivered by all those who engage in the clinical process. Explanatory models examine people's cognitive processes and are based on their cultural knowledge and idiosyncratic experiences. Popular culture and the media also inform explanatory models, as do the health care culture and the social network of the individual. These elements guide the interpretation and action concerning health care use.

Individuals form explanatory models to cope with a specific health problem. Explanatory models determine important clinical evidence and how it is organized and interpreted for treatment approaches. Explanatory models help patients and families make sense of illness episodes. Kleinman's explanatory model distinguishes between the idea of *disease* and *illness*. *Disease* refers to a malfunctioning of biological and/or psychological process, while *illness* refers to the psychosocial experiences and meaning of perceived disease. *Illness* also includes communication and interpersonal interaction within the family and social network. The experience of illness is considered within the context of social systems and rules for behavior; illness is also believed to have culture influences and to be culturally constructed.

The social context of the culture of health care contains three structural domains: (1) professional, (2) popular, and (3) folk. The *professional domain* consists of doctors and nurses or licensed practitioners. The *popular domain* includes family, the social network, and the community. The *folk domain* is the non-professional healers such as *curanderas* or herbalists. Each domain has it own explanatory systems, social roles, interaction settings, and institutions. When an individual is coping with an illness, they will utilize the popular domain to find a cure or alleviate the symptoms. They might consult with family, friends, or go to clergy in their community. If illness is unresolved, the individual will take recommendations from the popular domain to enter the professional domain either to visit a doctor or go to the hospital. On the other hand, the individual will visit a folk healer again based on recommendations from their popular domain.

Patient, family, and physician explanatory models follow five dimensions: (1) etiology, (2) onset of symptoms, (3) pathophysiology, (4) course of sickness including type of sick role–acute, chronic, and impaired–and the severity of the disorder, and (5) treatment (Kleinman, 1980, p.105). Explanatory models (EM) explore the cause or the origin of the illness. EMs explain when and how the symptoms started and the types of physical changes the individual has noticed since the onset of symptoms. EMs also explain the course of the illness whether it is acute, chronic or impaired and how severe the illness is. Treatment, the last dimension covered in the EM, is the actions that one can take to reduce symptoms or find a cure for the illness.

In an explanatory model, the patient-practitioner relationship is a transaction that negotiates the clinical realities of each participant. The negotiation centers on resolving the discrepancies between the patient and the practitioner explanations of care. The family's EM is also included in this discussion. This is an opportunity for the practitioner to understand the patient's EM and it is also an opportunity for the practitioner to educate the patient. This transaction also consists of the therapeutic values, expectations, and goals for the patient and the practitioner. Large discrepancies between the two EMs affect clinical management and can lead to inadequate or poor care. This negotiation is an important step in establishing trust with the patient, promoting patient satisfaction and compliance to agreed upon treatment actions.

Kleinman's Explanatory Model has been useful in studying how culture influences health beliefs, how health beliefs vary and are complex especially when it comes to language and expressing emotion, and the blending two cultures to understand illness (Guarnaccia, Rivera, Franco, & Neighbors, 1996; Callan & Littlewood, 1998; Williams & Healy, 2001; Jezewski & Poss, 2002).

Green's Adapted Model

Green (1999) adapted Kleinman's explanatory model (Figure 1) into a help seeking behavior model that further clarifies the client-provider relationship as a cross-cultural experience. Green takes the client explanatory model and labels it the *client culture* and he labels the practitioner explanatory model the *professional subculture*. The client culture includes problem recognition, problem labeling and diagnosis, indigenous help providers, utilization of help providers and problem resolution and the professional subculture.

Client problem recognition occurs when the client notices a change in their usual functioning or a problem. The *client labels and diagnoses his or her problem* is based on their knowledge of the illness which comes from their everyday experience, their cultural experience, and feedback from their social network including their families, friends, and other community members. Healers, or *indigenous help providers* in the client community, include herbalists, *curanderas*, or voodoo practitioners. This information influences *client utilization of help providers,* shaping the decision of whether to utilize formal or indigenous help providers. Hopefully, the use of help providers leads to *problem resolution.*

Minority professionals are significant to the client because they are included in both the client subculture and the professional subculture. They are professionals who are bicultural and sometimes bilingual. This role helps in decreasing cultural distance from the client. They can help the minority client navigate the barriers in the professional subculture in seeking problem resolution.

FIGURE 1. Kleinman's Explanatory Model

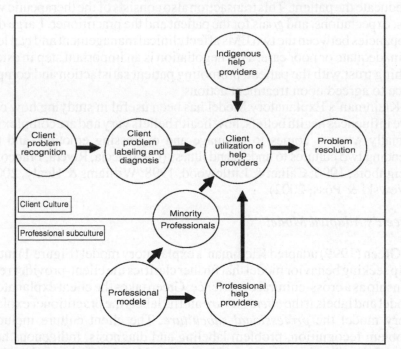

Adapted from: Green, J. (1995). Cultural awareness in the human services: A multi-ethnic approach. Needham Heights, MA: Allyn & Bacon.

The *professional subculture* includes minority professionals, professional models, and professional help providers. *Professional models* are the models that practitioners used to assess clients; some based on the medical model. Professionals create cultural distance between the professional and the client when they misuse culture in the model of assessment. Assuming that all clients of a similar culture are the same and stereotyping cultural behavior can be a misuse of culture. *Professional help providers* are physicians, nurses, social workers, licensed practitioners who assist the client in resolving their problem.

RECOMMENDATIONS AND IMPLICATIONS FOR PRACTICE

As older Latinos turn to mental health services, they often face several problems in the environment including language and cultural distance. In order to decrease this cultural distance, the social worker needs to take into account the factors that contribute to distancing, building an understanding of what is associated with cultural distance for *each* client and performing accurate assessments. Social workers providing treatment to older Latinos also need to understand the mechanisms of cultural distancing within themselves to treat older Latinos effectively.

With the current population growth, the barriers and needs of older Latinos will need ongoing assessment. Other recommendations for social work and healthcare providers are to increase education on mental illness and services to older Latinos and their adult children and families. For example, older Latinos and their families need education concerning the insurance benefits for which they qualify for mental health services. Healthcare providers also need continuing education on mental illness and services.

In working with older Latinos, social workers need to consider the degrees of acculturation, language and preference, as well as adherence to traditional customs, values, and norms of those being treated (Santiago-Rivera, 1995). Professionals need to move beyond holding a simplistic view of culture as creating a physical atmosphere and hiring people who speak the language to incorporate a more detailed way of understanding the multiple dimensions of culture (Bernal & Castro, 1994). For social work professionals, some suggestions include cultural competency training focused on the language and culture of the region. Professionals need to understand and learn that Spanish exists in different dialects, that Latinos come from different countries, and that Latinos have lived different lifestyles and have different life experience. There is also a need for more bilingual/bicultural social workers and a need to recruit students of color to social work. These are considerations for developing policy and programs that will service older Latinos.

REFERENCES

Administration on Aging (2001). *Cultural Competency.* Retrieved on February 1, 2002 from www.aoa.gov/may2001/factsheets/Cultural-Competency.html

Alegria, M., Canino, G., Rios, R., Vera, M., Calderon, J., Rusch, D. & Ortega, A. (2002). Inequalities in use of speciality mental health services among Latinos, African Americans, and Non-Latino Whites. *Psychiatric Services, 53,* 12: 1547-1555.

Angel, J. L., Angel, R. J., & Markides, K. S. (2002). Stability and change in health insurance among older Mexican Americans: Longitudinal evidence from the Hispanic established populations for epidemiology study of the elderly. *American Journal of Public Health, 92* (8): 1284-1272.

Angel, J. L., Angel, R. J., McClellan, J. L., & Markides, K. S. (1996). Nativity, declining health and preferences in living arrangements among elderly Mexican Americans: Implications for long-term care. *The Gerontologist 36*(4): 464-473.

Angel, R. & Angel, J. (1997). *Who will care for us? Aging and long-term care in multicultural America.* New York: New York University Press.

Bernal, M. & Castro, F. (1994). Are clinical psychologists prepared for service and research with ethnic minorities? *American Psychologist, 49* (9): 797-806.

Black, S. A., Goodwin, J. S., & Markides, K. S. (1998). The association between chronic diseases and depressive symptomatology in Older Mexican Americans.

Bureau of the Census (2000). The Hispanic Population: Census 2000 Brief http://www.census.gov/prod/2001pubs/c2kbr01-3.pdf

Bureau of Census (2002). American Community Survey Profile. Retrieved 10/02/03 http://www.census.gov/acs/www/Products/Profiles/Single/2002/ACS/Tabular/010/01000US1.htm

Callan, A. & Littlewood, R. (1998). Patient satisfaction: Ethnic origin or explanatory model? *International Journal of Social Psychiatry, 44*, 1-11.

Carrillo, E. (2001). Assessment and treatment of the Latino patient. In, *The Latino psychiatric patient: Assessment and treatment.* Lopez, A. G. & Carrillo, E. (Eds.). American Psychiatric Publishing, Inc.: Washington, DC.

Center for Disease Control and Prevention (CDC). (2004). *The state of aging and health in America.* www.cdc.gov/aging

Choi, N. G. & Gonzalez, J. (2005a). Barriers and contributors to minority older adults' access to mental health treatment: Perceptions of geriatric mental health clinicians. *Journal of Gerontological Social Work, 44*(3/4): 115-135.

Collins, K. S., Hughes, D. L., Doty, M. M., Ives, B. L., Edwards, J. N., & Tenney, K. (2002). *Diverse communities, common concerns; Assessing health care quality for minority Americans.* Findings from the Commonwealth Fund 2001 Health Care Quality Survey. New York, NY.

Crimmins, E. M., Hayward, M. D., & Saito, Y. (1994). Changing mortality and morbidity rates and the health status and life expectancy of the older population. *Demography, 31*, 159-175.

Davis, K., Leijenaar, M., & Oldersma, J. (1991). *The gender of power.* Newbury Park, CA: Sage Publications.

Espino, D. V. (1990). Mexican-American elderly: Problems in evaluation, diagnosis, and treatment. In M. S. Harper (Ed.), *Minority aging: Essential curricula content for selected health and allied health professions.* (DHHS Publication No. HRS (P-DV-90-4). Washington, DC: Government Printing Office.

Espino, D. (1993). Hispanic elderly and long term care: Implications for ethnically sensitive services. In C. Barresi & D. Stull (Eds.), *Ethnic elderly and long-term care.* New York: Springer, 101-112.

Federal Interagency Forum on Aging Related Statistics (2000). *Older Americans 2000: Key indicators of well-being.* Retrieved February 1, 2002 from www.agingstats.gov/chartbook2000/population.html

Freimen, M. P. & Cunningham, P. J. (1997). Use of health care for the treatment of mental problems among racial/ethnic subpopulations. *Medical Care Research and Review 54*: 80-101.

Garcia, R. A. (1977). *The Chicanos in America 1540-1974*. Oceana Publications Inc.: New York.

Goldenberg, I. (1978) *Oppression and social intervention*. Chicago: Nelson-Hall.

Green, J. (1999). *Cultural awareness in the human services: A multi-ethnic approach*. Allyn and Bacon: Boston.

Guarnaccia, P. J., Rivera, M., Franco, F., & Neighbors, C. (1996). The experience of *Ataques de nervios*: Towards an anthropology of emotions in Puerto Rico. *Culture, Medicine and Psychiatry, 20*, 343-367.

Guarnaccia, P. J. & Rodriguez, O. (1996). Concepts of culture and their role in the development of culturally competent mental health services. *Hispanic Journal of Behavioral Sciences, 18* (4) pp. 419-444.

Hazuda, H. P. & Espino, D. V. (1997). Aging, chronic disease, and physical disability in Hispanic elderly. In K. S. Markides & M. R. Miranda (Eds.), *Minorities, aging and health*. Thousand Oaks, CA: Sage, 127-148.

Health Care Financing Administration. (2000). Office for civil rights' policy guidance on limited English proficient persons. Retrieved October 2, 2003, from http://www.hcfa.gov/medicaid/smd83100.htm

Henry J. Kaiser Family Foundation (1999). *The Faces of Medicare*. Retrieved on January 24, 2002 from http://www.kff.org/medicare/1481-index.cfm

Jezewski, M. & Poss, J. (2002). Mexican Americans' explanatory model of type 2 diabetes. *Western Journal of Nursing Research, 24* (8): 840-858.

Johnson, R. J. & Wolinsky, F. D. (1994). Gender, race, and health: The structure of health status among older adults. *The Gerontologist, 34*, 3, 282-284.

Juarbe, T. (1995). Access to health care for Hispanic women: A primary health care perspective. *Nursing Outlook, 43*(1), 23-28.

Kart, C. S. (1985). *The realities of aging: An introduction to gerontology*. Boston: Allyn and Bacon.

Kleinman, A. (1980), *Patients and healers in the context of culture*. Berkeley: University of California Press.

Lago, C. & Thompson, J. (1996). *Race, culture, and counseling*. Buckingham: Open University Press.

Lantican, L. S. M. (1998). Mexican American clients' perceptions of services in an outpatient mental health facility in a border city. *Issues in Mental Health Nursing, 19, 125-137.*

Markides. K. S. & Black, S. A. (1996). Race, ethnicity, and aging: The impact of inequality. In R. H. Binstock & L. K. George (Eds.), *Handbook of aging and the social sciences* (4th ed.). San Diego, CA: Academic Press, pp. 153-170.

Mutchler, J. E. & Burr, J, A. (1991). Racial differences in health and health care service utilization in later life: The effect of socioeconomic status. *Journal of Health and Social Behavior, 32*, 342-356.

Magilvy, J. K., Congdon, J. G., Martinez, R. J., Davis, R., & Averill, J. (2000). Caring for our own: Health care experiences of rural Hispanic elders. *Journal of Aging Studies, 14* (2) pp. 171-191.

Malgady, R. G., Rogler, L. H., & Marcos, L. R. (1997). *Culture and behavior in psychodiagnosis of Puerto Ricans* (Report prepared under Grant No. R01MH45939). Rockville, MD: National Institute of Mental Health.

McLemore, S. D., Romo, H., & Gonzalez Baker, S. (2001). *Racial and ethnic relations in America, 6th edition.* Allyn & Bacon: Boston.

Miranda, A. O. & Matheny, K. B. (2000). Socio-psychological predictors of acculturative stress among Latino adults. *Journal of Mental Health Counseling, 22* (4): 306-317.

O' Hagan, K. (2001). *Cultural competence in the caring professions.* Jessica Kingsley Publishers: Philadelphia, PA.

Padgett, D. K., Patrick, C., Burns, B. J., & Schlesinger, H. J. (1994). Ethnicity and the use of outpatient mental health services in a national insured population. *American Journal of Public Health, 84* (2): 222-226.

Pinderhughes, E. (1989). Understanding race, power, ethnicity, and power: The key to efficacy in clinical practice. The Free Press-A Division of Macmillan, Inc.: New York.

Saleebey, D. (1997). The strengths perspective in social work practice. Longman Publishers: White Plains, New York.

Santiago-Rivera, A. L. (1995). Developing a culturally sensitive treatment modality for bilingual Spanish-speaking clients: Incorporating language and culture in counseling. *Journal of Counseling and Development, 74*: 12-17.

Sarrett, R. A., Todd, A. M., Decker, J. T., & Walters, G. (1989). The use of formal helping networks to meet the psychological needs of the Hispanic elderly. *Hispanic Journal of Behavioral Sciences, 11* (3): 259-273.

Smart, J. F. & Smart, D. W. (1995). Acculturative stress: The experience of the Hispanic immigrant. *The Counseling Psychologist, 23*: 25-42.

The Center for Mental Health Services (1999). *Facts Sheets–Latinos/Hispanic Americans.* Retrieved January 9, 2002 from http://www.mentalhealth.org/cre/fact3.asp

Timmins, C. L. (2002). The impact of language barriers on the health care of Latinos in the United States: A review of the literature and guidelines for practice. *Journal of Midwifery & Women's Health, 47* (2): 80-96.

Torrez, D. J. (1998). Health and social service utilization patterns of Mexican American older adults. *Journal of Aging Studies, 12* (1): 82-99.

Trevino, F. M. (1999). Quality care for health care for ethnic/racial minority population. *Ethnicity & Health 4*(3) pp. 13-25.

Tulane Hispanic Health Initiative (2002) *Hispanics/Latinos in the United States General Health Status.* http://www.som.tulane.edu/thhi/hstatus1.htm

U.S. Department of Health and Human Services (2003). A Statistical profile of Hispanic older Americans aged 65 +. Administration on Aging.

U.S. Department of Health and Human Services. (1999). *Mental Health: A Report of the Surgeon General.* Rockville, MD: U.S. Department of Health and Human Services, Substance Abuse and Mental Health Services Administration, Center for Mental Health Services, National Institutes of Health, National Institute of Mental Health.

U.S. Department of Health and Human Services, Health Care Financing Administration (HCFA). (1999). *Medicare and you, 2000.* Washington, DC: HCFA.

Vasquez, C. I., & Clavijo, A. M. (1995). The special needs of minorities: A profile of Hispanics. In *Mental Health Services for Older Adults: Implications for Training and Practice in Geropsychology*, Knight, B.G., Wohlford, L. T., & Santos, J. (Eds) American Psychological Association, Washington, DC.

Vega, W. A., Kolody, B., & Aguilar-Gaxiola, S. (2001). Help Seeking for Mental Health Problems Among Mexican Americans. *Journal of Immigrant Health, Vol. 3,* No. 3: 133-140.

Villa, V. M. & Aranda, M. P. (2000). Demographic, economic, and health profile of older Latinos: Implications for health and long-term care policy and the Latino family. *Journal of Health and Human Services Administration, Vol. 23,* No. 2: 161-180.

Warda, M. (2000). Mexican Americans' Perceptions of Culturally Competent Care. *Western Journal of Nursing Research,* 22(2), 203-224.

Williams, B. & Healy, D. (2001). Perceptions of illness causation among new referrals to a community mental health team: Explanatory model or exploratory map? *Social Science and Medicine, 53,* 465-476.

Zuniga, M. E. (1987). Mexican-American clinical training: A pilot program. *Journal of Social Education, 23,* 11-20.

doi:10.1300/J137v14n01_04

Chapter 5

Self-Care in Caregiving

Sally Hill Jones

SUMMARY. This chapter discusses strategies to facilitate caregiver self-care from a social work perspective. The functional age model of intergenerational treatment (Greene, 1986, 1994, 2000) is used to explore the context of caregiving, including the developmental course, challenges, rewards, coping methods, and consequences of caregiving for a variety of clients, followed by an exploration of the process of assessing and intervening with the caregiver to foster healthy self-care practices. doi:10.1300/J137v14n01_05 *[Article copies available for a fee from The Haworth Document Delivery Service: 1-800-HAWORTH. E-mail address: <docdelivery@haworthpress.com> Website: <http://www.HaworthPress.com> © 2006 by The Haworth Press, Inc. All rights reserved.]*

KEYWORDS. Self-care, coping methods, caregiving rewards

INTRODUCTION

Social workers who assist caregivers have the exceptional opportunity of witnessing courage, resilience, creativity, dedication, and love in the face of sometimes daunting obstacles. Many caregivers manage the challenges of caregiving without outside help. Social workers are generally

---

[Haworth co-indexing entry note]: "Self-Care in Caregiving." Jones, Sally Hill. Co-published simultaneously in *Journal of Human Behavior in the Social Environment* (The Haworth Press, Inc.) Vol. 14, No. 1/2, 2006, pp. 95-115; and: *Contemporary Issues of Care* (ed: Roberta R. Greene) The Haworth Press, Inc., 2006, pp. 95-115. Single or multiple copies of this article are available for a fee from The Haworth Document Delivery Service [1-800-HAWORTH, 9:00 a.m. - 5:00 p.m. (EST). E-mail address: docdelivery@haworthpress.com].

called on to assist those caregivers for whom the challenges overwhelm their external and/or internal resources. Feeling strongly that they should be the one to care for their family member or friend, caregivers can find themselves choosing between their caregiving obligations and their own health and well-being. Therefore, when assisting a person with a chronic or terminal illness, the social worker must understand the importance of also attending to the needs of their caregiver(s). By viewing the family unit as the client, geriatric social workers can empower caregivers to attend to his or her own self-care and well-being.

This chapter discusses strategies that social workers can use to facilitate caregiver self-care. The functional age model of intergenerational treatment (Greene, 1986, 1994, 2000) provides a framework to explore the context of caregiving, including the developmental course, challenges, rewards, coping methods, and consequences of caregiving for a variety of clients. The chapter continues with a description of the process of assessing and intervening with caregivers to foster healthy self-care practices.

CHALLENGES

As there are risks as well as rewards inherent in the caregiving role, social workers often address the balance of these factors to prevent or diminish the risks to a caregiver's health and to promote their well-being and resilience. Because a caregiver's self-care is affected by the types of challenges he or she must face, social workers and clients initiate the intervention process by identifying those issues unique to a specific situation.

Although the types of caregiving challenges vary, there are some general themes: For example, when a care recipient exhibits difficult behaviors, this can be a severe source of distress for the caregiver (Ford et al., 1997; Gottlieb & Gignac, 1996; Struening et al., 1995). Problem behaviors can include wandering, night disruptions, incontinence, refusal to bathe, aggressive verbalizations and behaviors, unremitting repetitive questions, embarrassing or dangerous behavior, and agitation. Other challenges include undergoing a lengthy caregiving period, having insufficient supports, and facing end-of-life issues.

The result of these types of challenges can overwhelm the caregiver's resources and may result in physical and mental difficulties. Studies have found that the stress of caregiving is related to depression, anxiety, health problems, compromised immunity, and an exacerbation of existing health issues (Cannuscio et al., 2002; Vitaliano, Zhang, & Scanlon,

2003). Previous psychiatric issues can also interact with caregiver stress. In such situations there is a higher likelihood of a recurrence of mental illness (Russo et al., 1995).

An extensive meta-analysis of research on the risk of illness in caregivers revealed that caregivers reported poorer global health and took more medications for physical problems than noncaregivers (Vitaliano, Zhang & Scanlan, 2003). Caregivers had 23 percent higher levels of stress hormones and 15 percent lower level of antibody responses, increasing risks for hypertension and diabetes, as well as lowering resistance to viruses.

Social workers should also consider positive caregiving experiences as a vital part of the self-care picture. Kramer (1997) uses the term *gain* as "the extent to which the caregiving role is appraised as enhancing an individual's life space and is enriching" (p. 219). Gains or rewards reported include:

- a heightened sense of self and self-worth,
- feeling privileged to be a caretaker,
- feelings of competence and pride in the ability to meet the challenges of the role,
- an increased spiritual connection,
- the opportunity to learn new skills,
- the chance to have a closer relationship with a loved one, family or friends,
- an enhanced sense of meaning,
- warmth and pleasure,
- the knowledge that a loved one is getting the best care, and
- appreciation from a loved one (Berg-Weger et al., 2001; Kramer, 1997; Noonan & Tennstedt, 1997).

To fully understand the caregiving experience, the social worker must grasp the often intangible rewards of that experience, which may serve as buffers against or ways of coping with caregiving challenges.

DEVELOPMENTAL COURSE OF CAREGIVING

Caregiving is a dynamic developmental process that does not progress in stepwise fashion. The needs of the care recipient and the caregiver change over time, as does the caregiver's role expertise. There are wide variations in the timing and order of each phase, depending on the numerous factors that enter into each situation. Several authors discuss overlapping stages or key transition points in the developmental course for various types of caregiving (Aneshensel et al., 1995; Bowers, 1987, 1988; Montgomery & Kosloski, 2005; Nolan, Keady, & Grant, 1995; Seddon, 1999). Table 1 summarizes these conceptualizations, incorporated in the subsequent discussion.

In assessing the caregiver's needs, the social worker considers the timing of the client's developmental caregiving course, tailoring interventions to his or her needs at a specific point in time. Since many caregivers, especially spouses, request help late in the course of caregiving, outreach and prevention are needed to identify problems early before a crisis arises. That is, early intervention can avert more severe problems later in the caregiving developmental course (Berg-Weger & Tebb, 2003-2004).

Anticipatory Care

As transition times occur over the course of care, difficulties may emerge and be a time for intervention (Berg-Weger & Tebb, 2003-2004). The first transition point comes when there are indications of a potential for caregiving, either from the aging process, early signs of a disability, or knowledge of potential risks such as hereditary factors that may come into play. Families may begin to consider future needs in making life deci-

TABLE 1. Developmental Course of Caregiving

Author	Anticipatory Care	Diagnosis	Manifest Caregiving	Advanced Caregiving	Ending	Post-Caregiving
Bowers	Anticipatory	Preventative	Supervisory and instrumental	Protective and preservative		
Nolan	Building on the past	Recognizing the need	Taking it on	Working through it	Reaching the end	New beginning: preservative and reconstructive
Seddon	Managing uncertainty	Trial and error	Coming to grips	Establishing the upper hand		Keeping going
Aneshensel		Role acquisition	Role enactment		Role disengagement	
Montgomery and Kosloski		Performing initial caregiving task	Providing personal care; child seeking services	Spouses seeking services	Considering placement in facility and placement	Continuing care after placement

sions. Preventive work can begin at this stage, preparing for what lies ahead: Resources can be put in place, information gathered and integrated, and plans made. An example might involve facilitating a family's discussion of end-of-life issues while death is still "down the road." Although what is decided may change considerably over time, the process of becoming comfortable with such a discussion can be an important first step.

Diagnosis

When a diagnosis of a threatening condition or illness is made, the family begins to deal with the facts and the meaning of new, life-altering knowledge. Many times the diagnosis precipitates a crisis for the family. How the family is informed of a threatening condition may or may not exacerbate the shock. The family may also be affected by the uncertainty of the course of the illness, its treatability and eventual outcome. These feelings are particularly true for potentially terminal illnesses such as cancer or AIDS or during the treatment phase when outcomes are unclear.

Caregiving may be said to begin at the point of diagnosis. Care at that time might involve accommodating to treatment regimens or making adjustments for safety issues, such as deciding whether the dementia care recipient can safely be left alone. Interventions in this phase often focus on helping the caregiver to manage the shock, denial, and grief processes. In addition, caregivers may be helped to explore and integrate the implications of the diagnosis, as well as to begin to adjust to the disruptions they may face in their normal course of life. In addition, caregivers may need skills to navigate the emotional ups and downs of treatment.

Self-care assistance at this point includes helping caregivers factor in how they can meet their own needs as they grapple with the news of the diagnosis. For example, caregivers need to understand and process their emotions and identify supportive persons in their networks. Considering self care at an early point in the caregiving process may promote receptivity to support and assistance as challenges increase. Caregivers sometimes feel they must conceal their negative emotions to protect the care recipient. As a result, the caregiver may feel alone, particularly if the care recipient has been their confidante. The social worker can explore with the family the possibility of learning to express their emotions with each other to prevent distancing and to promote supportive behaviors.

Self-Identification

Thinking of oneself as a caregiver is a significant turning point in the care developmental process, reoccurring at several points along the caregiving route. Adult children often define themselves as caregivers and seek services more readily and earlier (at diagnosis) than spouses, who wait until the manifest or even advanced stages of caregiving (Dobrof & Ebenstein, 2003-04).

When an individual does not identify as a caregiver, he or she is less likely to ask for available assistance (Kutner, 2001). Therefore, social workers may need to do outreach work to assist the caregiver in this transition in order to make needed help available. This may involve exploring the reasons for not identifying as a caregiver and finding ways that services and self-care fit in the caregiver's view of their evolving role. Services may also need to be defined and marketed in a way that complement the culture of the caregiver.

Manifest Caregiving

The manifest caregiving phase involves a progression of increasing involvement in caregiving tasks from management of care to heavy involvement in the day-to-day matters. Social workers tend to be more involved during this phase and the next phase–when challenges can overwhelm resources. This is a time, for example, when more caregivers for ill children, particularly European-Americans, consider the possibility of institutionalization or placement outside the home. Because the negative effects on the caregiver's physical and emotional health, relationships, employment, and connection to community and spirituality can accumulate, the social worker may need to make renewed efforts to find and supplement resources. In addition, caregivers may find that their feelings of anticipatory grief wax and wane necessitating adequate space and time to process.

At this time, it is crucial to focus on assisting caregivers in finding ways to maintain their own physical and mental health, while meeting caregiving goals as fully as possible. Interventions must be tailored to each situation, developing a variety of self-care strategies that can be used as needs change, finding or developing resources, and learning specific skills.

Advanced Caregiving

In the advance caregiving stage several directions are possible: The caregiver may reach the point where he or she may need to explore placement of the care recipient; or additional resources may be required in the home. Because spousal caregivers and caregivers of color tend to wait until very late in the caregiving process to access resources, services may not be adequate to prevent placement. If placement in an institution is considered necessary due to the impossibility of continuing home care, the social worker's task is to support the caregiver in making the decision that best fits the situation.

Another direction possible in this phase is that the caregiver feels more competent about caregiving, continuing to work hard to maintain stability. She may become more proactive in meeting challenges and experience more rewards. In addition, she may experience more confidence in her abilities, yet self-care continues to be needed. Intervention focuses on assisting the caregiver to maintain stability. Advocacy for continuation of services may be required.

Ending

Finally, the caregiving situation progresses to the point where the end is in sight. This can be due to the care recipient's approaching death or their move into another living situation. The focus of interventions at this phase is assisting caregivers in managing their emotions and the tasks associated with this life transition. With death, the task is to facilitate the opportunity for the caregiver to process grief, resolve unfinished business with the care recipient, and plan for life's end. When the care recipient moves out of the home, practical and emotional assistance may be needed.

Post-Caregiving

After caregiving ends, it is important to recognize that this as another significant transition for the caregiver. There can be a sense of loss and grief for the care recipient, for the caregiving role, and for the support network. When caregiving ends due to the death of the care recipient, the major concern is bereavement. Several studies show that physiological impairment and depressive symptoms continue after the caregiving ends, especially with bereaved spousal caregivers (Bodnar & Kiecolt-Glaser, 1994; Esterling et al., 1996). In addition, several factors of the caregiving experience affect the adjustment after the death of the care recipient such as unresolved feelings about the relationship or continued conflictual feelings about a nursing home placement (Aneshensel et al., 1995;

Kasl-Godley, 2003; Pruchno et al., 1995). Older widowed men are especially vulnerable to the risk of depression and suicide (Collins et al., 1994; Templer & Cappelletty, 1986). Therefore, the self-care of the caregiver continues to be a concern. Interventions focus on grief and loss, as well as helping the client begin to construct a life without the caregiving role and the care recipient's physical presence.

THE PROCESS OF SELF-CARE PLANNING WITH CAREGIVERS

Fostering the self-care of the caregiver requires grasping the scope of the caregiving system, building a trusting relationship, assessing needs and assets, and collaboratively developing an intervention plan. Based on the assessment, the social worker and caregiver(s) develop a self-care plan, a dynamic agreement that changes over time as the situation changes, as methods are tried and found effective or ineffective, and as the trust develops between the social worker and the caregiver/family.

Identifying the Caregiving System

Getting a grasp of the caregiving network is an initial assessment task. Caregiving networks range from one primary caregiver to the nuclear family to a broad network that includes many natural helpers, families of choice, and long-distance family members. When there is a large network of natural helpers, the social worker views this as the caregiving system and determines the roles each person plays. It may be helpful to develop rapport with one or two key informants who serve as liaisons with other family members (Gallagher-Thompson et al., 2003).

Developing a Trusting Relationship with the Caregiver

As in any helping relationship, the development of trust is vital. In gaining trust, it is essential for social workers to communicate that they understand how the caregiver is experiencing her role. Until trust is developed, caregivers may give underestimates of the amount of stress they are experiencing. The practitioner explores the context of caregiving by viewing her client as a person who has had a life and relationships before her caregiving role began. As trust develops, the social worker then delves into the caregiver's views on self-care. Often, concerned family members and friends say to caregivers, "you have to take care of yourself too" without a full understanding of what this would mean. The social worker takes the time to do this and to communicate this understanding.

Understanding the Culture

When the caregiver and social worker have significantly divergent experiences due to differences in race, gender, age, ability, sexual orientation, socioeconomic level, culture or religion, extra effort is needed to build trust. As part of a health care team, the social worker needs to obtain an understanding of the client family's history of oppression and lack of medical access. When the social worker and caregiver share the same culture, the social worker may use those similarities to help the client, while not assuming similarities before they are explored. In addition, the practitioner must recognize that expectations for self-disclosure vary among different cultures. Therefore, it is important to establish the level of openness with which the caregiver is comfortable. That is, interventions must fit within the caregiver's cultural framework to be relevant and effective. As trust develops, the client(s) more fully participate in the assessment and planning process.

Culture and Challenge

Understanding the culture of caregivers is a key to effective social work practice. However, research on how culture influences caregiving practices is not conclusive. For example, some research shows that African-American and Hispanic caregivers experience less distress from caregiving than white counterparts, while other conflicting studies find no differences (Dilworth-Anderson, Williams, & Gibson, 2002). In another example, depression has been found higher in Caucasian and Hispanic caregivers than in African-Americans. Yet, Fox, Hinton, and Levkoff (1999) contend that researchers fail to capture the distress of caregivers of color. Whereas Chadiha et al. (2004) suggest a balanced view, stating that female African-American caregivers actually experience two realities: (1) their strong coping and personal strength that results in reports of high rewards and low strain, and (2) their vulnerability, at-risk of poor health, family destabilization, and impoverishment.

Research shows that U.S. Latino dementia caregivers are younger, poorer, less educated, underemployed, and in significantly worse mental and physical health than white counterparts (Cox & Monk, 1990; Polich & Gallagher-Thompson, 1997). They also underutilize formal services and their care recipients remain living in the community longer (Aranda & Knight, 1997). Thus, different aspects of the caregiving experience may be perceived as stressful by those of different cultures. For example, Mui (1992) found that although black daughters had less overall role strain, both black and white daughter caregivers experienced role strain but from different sources. Cox (1995) found that, for black caregivers, stress resulted from perceived lack of informal supports and a sense of incompetence. For white caregivers, the stress came mostly from the impairment of the care recipient. These contradictory study findings suggest that practitioners need to appreciate how specific cultural expressions affects caregiving practices.

A social worker may want to begin the process of self-care planning by exploring the particular views of the caregiver including:

- Views of disease or disability–Do clients prescribe to a Western medical model in which illness is a normal part of life? Or is illness thought to be due to fate, the will of God, or a source of shame or stigma?
- What language does a client speak? Do translations of words related to the disease or disability give clues to their cultural meaning?
- What is viewed as a problem? When social roles are not fulfilled or when a person is no longer able to care for themselves, what are family members expected to do?
- What are the views about seeking outside help? Is outside help acceptable or is it perceived as a failure in caregiving obligations?
- What is the cultural view of caregiving? Is the caregiver repaying a debt or continuing a tradition of family mutuality? Is caregiving a duty or obligation in one's family? Is it valued and expected? Or is caregiving disruptive to an individual caregiver's life goals?
- What is the cultural view of self-care? Is it an expected, natural part of caregiving? Or is the caregiver expected to provide care alone, submerging his or her own needs?

THE ASSESSMENT

Assessment of the caregiver's self-care is done within a biopsychosocial and spiritual framework. To arrive at an effective care plan, the social worker assesses each area of functioning, considering internal and external needs and assets. (This may be thought of as a grid.)

The Physical Self

It is well-documented that the "maintenance of physical health and function [is] essential to the ability of older adults to begin and continue caregiving" (McCann et al., 2004, p. 1800). Thus, the social worker first obtains an overall picture of the caregiver's physical health, including any past or current physical illnesses, medications, treatments, and indications of lowered immunity. In addition, the social worker explores the caregiver's physical self-care, such as attending to physical illnesses, taking medications as needed, getting medical care, and following recommended dietary and exercise regimens. This allows the practitioner to identify specific caregiver physiological vulnerabilities and address needs for prevention and treatment.

Research suggests physical vulnerabilities of which social workers should become aware:

- Caregivers with high caregiving demands, with little respite, are more vulnerable to physiological difficulties (Irwin, Hauger & Patterson, 1997).
- Caregivers with an existing illness are more likely to decline physically due to caregiving challenges (McCann et al., 2004).
- Clients from lower socioeconomic levels or from oppressed groups generally are more likely to receive lower quality medical care, or to neglect medical care because of lack of access.
- Caregivers in the post-caregiving phase are physiologically vulnerable, and may experience fatigue, lowered immunity, accident-proneness, sleeping and eating difficulties, and for some, suicidal ideations.

The social worker expands the assessment beyond physical illness into the realm of physical wellness and stress. The purpose here is to pinpoint how the caregiver physiologically experiences stress. Specifically, the caregiver is asked where she feels stress in her body (shoulders, back, stomach, head, jaw, and so forth). How is stress affecting any existing physical problems? Are there any sleeping or eating difficulties resulting from the stress of caregiving tasks? With caregivers who are less aware of their physiological stress symptoms, the social worker may suggest they keep a log to determine frequency and context of stress symptoms.

Equally important information to obtain is the caregiver's current and past methods of relieving or reducing stress. Again, the caregiver may not be aware of small ways she reduces stress, such as taking a hot shower or a deep breath, or listening to music.

In some cultures, physical, mental, and emotional symptoms are not as distinct from one another as they are in the Western medical paradigm. Therefore, the social worker recognizes that there are various views about physical stress and illness and their causes and solutions, and seeks information congruent with the caregiver's cultural and community frameworks.

Specifying External Needs and Assets. Using the information gathered, the social worker and caregiver determine what the external needs and assets are in the physical arena. Examples are transportation to the doctor or to an exercise class, equipment such as wheelchairs, walkers, ramps, an uncluttered space, or someone to stay with the care recipient. Additionally, the caregiver may need help finding or paying for appropriate medical care, medications, or a nutritionist to attend to her dietary needs. Exploration of external assets in this area includes a thorough search for needed informal and formal resources. The caregiver's cultural and community supports for physical wellness are included as assets, as well as valued indigenous healers and practices.

Specifying Internal Needs and Assets. Beyond concrete needs, the social worker looks at the caregiver's internal needs and assets and how he or she deals with her own physical health. Specifically, the social worker and caregiver consider the client's attitudes toward health and wellness. What value does the client place on her health? To what extent does she accept and integrate health information? Is her knowledge of the physical aspects of stress and relaxation used to promote well-being or does she need help moving forward with a program to reduce stress? When the caregiver recognizes his or her body's signals of distress, does she attend to these warning signs? In this way, the caregiver's ability to communicate her needs is assessed.

The information gathered leads to the *physical aspect of the self-care plan.* The plan can include teaching the client the knowledge and skills needed to foster well-being, such as information about how stress affects the body, or how relaxation counters these effects (Benson, 1975; Davis, Eshelman, & McKay, 2000). Resource referrals on stress reduction methods may be made including those to increase body awareness, promote muscle relaxation, and increase exercise.

The Psychological Self

The caregiver's psychological health and well-being are crucial areas of assessment. As trust develops, the social worker is particularly interested in how the client's emotional well-being has changed since caregiving process began. As this story unfolds, the social worker learns how the caregiver views herself in the caregiving role. Cognitive processes or thought patterns related to caregiving are important to delve into here. To that end, the social worker and caregiver identify common self-statements and cognitive schema that contribute to or harm the caregiver's coping style. To facilitate this process, the caregiver can keep a log or journal of his or her internal dialogue about caregiving. If the log is kept for a period of time, the caregiver can discover patterns important to a self-care plan. The social worker and the caregiver can also look for thoughts that are not helpful such as having to be a perfectionist to succeed or being too self-critical about caregiving tasks. An example of a common difficulty is the caregiver allowing herself to use respite care when needed. As the social worker and caregiver explore the caregiver's internal dialogue or debate about respite, the issue is sometimes resolved.

There are additional common psychological issues for social workers to explore:

- Depression and anxiety have major negative effects on caregiving. Therefore, the social worker must determine what aspects of the caregiving situation contribute to such symptoms.
- Conflict, guilt, irritability, and anger are common feelings for caregivers. Anger that the care recipient has put the caregiver in a taxing position is a common emotion that can begin a cycle of guilt and antagonism. This can be exacerbated if the caregiver's family, community, or culture supports the view that it is unacceptable to express anger in the caregiving situation.
- Many caregivers experience grief in anticipation of the death of the care recipient. Grief often comes in stages as the care recipient's functioning declines and s/he is increasingly unable to participate in the relationship previously enjoyed with the caregiver.
- Complicated grief can make the care process even more difficult. One example is disenfranchised grief, when the loss involves a situation that is typically shameful or overlooked by society. For example, with a loss of someone to AIDS, the caregiver's grief may be complicated by feelings of shame and a lack of support from others.

Positive emotions are also experienced by caregivers. These can be affirmed by the social worker by inviting the client to talk about the times that caregiving made them feel rewarded, inspired, fortunate, or appreciated, as well as closeness to the care recipient. By learning what coping methods a caregiver uses, the social worker can assist the client in identifying her emotional needs. It is important to also explore current and past successes in managing emotions (Farran, 1991). For example does he or she write, enjoy music, talk to friends or family, garden, laugh, or seek amusement? Does he or she use humor to ease the situation? Does the caregiver engage in meaning making to normalize experiences and feelings (see Table 2)?

Specifying External Needs and Assets. The social worker and caregiver come to a mutual agreement about the external needs and assets available to allow for emotional expression and relative psychological well-being. The client may need practical help such as someone to stay with her, transportation to visit with friends, go to choir practice, bingo, or an art class.

TABLE 2. Classification Scheme of Caregiving Coping

Making Meaning	Causal attribution for symptoms/events/disease "Reads" cognitions/internal states of care recipient Searches for meaning of adversity Normalizes experience/feelings
Acceptance	Accepts or strives to accept disease/behavior/deprivation/the necessity of continuing involvement
Positive Framing	Focuses on positives Makes downward comparison (social or situational) Minimizes negative repercussions
Wishful Thinking	Wishes about disease and about easing of caregiving
Avoidance/Escape	Withdraws from behavior episode Respite from caregiving Cognitive avoidance Ignores while physically present Escape through fantasy Mental distraction
Vigilance	Continuously watchful Mental preoccupation
Emotional Expression/ Inhibition Expression	Expresses emotions openly Inhibits open expression of emotions Admonishes self not to experience or express emotions
Future Expectancies	Optimism: optimistic/hopeful; open toward future Pessimism: pessimistic/fearful; fears similar fate
Humor	Laughs; teases
Help-Seeking	Talking to or practical help from professionals Talking to or practical help from lay associates
Symptom Management: Verbal, Behavioral	*Verbal:* requests, commands, threatens, instructs, directly confronts, rationally explains, changes subject, comforts/reassures/calms, avoids topic that arouses distress *Behavioral:* arranges environment, physically assists/steers/controls, takes over tasks/decisions, uses distraction to interrupt behavior, allows behavior to play out, avoids behavior that arouses distress, comforts/reassures/calms, administers medication

Adapted from: Gottlieb & Gignac (1996) *Journal of Aging Studies, 10,* 137-155.

Referrals needed for psychiatric treatment or support groups should also be addressed.

Specifying Internal Needs and Assets. Internal needs and assets in the emotional and coping area are important to spell out. This is accomplished by taking into account what the caregiver, her community, and culture view as appropriate emotional expression. Does the caregiver need knowledge about common emotions caregivers experience such as depression, anxiety, and grief? This information is used to develop *a self-care plan related to her psychological or emotional self.*

The Sociocultural Self

Assessment of the relational aspects of well-being involves a consideration of the overall pattern of the caregiver's relationships, both before and after caregiving began, as well as through out the developmental course of caregiving. The areas explored are the relationships with the care recipient, family, peers, community, and spirituality:

- The *caregiver's relationship with the care recipient* and how care has affected it is a critical area of assessment. Are there feelings of resentment, burden, or irritability? Maintaining closeness with the care recipient is often very important to the caregiver, with valiant efforts made toward this end. Many caregivers are successful in accomplishing this despite all the changes brought about by the need to perform caregiving tasks (Bull, 1998). The quality of the relationship prior to caregiving is a significant predictor of level of caregiver distress (Lindgren, Connelly, & Gaspar, 1999; Morgan & Laing, 1991). However, as the care recipient becomes more dependent or nears the end of life, caregivers can sometimes find new closeness with the care recipient, using this opportunity for healing or moving past old hurts.
- Family dynamics in the caregiving situation are vital determinants of the quality of self-care for the caregiver. Therefore, the social worker explores the caregiver's *relationship with other family members.* Because family may be defined in many ways, the social worker needs to determine who the caregiver identifies as family, allowing for a broad range of definitions. The strain of the caregiving situation can bring out old harmful family dynamics as well as strengths in pulling together to care for a loved one. The caregiving situation requires some families to use abilities in working together and problem-solving in ways not previously

needed. Social workers often hear many versions of the family story and must be able to gradually pull together a useful narrative from which to work with the caregiver.

* *Relationships with peers* are a very important resource for the caregiver, providing support in ways that family and professionals cannot. Peer support can include friends, neighbors, coworkers, and fellow worshippers. The literature discusses the tendency for some caregivers to isolate themselves, especially as the needs of the care recipient tie them increasingly to the home or if the caregiver views the care recipient's illness/disability as bringing shame onto the family. The social worker learns from the caregiver her previous level and quality of peer support. How has the support changed? What are current support needs and the opportunities available to her for peer connection?

* The social worker also needs to learn from the caregiver how her caregiving and self-care is affected by her *interaction with community agencies*. By understanding the varying levels of involvement a caregiver has with community agencies, the social worker can better match services with client needs. For example, adequate, accessible medical services can be a significant difficulty. Therefore, the ability of the caregiver to advocate for herself in this regard as well as the response to her needs is assessed.

* A *spiritual connection* is recognized as a major resource for many clients that social workers serve. A spiritual connection can range from religious involvement to a more general spiritual connection to something larger than the self. For the caregiver, this connection can provide a framework for addressing the meaning of the caregiving situation. Making meaning of caregiving situations may foster growth and resilience among caregivers. The social worker needs to be comfortable inquiring about the caregiver's spiritual resources in a way that does not impose or judge, but also acknowledges what is significant in the caregiver's life.

Specifying External Needs and Assets. As in the other areas assessed, external needs often depend on access to or reaching out to informal and formal care providers such as a spiritual or religious community of supportive people.

Specifying Internal Needs and Assets. The internal needs may include the empowerment of the caregiver to take the time for his or her relational needs. The caregiver's abilities to cognitively reframe care recipient negative behaviors can also assist in the relationship with the care recipient.

Learning assertiveness skills to use with community agencies is an asset that the caregiver can develop. The caregiver's ability to access her internal spiritual resources is another strength that can be enhanced. The integration of this assessment information leads to a *sociocultural plan of self-care* that supports healthy relationships.

TOTAL PLAN OF CARE

The various self-care plans in the physical/biological, psychological, and sociocultural domains result in a comprehensive assessment. The social worker and caregiver then develop a plan consisting of goals, objectives, timelines, and outcome evaluation measures. It is extremely important, given the likelihood that a caregiver needing assistance will already feel overloaded with demands, that she be helped to prioritize the goals and formulate small, realistic action steps that do not significantly contribute to her day's work.

Generally, interventions begin with the goal of increasing external supports and resources so that caregiving demands are reduced or relief is set in motion. Specific skills to deal with challenging care recipient behavior may also be an early intervention in order to reduce distress, along with simple relaxation techniques. Altering the internal experience of the caregiver by way of cognitive/behavioral techniques or expressive psychotherapies may not be effective until the immediate distress is relieved.

Family interventions can also be offered. During these meetings conflicts around caregiving and the need for the primary caregiver to engage in self-care can be discussed. At times, the social worker and the family decide to work on underlying or old family issues that interfere with caregiving. At other times, this is not possible or desired, and the interventions are designed to work around the conflicts, minimizing their effect.

Depending on the openness on the part of the caregiver to attending a group, support groups can be offered, with the knowledge that this will require the primary caregiver receiving substitute care and transportation. The type of support groups is chosen based on the caregiver's preference, whether it be an education focus, or an opportunity to vent and share with others experiencing similar situations. Research suggests that support groups are more effective for men, people of color, and GLBT caregivers if they are homogeneous. Outreach is often needed to get members for these groups, since they have not been typically oriented to their needs and cultures, or been held in inaccessible locations. Finally, the caregiver may want time to attend religious services, time alone to appreciate nature, a referral to a spiritual advisor, or other forms of spiritual connection.

At times, social workers engage in case management services to coordinate care, obtain access to care, and negotiate for services that meet the client's needs. Another part of many intervention plans can be advocacy for the caregiver. This often takes the form of obtaining services that meet the needs of the caregiver, such as adequate and responsive medical services, culturally responsive services from agencies and organizations, or recognition of a gay or lesbian partner as the decision-maker. The social worker may also teach assertiveness skills through modeling and rehearsal, so that the caregivers learn to advocate for themselves.

Caregivers who are members of oppressed groups face not only the difficulties of caregiving, but may encounter barriers to resources and respectful treatment due to prejudice and discrimination. Finally, the self-care plan is modified as the needs and opportunities for self-care change. As with any intervention plan, it is a work in progress, changing to fit the needs of the client. Therefore, it is helpful for the social worker to prepare the client for some trial and error in the process, as they work together to find the self-care plan that is tailored to fit current and ongoing needs.

CONCLUSION: SELF-CARE OF THE SOCIAL WORKER

Included in the caregiving ecology is the social worker, whose self-care is also a necessary element to a well-functioning system. There are many rewards for social workers who help caregivers. However, there are also continuous exposure to clients' life crises, including trauma, chronic illness and death. Even as the social worker expresses empathy with clients in these situations, he or she is vulnerable to burnout and secondary or vicarious traumatization, sometimes called *compassion fatigue*. This can take the form of posttraumatic stress symptoms that challenge even well-established beliefs systems. Therefore, it is the responsibility of the social worker to plan her own self-care. Using the content areas suggested for the caregiver, the social worker, with the help of supervisor and peers can assess her own physical, psychological, and sociocultural needs and assets. She can identify her vulnerabilities and strengths, track her coping styles, and make plans to seek respite or to try new methods of coping.

REFERENCES

Aneshensel, C. S., Pearlin, L. I., Mullan, J. T., Zarit, S. H., & Whitlatch, C. J. (1995). *Profiles in caregiving: The unexpected career.* San Diego: Academic Press.

Aranda, M. P., & Knight, B. G. (1997). The influences of ethnicity and culture on the caregiver stress and coping process: A sociocultural review and analysis. *Gerontologist, 37*:342-354.

Benson, H. (1975). *The relaxation response.* New York: Morrow.

Berg-Weger, M., Rubio, D. M., & Tebb, S. S. (2001). Strengths-based practice with family caregivers of the chronically ill: Qualitative insights. *Families in Society: Journal of Contemporary Human Services, 82* (3):263-272.

Berg-Weger, M., & Tebb, S. S. (2003-2004). Conversations with researchers about family caregiving: Trends and future directions. *Generations* (Winter):9-16.

Bodnar, J. C., & Kiecolt-Glaser, J. K. (1994). Caregiver depression after bereavement: Chronic stress isn't over when it's over. *Psychology and Aging, 9:*372-380.

Bowers, B. J. (1987). Inter-generational caregiving: Adult caregivers and their ageing parents. *Advances in Nursing Science, 9:*20-31.

Bowers, B. J. (1988). Family perceptions of care in a nursing home. *Gerontologist, 28:*361-367.

Bull, M. A. (1998). Losses in families affected by dementia: Coping strategies and service issues. *Journal of Family Studies, 4:*187-199.

Cannuscio, C. C., Jones, C., Kawachi, I., Colditz, G. A., Berkman, L., & Rimm, E. (2002). Reverberations of family illness: A longitudinal assessment of informal caregiving and mental health status in the Nurses' Health Study. *American Journal of Public Health, 92:*1305-1311.

Chadiha, L. A., Adams, P., Biegel, D. E., Auslander, W., & Gutierrez, L. (2004). Empowering African American women informal caregivers: A literature synthesis and practice strategies. *Social Work, 49*(1):97-109.

Collins, C., Stommel, M., Wang, P., & Given, C. W. (1994). Innovative intervention approaches for Alzheimer's disease caregivers. In D. E. Biegel & A. Blum (Eds.), *Innovations in practice and service delivery across the lifespan.* New York: Oxford.

Cox, C. (1995). Comparing the experiences of black and white caregivers of dementia patients. *Social Work, 40:*343-349.

Cox, C., & Monk, A. (1990). Minority caregivers of dementia victims: A comparison of Black and Hispanic families. *Journal of Applied Gerontology, 9:*340-354.

Davis, M., Eshelman, E. R., & McKay, M. (2000). *The relaxation, & stress reduction workbook* (5th ed.). Oakland, CA: New Harbinger.

Dilworth-Anderson, P., Williams, I. C., & Gibson, B. E. (2002). Issues of race, ethnicity, and culture in caregiving research: A 20-year review (1980-2000). *Gerontologist, 42*(2):237-273.

Dobrof, J., & Ebenstein, H. (2003-2004). Family caregiver self-identification: Implications for healthcare and social service professionals. *Generations* (Winter):33-38.

Esterling, B. A., Kiecolt-Glaser, J. K., Glaser, R. (1996). Psychosocial modulation of cytokine-induced natural killer cell activity in older adults. *Psychosomatic Medicine, 53:*264-272.

Farran, C. J., Keane-Hagerty, E., Salloway, S., Kupferer, S., & Wilken, C. S. (1991). Finding meaning: An alternative paradigm for Alzheimer's disease caregivers. *Gerontologist, 31:*483-489.

Ford, G. R., Goode, K. T., Barrett, J. J., Harrell, L. E., & Haley, W. E. (1997). Gender roles and caregiving stress: An examination of subjective appraisals of specific primary stressors in Alzheimer's caregivers. *Aging, & Mental Health, 1*(2):158-166.

Fox, K., Hinton, W. L., & Levkoff, S. (1999). Take up the caregiver's burden: Stories of care for urban African American elders with dementia. *Culture, Medicine, and Psychiatry, 23:*501-529.

Gallagher-Thompson, Hargrave, R., Hinton, L., Arean, P., Iwamasa, G., & Zeiss, L. M. (2003). In D. W. Coon, & D. Gallagher-Thompson, & L. W. Thompson (Eds.), *Innovative interventions to reduce dementia caregiver distress: A clinical guide.* New York: Springer.

Gottlieb, B. H., & Gignac, M. A. M. (1996). Content and domain specificity of coping among family caregivers of persons with dementia. *Journal of Aging Studies, 10:*137-155.

Greene, R. R. (1986). The functional-age model of intergenerational therapy: A social casework model. *Clinical Gerontologist, 5:*335-346.

Greene, R. R. (2000). Serving the aged and their families in the 21st century using a revised practice model. *Journal of Gerontological Social Work, 34*(1):43-62.

Greene, R. R., Kropf, N., & MacNair, N. (1994). A family therapy model for working with persons with AIDS. *Journal of Family Psychotherapy, 5*(1): 1-20.

Irwin, M., Hauger, R., Patterson, T. L. et al. (1997). Alzheimer caregiver stress: Basal natural killer cell activity, pituitary-adrenal cortical function, and sympathetic tone. *Annals of Behavioral Medicine, 19* (2):83-90.

Kasl-Godley, J. (2003). Anticipatory grief and loss: Implications for intervention. In D. W. Coon, & D. Gallagher-Thompson, & L. W. Thompson (Eds.), *Innovative interventions to reduce dementia caregiver distress: A clinical guide.* New York: Springer.

Kramer, B. J. (1997). Gain in the caregiving experience: Where are we? What next? *Gerontologist, 37:*218-232.

Kutner, G. (2001). *AARP Caregiver Identification Study.* Washington, D.C.: American Association of Retired Persons.

Lindgren, C. L., Connelly, C. T., & Gaspar, H. L. (1999). Grief in spouse and children caregivers of dementia patients. *Western Journal of Nursing Research, 21:*521-537.

McCann, J. J., Hebert, L. E., Bienias, J. L., Morris, M. C., & Evans, D. A. (2004). Predictors of beginning and ending caregiving during a 3-year period in a biracial community population of older adults. *American Journal of Public Health, 94*(10):1800-1807.

Montgomery, R., & Kosloski, K. D. (2005). Change, continuity, & diversity among caregivers. Administration on Aging website, www.aoa.gov/prof/aoaprog/caregiver/careprof/progguidance/background/program%5Fissues/Fin-Montgomery.pdf. Retrieved April 10, 2005.

Morgan, D. G., & Laing, G. P. (1991). The diagnosis of Alzheimer's disease: Spouse's perspectives. *Qualitative Health Research, 1:*370-387.

Mui, A.C. (1992). Caregiver strain among black and white daughter caregivers: A role theory perspective. *The Gerontologist, 32*: 203-212.

Nolan, M., Keady, J., & Grant, G. (1995). Developing a typology of family care: Implications for nurses and other providers. *Journal of Advanced Nursing, 21:*256-265.

Noonan, A. E., & Tennstedt, S. L. (1997). Meaning in caregiving and its contribution in caregiver well-being. *Gerontologist, 17:*785-794.

Polich, T., & Gallagher-Thompson, D. (1997). Preliminary study investigating psychological stress among Hispanic female caregivers. *Journal of Clinical Geropsychology, 3:*1-15.

Pruchno, R. A., Moss, M. S., Burant, C. J., & Schinfeld, S. (1995). Death of an institutionalized parent: Predictors of bereavement. *Omega, 31*(2):99-119.

Russo, J., Vitaliano, P. P., Brewer, D., Katon, W., Becker, J. (1995). Psychiatric disorders in spouse caregivers of care-recipients with Alzheimer's disease and matched controls: A diathesis-stress model of psychopathology. *Journal of Abnormal Psychology, 104:*197-204.

Seddon, D. (1999). Negotiating caregiving and employment. In Cox, S. & Keady, J. (Eds.), *Younger people with dementia: Planning, practice and development.* London: Jessica Kingsley Publishers.

Struening, E. L., Stueve, A., Vine, P., Kreisman, D. E., Link, B. G., & Herman, D. B. (1995). Factors associated with grief and depressive symptoms in caregivers of people with serious mental illness. *Research in Community and Mental Health, 3:*91-124.

Templer, D. I., & Cappelletty, G. G. (1986). Suicide in the elderly: Assessment and intervention. *Clinical Gerontologist, 5:*475-487.

Vitaliano, P. P., Zhang, J., & Scanlan, J. M. (2003). Is caregiving hazardous to one's physical health? A meta-analysis. *Psychological Bulletin, 129:*946-972.

doi:10.1300/J137v14n01_05

Chapter 6

Issues in Caregiving:
Elder Abuse and Substance Abuse

Mary Margaret Just

SUMMARY. Some 10 to 29% of persons over 65 in the United States are sufficently physically, cognitively, or emotionally impaired to need some level of caregiving from their informal and formal support systems. Unfortunately, there are still some older persons who need care, but care is either not provided, inadequate, or involves some form of mistreatment. This chapter discusses the difficulties of maltreatment and substance abuse. doi:10.1300/J137v14n01_06 *[Article copies available for a fee from The Haworth Document Delivery Service: 1-800-HAWORTH. E-mail address: <docdelivery@haworthpress.com> Website: <http://www.HaworthPress.com> © 2006 by The Haworth Press, Inc. All rights reserved.]*

KEYWORDS. Caregiving abuse and maltreatment, substance abuse

INTRODUCTION

For the past 30 years, inadequate care for older persons, particularly care that results in charges of abuse, neglect, or exploitation, has been recognized as an important social issue. Published accounts appear to sug-

[Haworth co-indexing entry note]: "Issues in Caregiving: Elder Abuse and Substance Abuse." Just, Mary Margaret. Co-published simultaneously in *Journal of Human Behavior in the Social Environment* (The Haworth Press, Inc.) Vol. 14, No. 1/2, 2006, pp. 117-137; and: *Contemporary Issues of Care* (ed: Roberta R. Greene) The Haworth Press, Inc., 2006, pp. 117-137. Single or multiple copies of this article are available for a fee from The Haworth Document Delivery Service [1-800-HAWORTH, 9:00 a.m. - 5:00 p.m. (EST). E-mail address: docdelivery@haworthpress.com].

Available online at http://jhbse.haworthpress.com
© 2006 by The Haworth Press, Inc. All rights reserved.
doi:10.1300/J137v14n01_06

gest that most persons over 65 are imperiled and defenseless. Stereotypes notwithstanding, the majority of older persons take care of themselves. However, some 10 to 29% of persons over 65 in the United States are sufficiently physically, cognitively, or emotionally impaired to need some level of caregiving (AoA, 2005). Most of those who need care receive adequate care from their informal and formal support systems. Unfortunately, there are still some older persons who need care, but care is either not provided, inadequate, or involves some form of mistreatment. Within the past three decades, all states have developed some form of adult protective services, but laws vary widely in the level of intervention permitted (AoA, 2005).

Literature on elder abuse indicates that only a small percentage of informal and formal caregivers perpetrate abuse, neglect, or exploitation upon those they are supposed to help. However, since the older population is growing as baby boomers enter it, the percentage does not have to be large to involve millions of men and women (Choi & Mayer, 2000). Estimates of substantiated elder mistreatment have varied from 3.2% (Pillemer & Finkelhor, 1988) to 5% of persons aged 65 and older, gained from international studies (Sijuwade, 1995). The United States Census Bureau estimates there were just over 48 million persons over 60 in 2003 (U.S. Census Bureau, 2005). A five percent rate of abuse would mean that perhaps as many as 2.4 million older persons suffer from some level of mistreatment.

The 1996 National Elder Abuse Incidence Study collected data in 20 counties in 15 states from a probability sample of Adult Protective Services agencies and specially trained individuals in community agencies called sentinels. The study estimated that almost one half million older persons were determined to be abused and neglected, but that for every mistreated older person reported to APS and substantiated, there were five mistreated older persons who were not reported (Cyphers, 1999). In 2000, a survey of Adult Protective Services agencies in 50 states, the District of Columbia, and Guam also found nearly half a million (472,813) elder/adult abuse reports (NCEA, 2002).

When elder abuse attracted attention in the mid 1970s (Butler, 1975, Quinn & Tomita, 1986), early studies looked at characteristics of those who were abused. However, later studies (Wolf & Pillemer, 1989) indicated that elder abuse was more likely to be associated with perpetrators' problems than those of the victims. Some studies found that the victim was involved in the abuse of alcohol or other drugs; others that the caregiver was drinking or using drugs (Choi & Mayer, 2000).

Estimates of older persons' alcohol abuse vary from 10 to 18% of the older population (Perkins & Tice 1999). Cohort effects–those born at a particular point in time–are highly likely (NIAAA, 1998). "Old," defined as those over 60, now includes those who survived Prohibition, the Great Depression, World War II, the Cold War, and most recently those who were young in the 1960s and 70s when attitudes toward alcohol and drug use changed for part of the population (O'Connell, Chin, Cunningham, & Lawlor, 2003).

Definitions abound for the types and levels of elder abuse, neglect, and exploitation (Lachs & Pillemer, 1995), and for abuse of alcohol and other drugs (McNeece & DiNitto, 2005). Pertinent national, state, and local laws and regulations, and the latest national, state, and local news regarding elder abuse and substance abuse are available on the Internet.

ASSESSMENT

Efforts to improve the care that human beings give themselves and receive from others depend on accurate assessment of the situation by all those involved. Assessment may be rooted in any of a number of models, including the problem-solving model (Pincus & Minihan, 1973), a strengths-based approach (Saleeby, 1996), a resilience-enhancing model (Greene, 2002), the Functional Age Model (Greene, [1986] 2000) presented in this volume, or some combination of models. The standards set for physical, mental, social, and spiritual well-being by older persons, their families and friends, and professionals in health care, medicine, psychology, counseling, social work, law or religion often differ from model to model, and always differ from individual to individual.

Protective service agencies, care management service agencies, and health care providers in hospitals, home health agencies, and nursing homes normally prescribe an assessment format that satisfies professional standards for evaluating relevant biological, psychological, social, cultural, legal, and religious factors. If efforts to reduce the mistreatment of older persons are to be successful, even carefully designed assessment formats demand application of the interviewer's knowledge, skills, and values.

Biological Factors

Although being old does not necessarily mean that a person will be visually impaired, hearing impaired, plagued by arthritis, or coping with consequences of illnesses and injuries, as any person ages the probability becomes greater that he or she will have some physical impairment (Bergeron, 2000). Those who hope to help vulnerable older persons receive appropriate care must assess older persons' physical status accurately.

Most studies of elder abuse find that mistreated older persons tend to be physically frail and dependent. Being over 80 and female are significant risk factors (Cyphers, 1999). Choi and Meyer (2000) found that 55% of those who were self-neglecting, financially exploited, or maltreated by others had physical health problems. Seventy percent of the mistreated persons were female. Lachs and Pillemer's (1995) review of studies indicated that frailty was not directly related to abuse, but may have diminished the victim's ability for self defense or escape. Abuse, neglect, and exploitation have been found to shorten survival rates even after services are provided (Lachs, Williams, O'Brien, Pillemer & Charleston, 1998).

Interdisciplinary geriatric assessments, when available, can be particularly helpful. Since passage of the Health Insurance Portability and Accountability Act of 1996 (HIPAA), potential helpers must be aware of the policies that govern gathering information and getting authorization from persons being assessed or their legal guardians (DHHS, 2005). The involvement of the person being assessed necessitated by HIPPA can contribute to their informed collaboration in the helping process. However, if the older person declines to cooperate, gathering accurate information and collaboration between formal and informal caregivers can be virtually impossible.

Only 6.7% of the maltreatment victims in the Choi and Meyer (2000) study abused alcohol or other drugs. Choi and Meyer found that those who abused alcohol or other drugs were much more likely to be involved in self-neglect than they were to be victims of financial exploitation or maltreatment by others. Some older persons have been involved in alcohol or drug misuse since early in their lives and survived. Others have misused sporadically over time, or begun late in life after some life crisis. Women are more likely than men to have concealed misuse. Men of any age are more likely to abuse substances than women. Single men including widowers and the never married are more likely to abuse alcohol than married men (Perkins & Tice, 1999).

The National Institute on Alcohol Abuse and Alcoholism Alcohol Alert (NIAAA) warns of potential interactions between alcohol and aging, particularly the risk of automobile accidents and the interaction between alcohol use and medications. The NIAAA recommends that persons over 65 limit themselves to only one drink a day. However, the practice of "don't ask, don't tell" is often followed by both older persons who drink and by those who take care of them. Both informal and formal caregivers sometimes have difficulty distinguishing between the effects of aging and the effects of substance abuse (NIAAA, 1998). Cognitive impairment, loss of balance, and hand tremors, for example, may have other causes than alcohol or drug abuse. Age-related health problems and alcohol or drug-related problems tend to feed upon one another, and studies indicate that older persons who have misused alcohol have more health problems than those who drink moderately or not at all (O'Connell, Chin, Cunningham, & Lawlor, 2003).

Given the physical and social consequences of alcohol or drug abuse, caring for someone who has misused alcohol or drugs can be difficult for either informal or formal caregivers. Unfortunately there are no longitudinal empirical studies addressing these problems (Choi & Mayer, 2000). Reid, Boutros, O'Connor, Cadariu, and Concato (2002) reviewed 84 research studies done between 1966 and 1998. The studies looked at the relationship between alcohol and falls, fall injuries, functional impairment, cognitive impairment, and mortality among older adults. They found that relationships remain uncertain, since the majority of studies found no association, and all had some methodological flaws.

Routine, consistent, documented assessments of alcohol and other drug use across the life span using screening instruments designed for older persons can limit detection and lead to misdiagnosis. The CAGE questionnaire, supplemented by further questions, is useful (O'Connell, Chin, Cunningham, & Lawlor, 2003).

Psychological Factors

Both cognitive impairment and mental illness make older persons more vulnerable to mistreatment. Older persons who are mentally competent by state standards may accept or decline offers of caregiving services. They are also free to continue their existing caregiving arrangements, even though others see those arrangements as abusive, neglectful, or exploitative. Standards for competency vary widely from state to state and are designed to protect individuals' right to self-determination, not their physical safety (Bergeron, 2000). Exploration of state laws and how they are enforced is wise when trying to determine whether intervention is needed or possible, particularly across state lines.

Depression, anxiety, bipolar disorders, and schizophrenia may occur or persist in older persons. Studies have indicated that older persons with severe mental illness are more vulnerable to abuse, and that abused older persons are more prone to depression than non abused older persons. Choi and Mayer (2000) found that a statistically significant portion (18%) of the maltreated older persons in their study showed signs of depression and/or anxiety. The "learned helplessness" associated with depression, fear, anxiety, delirium, and dementia affect how easily a person is victimized and how able the person is to envision alternatives.

The development of effective psychotropic medication has benefited some older persons (Hatfield, 1999). However, alcohol, prescription drugs, and nonprescription drugs are all too often used to ameliorate emotional or physical pain. That use tends to impair not only intellectual functioning, but common sense. "If some is good, more is better" is dangerous for persons of any age, but particularly problematic for older persons due to the increased risk of interactions between prescription drugs, nonprescription drugs, and alcohol and the high probability that physical injury may occur (Perkins & Tice, 1999).

Cognitive impairment may be independent of or related to alcohol and drug use. Over two thirds of the maltreated older persons in Choi and Meyer's (2000) study showed some impairment of cognitive ability, and nearly 13% were unable to understand consequences of their choices. Hendrie, Gao, Hall, Hui and Unverzagt (1996) found a consistent modest positive relationship between levels of alcohol consumption and cognitive test scores in their study of older black Americans in Indianapolis. Hazelton, Sterns, and Chisholm (2003) studied referrals made to psychiatrists from medical and surgical units in a Nova Scotia health center. The cognitive impairment of chronic alcoholics varied widely, but the authors emphasized that alcohol abuse or dependence alone did not make a person incapable of deciding how much support and assistance he or she required for daily living. In order to protect both the safety and autonomy of the older person whose status might improve or deteriorate over time, Hazelton, Sterns and Chisholm (2003) recommended assessing competence after at least 10 days of sobriety, doing a comprehensive cognitive examination, and scheduling reassessments. Planning and implementing services when the older person's competence varies can be problematic, and will be explored more fully later.

Social Factors

Some studies indicate that social isolation, lack of social support, and lack of financial resources leave older persons vulnerable to mistreatment. Choi and Mayer (2000) found that over 50% of the Adult Protect Services cases they reviewed "consisted solely of self-neglect, self-endangering behaviors, financial mismanagement, and/or environmental hazards that did not involve any perpetrator" (p.15). Nearly two-thirds of these older persons lived alone, and 10.4% had substance abuse problems.

When working with vulnerable older persons and their families, the older person, family members, and the social worker assess factors that may affect the family's ability to give care, and the older person's ability to accept that care. Lachs and Pillemer's (1995) review of elder abuse research found three important risk factors in caregivers: (1) mental illness or substance abuse problems, (2) a history of violence or antisocial behavior, and (3) financial dependence upon the older person. Basic to any caregiving arrangement that maximizes caregiver strengths, and minimizes challenges and stresses, is assessment of caregivers' physical health status, mental health, and cognitive status, past or present substance abuse, ability to cope with daily strain and occasional crisis, and caregivers' socioeconomic resources.

Informal Support Systems

In some families, in some cultures, "family values" include continuing to support other family members even when the demands are beyond the caregivers' physical, intellectual, emotional, or financial capacity. In other families, members habitually gain compliance or dominance through the use of physical force, intimidation, and withholding emotional support.

The National Elder Abuse Incidence Study of 1996 found that relatives or spouses, the usual primary caregivers for older persons, perpetrate 90% of abuse. The Adult Protective Service (APS) agencies' reports compiled in the study found that 85% of abusers were younger than the victims. APA and sentinel reports of abuse found men outnumbered women, but women were slightly more likely than men to have perpetrated neglect (Cyphers, 1999). A Canadian outreach program for seniors with substance abuse problems reported that 15 to 20% of those it served experienced elder abuse (Spencer, 2004).

There are indications that longstanding family problems and issues may lead to elder abuse (Perkins & Tice, 1999). Social workers are educated to avoid blaming the victim (Ryan, 1976), but sometimes care recipients and caregivers have history that leads to lingering trouble. Ramsey-Klawsnik (2000) offers a typology that takes into account factors that contribute to elder maltreatment. She postulates that there are five groups likely to perpetrate elder abuse.

1. The overwhelmed mean well, but their capabilities are not adequate to provide the care needed. Supportive services for the caregiver, offered without blame may be helpful. The impaired have physical or psychological conditions that limit their capacity for giving care. Treatment for their conditions and provision of support services may be helpful.
2. Narcissistic caregivers meet their own needs with others' resources, often covering up mistreatment with a veneer of charm.
3. Domineering or bullying caregivers stay angry, and may hurt not only those in their power, but also those who confront them.
4. Sadistic caregivers gain power and importance from inflicting harm.
5. Paid caregivers can be fired, but Ramsey-Klawsnik (2000) cautions that separating victims from a narcissistic, domineering, or sadistic family member or friend is difficult. She recommends counseling, support, and services for the victim so that their dependency on the caregiver is reduced or eliminated.

Counseling, support, and services for the caregiver may be helpful, if the caregiver will accept and use them. Like elder abuse, alcohol abuse is often a shameful secret, carried on in the privacy of homes. For both elder abuse and alcohol abuse, those involved may not know where to get help, or may be repelled by the organizations, agencies, and institutions that might detect trouble and intervene. In studies of domestic violence involving younger persons, substance abuse can remove inhibitions to expression of hostility, impulsiveness, and aggression, in some cases incidentally, in others deliberately (Spencer, 2004).

Some studies have found that caregiver stress is a risk factor for mistreatment. The so-called sandwich generation, middle aged persons who are providing care for older relatives while still raising children, often could use services such as financial and psychological counseling, support groups, and respite. Unfortunately services are sometimes unavailable or uncoordinated and overburdened family members handle problems without help (Hatfield, 1999).

Caregivers' ability to support themselves and contribute to the older person's financial support can be a factor in elder mistreatment (Lachs & Pillemer, 1995). Risk is higher when money is tight, the older person needs prescription drugs, and the caregiver is misusing alcohol, prescription, or nonprescription drugs.

The possibility of spouse abuse should be taken into consideration when assessing an older person's situation (Pillemer & Finkelhor, 1988).

Beach, Schulz, Williamson, Miller, Weiner, and Lance (2005) found that risk of harmful behavior is higher when care recipient needs are great, and when caregivers, particularly spouses, themselves have more physical symptoms, depression, or cognitive impairment.

Assessment of the role that nonrelatives play in caregiving involves many of the same physical, psychological, socioeconomic, moral and ethical factors involved in family caregiving. Sometimes older persons will attempt to preserve their independence or their sense of being a valued member of a community by claiming that their friends and neighbors would help them if help were needed. The older person's picture of what friends and neighbors can and will provide may be unrealistic (Bergeron, 2000). On the other hand, the older person's picture may be absolutely accurate, but he or she may not be willing to share that picture with others, including family and persons who are attempting to arrange care, until the others demonstrate a genuine commitment to partnership and respect for the older person and his or her perceptions.

Financial exploitation by nonrelatives is common. News accounts of the most recent con game perpetrated upon vulnerable older persons appear regularly. Choi and Mayer (2000) found that 38.8% of the financial exploitation discovered by APS workers in Erie County, NY, over a five year period was perpetrated by nonrelatives. Victims of financial exploitation had smaller social support networks than those who were victims of others abuse or neglect, and those who neglected or endangered themselves. Some cases reported that the perpetrators used alcohol to befuddle their victims.

Some studies indicate that minority older persons, particularly African-Americans are at higher risk of elder abuse (Choi & Mayer, 2000). The National Elder Abuse Incident Study (NEALS) found that a disproportionate number of African-American older persons were victims in substantiated APS investigations. However, NEAIS data from the sentinels in communities indicated that less than 10 percent of victims of mistreatment were members of any minority group (Cyphers, 1999).

Abuse, neglect, exploitation, and mistreatment associated with substance misuse are not confined to heterosexuals. Gay men, lesbians, bisexuals, and transsexuals are more often victims of abuse than perpetrators, but no group is free of persons who are incapable of or unwilling to give adequate care. The roles of lesbian partners in caregiving are explored in this journal. Gay men and lesbians who want to provide care for their partners must utilize powers of attorney, living wills, and other creative legal strategies to have any legal role in providing care. Creative legal strategies can become particularly relevant when persons related to either partner by blood, marriage, or adoption are actively homophobic, or when economic assets are involved.

Formal Support Systems

True respect for the older person's values, beliefs, and right of self determination includes asking about those values and beliefs, attending to the older person's responses, and offering several alternatives from which the older person can make a choice (Bergeron, 2000). Some older persons are extremely reluctant to accept outside help, particularly when that help comes from tax-supported agencies. Protective service workers often hear "I don't need Welfare," particularly if the protective service agency is sited in the state Department of Human Services. Another common statement is, "Promise you won't put me in the nursing home." However, the availability of alternatives to inadequate care or mistreatment depends upon the older person's informal and formal support systems values, beliefs, and willingness to invest resources. Informal resources must be assessed on a case by case basis. State agencies are the most widely available formal resources, and states do pay for nursing home care.

Older persons' vulnerability to mistreatment increases when under funding limits service staff and service availability. Despite the potential for promoting family preservation and well-being, service delivery systems that meet the needs of caregivers for older persons are limited. Unlike provisions in the child welfare system for subsidized care by relatives or foster parents, or inclusion of caregivers' needs in a public assistance check, caregivers for older persons usually serve at their own expense, or the expense of the older person (Bergeron, 2000).

States have taken responsibility for providing some services, but the federal government has a long history of holding hearings, mandating services and not appropriating funds. Deficiencies in public education, lack of research into the incidence of elder abuse, little consensus among states on definitions of mistreatment and services to address problems, ineffective lobbying, and limited real support from the White House have been problems for decades (Olinger, 1991).

All 50 states, the District of Columbia, and Guam do have protective service offices. In Louisiana and Oregon, responsibility for protective services to disabled adults and elder abuse victims is divided between two offices (NCEA, 2002). Those who hope to improve caregiving for older persons in general or any particular older person must be prepared to assess the local situation. Regulations, resources, and administration of programs vary widely from state to state, between urban and rural areas within states, and in different local cultures and economies.

Agencies and organizations that provide support services for older persons are not normally well-equipped to deal with abuse, neglect, and exploitation. Volunteers for Meals on Wheels, staff at congregate meal sites, paraprofessionals and professionals in home health agencies can be educated to become mistreatment-aware "sentinels," like those involved in the National Elder Abuse Incident Study (NCEA, 1998), and trained in techniques that will help protect older persons and those who serve them (Bergeron 2000).

Some professionals may not be aware of issues in elder abuse and the interventions that will alleviate problematic situations, despite a recent American Medical Association suggestion that physicians routinely ask about family violence (Lachs & Pillemer, 1995). A survey of physicians in Hamilton-Wentworth, Ontario, Canada, revealed that less than half (45.1%) were confident about assessing elder abuse, and less than a quarter (22.1%) were confident in their knowledge of relevant community services (Kruger & Patterson, 1997). A five year literature review of articles in major medical journals found only four articles containing primary data about elder abuse, compared to 248 child abuse-related articles (Lachs & Pillemer, 1995). Assessing the awareness level of local professionals and encouraging awareness of issues and available interventions are ongoing tasks for protective service agencies, and those who address mental health and substance abuse treatment needs in the community.

Values and Spiritual Factors

Caregivers, protective service workers, and those who arrange care are well advised to explore what the older person believes if they are to make sense of what the older person says he or she needs or wants. All too often potential caregivers and those who would protect older persons from mistreatment operate on assumptions about what the older person needs and wants, and even more often on assumptions about what the older person *should* need and want. A basic principle in assessment is asking the client/patient/consumer/target system what he or she thinks and feels he or she needs, and (somewhat distinct from need) what he or she thinks and feels he or she wants. Those who have kept lifelong vows of poverty, chastity, and obedience perceive needs and wants somewhat differently from those who have kept lifelong vows to travel first class, change partners when youth and beauty fade, and always take a leadership role.

Sophisticated assessment tools include appraisal of the older person's beliefs, values, ethical principles, perception of his or her relationship with God, a higher power, or the transcendent, and his or her appraisal of the meaning of events and life. Such assessment tools may also include an appraisal of the older person's caregivers' spiritual and religious orientation. Those who intend to protect older persons from mistreatment and arrange services to insure that their needs are met and wants satisfied to the extent possible are well advised to assess the extent to which the older person's spiritual and religious orientation is congruent with that of his or her caregivers.

Art Miles, a hospital chaplain, wrote, "Most victims of domestic violence are blamed by their perpetrators or others for their own abuse, or they fault themselves–a problem that's often exacerbated by skewed religious teachings" (Miles, 1999, p. 34). When a couple's children, friends, neighbors, or fellow church members think that an older person is mistreated, assistance from a trustworthy religious leader who can help the victim believe that mistreatment is not divinely ordained can be critical.

Cunradi, Caetano and Schafer's (2002) study of the relationship between religion and intimate partner violence found that men and women who attended church regularly had significantly lower rates of perpetration and victimization. Weekly attendance at religious services was associated with lower rates of intimate partner violence, and alcohol-related problems elevated the risk of violence. Although the study found that the association between religious factors is not strong when other factors such as age, education, race/ethnicity, and alcohol misuse are taken into account, the authors suggest that participation in a faith community may make mistreatment less likely.

CARE PLANNING

Access to Payment for Care

If older persons need treatment for physical illness, injury, mental health care, or treatment for misuse of alcohol and other drugs, they are often dependent upon some combination of Medicare and Medicaid. Some care is covered, some care is not reimbursed, and even professional health care, mental health care, and substance abuse treatment providers often have difficulty in dealing with intermediaries, the corporations that actually handle tax-supported payment for care. Despite policy makers' rhetoric about intervention in the least restrictive environment, Medicare part "A" will pay for inpatient mental health care but will only pay for 50% of approved outpatient mental health care costs. Rising prescription drug costs create major problems for older persons and caregivers, some of which may be addressed by the new Medicare prescription drug plan, but its effects as yet unknown (DHHS, 2005). States' Medicaid budgets are strained, and many states are rewriting plans to exclude all but the lowest-income households and radically reducing the amount of service covered. Medicaid continues to pay for much of the long term care provided in nursing homes, often the only available source of long term care for abused, neglected, or exploited older persons and for those whose alcohol or drug use makes them incapable of self care.

Planning with the Older Person

There are persons whose willingness to work toward change of behaviors involving drug or alcohol use varies with whether or not they are able to continue using alcohol or other drugs. Spike's (1997) analysis of the ethics of balancing decisions made when a person is capable of thinking in terms of long term gain (when he or she is in his or her usual state of mind) and decisions made when the person is thinking in terms of short term gain (when he or she is longing for a drink, a smoke, the drug of choice). Spike suggests collaborating with the person to determine what the person's long term goals are when the person is in his or her usual state of mind and agreeing upon a treatment plan that provides for alleviating anxiety and withdrawal symptoms when the person might focus on short term gain.

Abused older persons are often slow to trust, reluctant to change, and particularly wary of being sent to a nursing home. Unlike younger persons who survive domestic violence, building a new life over a span of years is not likely to seem like a feasible goal for most mistreated older persons. Changing living arrangements is likely to strain the emotional and financial resources of any domestic violence survivor, no matter what his or her age. Agreeing upon a plan that truly represents the older person's goals is likely to involve building a relationship over time (Bergeron, 2000).

Some service providers find that help for substance misuse is sometimes more acceptable to older persons when help is needed for physical problems (Spencer, 2004). However, it is seldom easy to create plans with a person who misuses alcohol, prescription drugs, or nonprescription drugs. Denial is a prominent feature of substance abuse and a common barrier to plans designed to prevent elder abuse and substance abuse or remedy their effects (McNeece & DiNitto, 2005).

Planning with Family, Friends, and Neighbors

Planning with the older persons' support network can be complex, even when members of the support network are not parties to mistreating the older person. If the older person, his or her support network, and the social worker have arrived at a mutually satisfactory definition of the available instrumental or emotional support, goal setting is simpler. In situations where the caregivers have been involved in mistreatment, respectful treatment, knowledge of family system dynamics and services for the caregiver are appropriate (Bergeron, 2000; Choi, 2000; Spencer, 2004).

Planning with Community Agencies and Organizations

Because elder mistreatment is illegal and can be lethal, law enforcement agencies and the courts may become involved. Particularly when mistreatment of an older person involves the sale or use of illegal drugs, or alcohol abuse, workers may have concerns for older persons' safety and their own. Those who work with battered women and their children stress secrecy and provide safe houses but these approaches are not generally used with older persons. Older victims of domestic violence are even less likely than battered women with children to prefer charges against their abusers, leave for a protected environment, and sever ties through protective orders or divorce (Bergeron, 2000).

A degree of cynicism is often present when planning for alcohol treatment for the older person or his or her caregivers. Studies indicate that older persons do benefit from alcoholism treatment, particularly the older persons who have shorter histories of alcohol misuse. Some studies suggest that older persons benefit from treatment in age-segregated settings (NIAAA, 1998).

Planning with an older person and his or her informal and formal caregivers should involve enhancing the resilience of all concerned, including the social worker who is arranging care to solve problems, address issues, and eliminate or minimize mistreatment. The resilience-enhancing model offered in the introduction to this volume (Chapter 1, Table 4) can be included in the planning process to the benefit of older persons, caregivers, and workers who intervene in situations where abuse has occurred.

IMPLEMENTATION

Access Issues

Most studies reviewed for this article strongly recommend that comprehensive detection, treatment, and follow up programs be developed to reduce older persons' vulnerability (Choi & Mayer 2000; Cyphers, 1999; Hazelton, Sterns, & Chisholm, 2003; Hatfield, 1999; NCEA, 1998; NCEA, 2002; O'Connell, Chin, Cunningham, & Lawlor, 2003). Accurate assessment and collaborative planning are not effective when services for mistreated elders are inadequate or simply unavailable.

Since the Older American's Act of 1965, the Administration on Aging's Area Agencies on Aging (AAA) have been mandated to provide information and referral services for older persons, but the AAAs can only inform and refer if services exist. Some public and private funds support nutrition, transportation, and recreation services. Specialized protective services units, tax supported and self help drug and alcohol treatment resources are limited in urban areas and extremely limited in rural areas. Even when services are available, and responsive to the needs and preferences of older persons, a combination of stigma and stereotyping may keep older persons and their support networks from accessing the services (Hatfield, 1999).

Adult Protective Services (APS) have been funded since Title XX of the Social Security Act was passed in 1975, but changes in funding over the past three decades have left APS across the United States with fewer dollars for an increasing number of older persons and other vulnerable adults. Adult Protective Services case workers' approaches are dictated by state law and agency policy and procedure. In most states, mentally competent adults may decline intervention and implementation of a service plan. In some states, APS may intervene only if alleged victim is physically or mentally vulnerable. Like child abuse and domestic violence, the extent to which mistreatment of older persons is detected, reported, and addressed with appropriate services varies widely, depending on local and state public policy and practice (Cyphers, 1999).

Although vulnerable older persons may say "I don't want Welfare," one seldom hears anyone say "I don't want health." Health care providers are in a particularly good position to recommend needed hospitalization, enhanced treatment for acute or chronic conditions, support groups for patients and caregivers, and the possibility of alternative living arrangements for the older person or the caregiver. In addition to awareness of the legal responsibility to report abuse that applies in any given location, health care providers should be aware of services which can be provided. Older persons are likely to be more willing to accept beneficial services than they are to leave themselves without care by turning an inadequate caregiver over to the legal system (Lacks & Pillemer, 1995).

Health care providers are, in most cases, alert to multiple injuries and implausible explanations when older persons seek treatment. Through training and experience, they become aware that inadequately explained bruises, lacerations or abrasions, or fractures and dehydration and malnutrition can be manifestations of abuse or neglect. Lachs and Pillemer (1995) strongly recommend protocols for the detection of mistreatment and documentation of findings in the medical record. Even if the older person is unready to address mistreatment problems, documentation allows the older person, caregivers, and the person arranging care or attempting to provide protective services to revisit reality at some future time.

As Perkins and Tice (1999) point out, many of the existing approaches to older persons' alcohol abuse emphasize deficits, problems, limitations, and pathology. Increasingly substance abuse treatment literature promotes a strengths perspective (Saleebey, 1997) that focuses on collaborative development of abilities, competencies, and resources. O'Connell, Chin, Cunningham, and Lawlor (2003) recommend inpatient detoxification for older persons, in view of the likelihood of other physical health problems. They also recommend psychoeducation, counseling, and motivational interviewing in age-homogenous settings. Some older persons benefit from residential treatment, some from community based programs, some from participation in self-help groups including Alcoholics Anonymous and Narcotics Anonymous.

Even when programs that serve and monitor vulnerable older persons exist, the programs themselves are vulnerable to changes in management priorities and the exigencies of funding. For example, nearly 25 years ago the Oklahoma Alliance on Aging worked to get a legislative appropriation for in-home/community-based care services. The Eldercare program offered a comprehensive assessment for anyone over 60 years old who lived in a county served by the program. In collaboration with the older person and his or her informal and formal support system, services were planned, provided, and reevaluated regularly. Between 1982 and 2003, the program expanded to serve 75 of Oklahoma's 77 counties. Giving potential 2004 state budget cuts as its reason, the Oklahoma Board of Health closed down the Eldercare program, indicating that it intended to spare its Children First and Child Guidance programs. Adult protective services and some services for low income older persons are provided by the Oklahoma Department of Human Services, but decades of staff experience and established networks of service for all income levels of older persons vanished within days (Beitsch, 2003; Killackey, 2003).

Every state but Arizona had at least one home and community based Medicaid waiver program in 2004. The waiver programs limit services to persons at risk of nursing home placement, and states may limit programs to those with specific problems in specific geographic areas. Even if the person is eligible for the state program, he or she may be placed on a waiting list. Only 27 states offer a personal care program that provides assistance with activities of daily living (AARP, 2005).

Choi and Meyer (2000) recommend outreach services for isolated, frail, cognitively impaired older persons. Provision of support services and financial management services to both older persons and caregivers can reduce abuse, neglect and exploitation. Choi and Meyer strongly recommend assessment and treatment for misuse of alcohol and other drugs since misuse not only puts older persons at higher risk of mistreatment but may have lethal results in combination with some medications.

MONITORING AND EVALUATION

Monitoring and evaluation are critical elements in preventing mistreatment of older persons by themselves and others. Through monitoring and evaluation all concerned can see if they are actually addressing the problems created by elder abuse, neglect, and exploitation. Monitoring and evaluation can also measure whether or not providing services for substance abuse by older persons and caregivers is effective.

Much of what must be monitored depends upon information reported by the older person. The AA program's tenth step, "Continued to take personal inventory and when we were wrong promptly admitted it" (Alcoholics Anonymous, 2002) summarizes what individuals can do for themselves after they have addressed alcohol-related and other problems. Information from the older person's initial biological, psychological, social, and spiritual assessment provides a baseline measure for improvement or decline over time. To the extent possible the older person monitors and evaluates his or her own physical health, recovery from illness or injury, mental health, recovery from substance abuse, ability to cope with life's stresses and strains, cognitive status, the quality and quantity of support received from informal and formal sources, his or her spiritual well-being and relationship with his or her faith community. Reclaiming responsibility can help maintain behaviors that are advantageous for the older person and decrease or eliminate behaviors that are harmful.

Both informal and formal caregivers benefit from planning their work and working their plan. Particularly when elder abuse and substance abuse have occurred, family, friends, neighbors and other sources of informal support are well-advised to assist the older person as they have agreed, but maintain vigilance for their own well-being. It is not difficult at all for caregivers to return to being overwhelmed, ignore their own impairments, or indulge any tendencies they may have to narcissism or bullying. Former caregivers found to be sadistic should be monitored by others to insure that they are no longer providing care.

Professionals, agencies and organizations that provide treatment and care for older persons are normally responsible to licensure boards, accrediting bodies, state and federal agencies charged with oversight, and their sources of reimbursement for services. The results of monitoring and evaluation are often matters of public record. Competent older persons, concerned family members, or professionals who arrange services for older persons are well-advised to monitor and evaluate those who provide treatment and care regularly and systematically, and give feed-back to the providers.

Advocates for older persons can also monitor and evaluate laws related to elder abuse. Again for example, in 2005, after six years of lobbying, Kentucky's advocates for laws that require prompt reporting of adult abuse, neglect or exploitation and better coordination between investigators and prosecutors saw the governor sign a bill into law (AARP, 2005). That only 27 perpetrators were convicted of adult abuse out of 6,000 reports since 2002 does not necessarily mean that Kentucky's adult protective service workers and prosecutors lacked diligence, since many older persons will not cooperate in prosecution of caregivers. Many reports are resolved without legal action, and even substantiated reports may not warrant prosecution of the person giving inadequate care.

Professionals, particularly those who teach and conduct research, are responsible for conducting, monitoring, and evaluating studies that look at who is affected by elder abuse and substance abuse, and what services enhance resilience and recovery. All too often studies conclude with "more research is needed," but that research never appears. Best practices and effective policies should be identified and disseminated.

REFERENCES

The information regarding elder abuse, neglect, and exploitation developed by the National Center for Elder Abuse (2005) is available at http://www.elderabusecenter. org. Extensive health and substance abuse information is available at http://www.nih. gov.

Administration on Aging. (2005). Elder Rights and Resources: Elder Abuse. Retrieved 3/24/2005 from http://www.aoa.gov/eldfam/Elder_Rights/Elder_Abuse/Elder_Abuse_ pf.asp.

Administration on Aging. (2005). Disability status of the civilian noninstitutional population. Retrieved 05/01/2005 from http://www.aoa.gov/prof/Statistics/Census2000/ SR3/Disabilities-State-65plus.xls.

The American Association of Retired Persons offers extensive access to information at http://www.aarp.org.

Alcoholics Anonymous. (1939, 1955, 1976, 2002). Alcoholics Anonymous: The story of how many thousands of men and women have recovered from alcoholism. New York: Alcoholics Anonymous World Services.

American Association of Retired Persons (2005). Midwest state news: Kentucky *AARP Bulletin 46* (5) 33.

Beach, S.R., Schulz, R., Williamson, G.M., Miller, L.S., Weiner, M.F. & Lance, C.E. (2005). Risk factors for potentially harmful informal caregiver behavior. *Journal of the American Geriatrics Society, 53,* (2) 255-261. Retrieved 05/01/2005 from http://www.aarp.org/research/ageline.

Beitsch, L. (March 31, 2003). Memo to Oklahoma State Department of Health Employees.

Bergeron, L.R. (2000). Servicing the needs of elder abuse victims. *Policy & Practice of Public Human Services,* 58 (3) 40-46.

Butler, R.N. (1975). *Why survive? Growing old in America.* New York: Harper & Rowe.

Choi, N.G. & Mayer, J. (2000). Elder abuse, neglect, and exploitation: Risk factors and prevention strategies. *Journal of Gerontological Social Work 33* (2) 5-25.

Coleman, B. & Kassner, E. (2004). Home and community-based long-term care services and supports for older people *American Association of Retired Persons Website.* Retrieved 05/01/2005 from http://www.aarp.org/research.

Cunradi, C.B., Caetano, R. & Shafer, J. (2002). Religious affiliation, denominational homogamy, and intimate partner violence among U.S. couples. *Journal of Religious Studies, 41* (1) 139-151.

Cyphers, G.C. (1999). Elder abuse and neglect. *Policy and Practice of Human Services 57* (3) 25-31.

Department of Health and Human Services (2005). Medicare and you 2005. Retrieved 4/21/2005 from http://www.medicare.gov.

Department of Health and Human Services (2005). Consumer rights under HIPAA. Retrieved 4/23/2005 from http://www.hhs.gov/ocr/hipaa/consumerrights.pdf

Greene, R.R. and Jones, S. (2006). The functional-age model of intergenerational treatment *Journal of Human Behavior in the Social Environment, 14* (1/2) 1-30.

Greene, R.R. (2002). Resiliency: An integrated approach to practice, policy, and research. Washington, D.C.: NASW Press

Hatfield, A. B. (1999). Barriers to serving older adults with a psychiatric disability. *Psychiatric Rehabilitation Journal, 22* (3) 270-277.

Hazelton, L.C., Sterns, G.L. & Chisholm, T. (2003). Decision-making capacity and alcohol abuse: Clinical and ethical considerations in personal care choices. *General Hospital Psychiatry 25* (2), 130-135.

Hendrie, H.C., Gao, S., Hall, K.S., Hui, S.L. & Unverzagt, F.W. (1996). The relationship between alcohol consumption, cognitive performance, and daily functioning in an urban sample of older black Americans, *JAGS 44* 1158-1165.

Killackey, J. (April 2, 2003). State eldercare program targeted for budget cuts. *The Oklahoman.*

Krueger, P. & Patterson, C. (1997). *Canadian Medical Association Journal, 157* (8) 1095-2001.

Lachs, M.S. & Pillemer, K. (1995). Abuse and neglect of elderly persons. *The New England Journal of Medicine, 332,*437-443.

Lachs, M.S., Williams, C.S., O'Brien, S., Pillemer, K.A., & Charlson, M.E. (1998). The mortality of elder mistreatment. *JAMA, 280* (5) 428-432.

McNeece, C.A. & DiNitto, D.M. (2005). Chemical Dependency: A Systems Approach (3rd ed.) Boston: Allyn & Bacon.

Miles, A. (1999). Issues in caregiving elder abuse and substance abuse. New York: The Haworth Press, Inc.

National Center on Elder Abuse (1998). *The National Elder Abuse Incidence Study* Retrieved 4/23/2005 from http://www.elderabusecenter.org.

National Center on Elder Abuse (2002) A response to the abuse of vulnerable adults: The 2000 survey of State Adult Protective Services. Retrieved 3/21/2005 from http://www.elderabusecenter.org.

National Center on Elder Abuse (2005). Website. Retrieved 4/23/2005 from http://www.elderabusecenter.org.

National Institute on Alcohol Abuse and Alcoholism. (1998). *Alcohol alert no. 40.* Bethesda, MD: NIAAA. www.niaaa.nih.gov/publications/aa40.htm retrieved 3/24/2005

O'Connell, H., Chin, A., Cunningham, C. & Lawlor, B. (2003). Alcohol use disorders in elderly people–redefining an age old problem in old age. *BMJ 327* 664-667.

Olinger, J.P. (1991). Elder abuse: The outlook for federal legislation. *Journal of Elder Abuse & Neglect, 3* 43-51.

Perkins, K. & Tice, C. (1999). Family treatment of older adults who misuse alcohol: A strengths perspective. *Journal of Gerontological Social Work 31* (3/4) 169-185.

Pillemer, K., & Finkelhor, D. (1988). The prevalence of elder abuse: A random sample survey. *Gerontologist, 20* (1) 51-57.

Pincus, A. & Minahan, A. (1973). *Social Work Practice: Model and method.* Itasca, IL: F.E. Peacock.

Quinn, M.J. & Tomita, S.K. (1986). Elder Abuse and Neglect: Causes, Diagnosis, and Intervention Strategies New York NY: Springer.

Ramsey-Klawsnik, H. (2000). Elder abuse offenders: A typology *Generations, 24* (2) 17-23.

Reid, M.C., Boutros, N.N., O'Connor, P.G., Cadariu, A. & Concato, J. (2002). The health-related effects of alcohol use in older persons: A systematic review. *Substance Abuse, 23* (3) 149-164.

Ryan, W. (1976). *Blaming the victim.* New York: Random House.

Saleeby, D. (1996). The strengths perspective in social work practice: Extensions and cautions. *Social Work, 41,* 296-306.

Sijuwade, P.O. (1995). Cross-cultural perspectives on elder abuse as a family dilemma. *Social Behavior and Personality 23* (3) 247-252.

Spencer, C. (2004). Alcohol and seniors: Alcohol and senior abuse cases. Retrieved 3/24/05 from http://aginaincanada.ca/Seniors%20Alcohol/1e6.htm

Spike, J. (1997). A paradox about capacity, alcoholism, and noncompliance. *The Journal of Clinical Ethics, 8* (3) 303-306.

United States Bureau of the Census (2005). Annual estimates of the population by sex and five-year age groups for the United States: April 1, 2000 to July 1, 2003. retrieved 4/22/2005 from http://www.census.gov/popest/national/asrh/ NC-EST2003/ NC-EST2003-01.xls

Wolf, J. & Pillemer, K. (1989). National survey on abuse of the elderly in Canada. *Journal of Elder Abuse & Neglect, 4* (2) 45-58.

doi:10.1300/J137v14n01_06

Chapter 7

The Hidden Population:
The Rural Female Elderly in Korea
and Their Economic Status

Eunkyung Kim

SUMMARY. The purposes of this chapter are to discuss the economic status of the rural elderly females in Korea and to examine factors related to poverty. It suggests that Korean rural female elderly, often windows, are faced with serious financial problems. Poverty is associated with age, educational attainment, marital status and living arrangement, and health. When these factors are considered together, it is apparent that rural female elders are facing more severe financial problems than urban female elderly and rural male elderly. doi:10.1300/J137v14n01_07 *[Article copies available for a fee from The Haworth Document Delivery Service: 1-800-HAWORTH. E-mail address: <docdelivery@haworthpress.com> Website: <http://www.HaworthPress.com> © 2006 by The Haworth Press, Inc. All rights reserved.]*

KEYWORDS. Korean elderly, poverty, widowhood

The number of Koreans age 65 and over is expected to triple by 2026 when the elderly will exceed 20% of the population. As a consequence,

---

This research was supported by Changwon National University, S. Korea, 2005.

[Haworth co-indexing entry note]: "The Hidden Population: The Rural Female Elderly in Korea and Their Economic Status." Kim, Eunkyung. Co-published simultaneously in *Journal of Human Behavior in the Social Environment* (The Haworth Press, Inc.) Vol. 14, No. 1/2, 2006, pp. 139-158; and: *Contemporary Issues of Care* (ed: Roberta R. Greene) The Haworth Press, Inc., 2006, pp. 139-158. Single or multiple copies of this article are available for a fee from The Haworth Document Delivery Service [1-800-HAWORTH, 9:00 a.m. - 5:00 p.m. (EST). E-mail address: docdelivery@haworthpress.com].

problems associated with the ageing of the population have emerged as some of the most serious social issues. Korea's population of rural elderly has been increasing, with the result that older females now comprise a numerically and disproportionately larger group of rural residents than ever before. The purposes of this paper are to discuss the economic status of rural elderly female in Korea and to examine factors related to poverty. This study shows that Korean rural female elderly, often widows, are faced with serious financial problems. Poverty is associated with age, educational attainment, marital status and living arrangements, and health. When these factors are considered together, it is apparent that rural female elders are facing more severe financial problems than urban female elderly and rural male elderly. Being old, female, and single living in a rural area represents a particular kind of "multiple jeopardy." To improve the economic status of rural female elderly, an income support policy is necessary. Also, it is clear that more research is needed to determine the nature and degree of economic status differences of the rural versus urban elderly by gender, and the particular characteristics and needs of rural female elderly, requiring a convergence of ageing policy and gender policy.

Using research to develop a demographic profile, this article discusses the economic status and needs of the rural female elderly in South Korea. In a time of cost containment and rapidly changing social service delivery systems, in the U.S. as well as globally, social workers will increasingly need to be able to respond to shifting environments by compiling such data for policymakers. Social workers will also have to make their case, as is done, here for a humane, coordinated and accessible range of health services for all citizens, and health/mental health care that recognizes and provides for the psychosocial needs of patients and families (Vourlekis & Leukefeld, 1989).

INTRODUCTION

Prolonged life expectancy and low fertility rates have contributed to a dramatic increase in both the absolute numbers and proportion of the elderly in the Korea's population of 44.7 million. The number of Koreans age 65 and over was about 3.4 million in 2000 and is expected to triple by 2026 when the elderly are projected to exceed 20% of the population (Korean National Statistical Office, 2005). As a consequence, problems associated with the ageing of the population have emerged as some of the most serious social issues that the country will have to deal with in the near future.

One indication of the ageing of the Korean population is the increase in the median age from 31.8 in 2000 to 34.8 in 2005. In 2000, the median age for the rural population was 31.8 for males and 33.8 for females in Eup, a Korean administrative district with a population between 20,000 and 50,000, and 37.5 for males and 44.7 for females in Myeon, a Korean administrative district where the population is less than 20,000. This compares to 31 for males and 33.1 for females in the urban population. The information about median age points to two important ageing issues. First, the rural population has an older age structure than the urban population. For example, the median age differences between urban and rural Myeon are 6.5 years for males and 11.6 years for females, respectively. While the general rural population decreased by 55.4% (15.5% - > 8.6%) between 1990 and 2000, that of the rural elderly aged 65 and over almost doubled, rising from 9.0% in 1990 to 14.7% in 2000. This is accounted for by a low birth rate and the out-migration of young people. As in other countries, urbanization is one of the most significant population trends of the last 50 years in Korea. Most of the out-migrants from rural areas have been young people. Thus, of the population remaining behind in rural areas, the proportion of elderly has increased greatly compared to the proportion of elderly living in urban areas (Kim & Choe, 1992).

The second implication of the changing median age is that the rural female population is the oldest age group. Women have a greater survival rate than men at all ages. In each age group over 65 years of age, women constitute a larger share of the population. In rural areas, women represent 59 percent of the population age 65 to 74 and 75.8 percent of the population age 85 and older. Because women live longer than men on average, their health and economic status are quite vulnerable at older ages.

A sizable amount of the gerontological literature has suggested that older rural elders have less income (Auerbach, 1976; Barusch, 1994; Kim, 1981; Minkler & Stone, 1985; Rogers, 1998), have poorer health (Barusch, 1994), live alone (Glasgow et al., 1993; McLaughlin & Jensen, 1993), and have access to less adequate transportation systems (Harris, 1978). It is very clear that rural elders have considerably lower incomes and higher poverty rates than their urban counterparts and that poverty rates are particularly high for the old-old, females, and those living alone.

The status of older rural adults is perhaps best captured by the phrase "double jeopardy" (Krout, 1986). Double jeopardy refers to the supposition that rural elders, in general, face challenges and problems based both on age and on other characteristics that are associated with older age, as well as disadvantages inherent in living in sparsely populated and geo-graphically remote rural areas with their lack of resources, opportunities, and services to meet those challenges (Krout & Coward, 1998). Indeed, female rural elders are said to suffer what is called "triple jeopardy," that is, in addition to known hazards of being old and rural, they may also face discrimination based on gender (Minkler & Stone, 1985).

Korea's population of rural elderly has been increasing, with the result that older females now comprise a numerically and disproportionately larger group of rural residents than ever before. Despite significant num-bers of rural female elderly, research on women, especially rural older women, has been underrepresented, and this relative lack of attention in-advertently helps to sustain older women's disadvantaged social, eco-nomic, and health status. Older rural females have to be one of the most hidden of all subgroups of seniors. Few studies have looked at older rural Korean women. Nor has a feminist perspective been brought to bear on how it is to be old and female and rural (Cape, 1987). Therefore, elderly rural women in Korea are remained largely out of sight and out of mind.

The purposes of this paper are twofold: to discuss the poverty status and the demographic silhouette of rural female elderly that can affect pov-erty in Korea and to add the dimensions of gender and place of residence as ageing issues relevant to ageing policy and programs in Korea. Be-cause governmental departments and the Korean National Statistical Of-fice do not analyze income and other demographic information by the place of residence and gender, this paper cannot report the direct national level data of income differences between rural and urban elderly by gen-der. Lack of adequate data is thus an important limitation of this study.

DEFINITION OF RURAL

Place of residence is one of many factors that can affect the well-being of the older population. Decisions about how to distinguish rural from ur-ban are necessarily somewhat arbitrary. One approach defines rural resi-dents as those people in areas that have low population size and density. Based on the definition of the Korean National Statistical Office used to guide this study, *urban* is defined as a total population of at least 50,000 or more. The *residual*–those who do not live in an urban area–are defined as rural. *Elderly* is defined as age sixty-five and over.

THE FEMINIZATION OF POVERTY AND OLDER WOMEN

Perhaps the most commonly used indicator of well-being is income and the economic status that accompanies it (Krout, 1986). Low income is associated with a plethora of needs such as housing, health and health care, and transportation, as well as more subjective factors such as life satisfaction. Problems stemming from lack of income have long been associated with being old. Numerous studies have noted that the incomes of the rural elders are substantially less than those of the elderly living in metropolitan places. It has been argued that the lifetime earnings of the rural elderly are lower due to the less adequate wage scale of such places in general (New York State Senate, 1980). According to Chung, Suk, Do, Kim, Lee, and Kim (2005), average monthly income was 529,000 won for urban elderly and 397,000 won for rural elderly. These rural/urban differences were especially notable for population subgroups based on gender.

While average individual monthly income was 1,248,000 won for male and 727,300 won for female, for those elderly sixty and over, males were receiving 879,600 won and females were receiving 433,000 won, which is about 1/2 of average female monthly income and less than half of male elders' monthly individual income (Table 1). Also elderly females represent 33.9% of the total female livelihood protection recipients in 2003 (Table 2). In addition, among older adults, 74.9% of the recipients of Basic Livelihood Security were female.

The figures in Table 1 and Table 2 suggest that the feminization of poverty is greater among the elderly in Korea. The term "feminization of poverty" has been used since the late 1970s to refer to those societal processes through which poverty is increasingly concentrated among women and children (Pearce, 1978).

Han (2002) reported that the average monthly income of rural male elderly was 585,000 won and 388,200 won for female elderly. In addition, it was reported that 22.9% of rural female elderly received Basic Liveli-

TABLE 1. Individual Monthly Income of the Elderly by Sex

	Total		Male		Female	
	Total	Over 60+	Total	Over 60+	Total	Over 60+
Income (won)*	936600	492100	1247900	879600	727300	433300

Adapted from: Korean National Statistical Office (2001): 2000 population and housing census report.
*$1 is equivalent to 1,020 won

TABLE 2. Percent of Basic Livelihood Security Recipients by Age and Sex

Age	Total	Male	Female
Total	1292690 (100.0)	541233 (100.0)	751457 (100.0)
18 Years & under	314580 (24.3)	159773 (29.5)	154807 (20.6)
18-30	129822 (10.0)	65649 (12.1)	64173 (8.5)
31-40	121517 (9.4)	48721 (9.0)	72796 (9.7)
41-50	198244 (15.3)	100245 (18.5)	97999 (13.0)
51-60	119979 (9.3)	57741 (10.7)	62238 (8.3)
61-64	68021 (5.3)	23499 (4.3)	44522 (5.9)
65 years and over	340527 (26.3)	85605 (15.8)	254922 (33.9)

Adapted from: Ministry of Health and Welfare (2004): 2004 Yearbook of Health & Welfare Statistics.

hood Security but only 10.6% of male elderly received Basic Livelihood Security. Research conducted by Mo (2002) in rural areas reported that the percentage of Medicaid beneficiaries for females were almost twice that of male respondents (18.4 % as opposed to 10.6%). In essence, rural female elderly, often widows, are faced with serious financial problems.

Among rural female elderly, 31.4% reported they did not receive any financial support from children or from others, compared to 17.3% of urban elderly female (Table 3). Therefore, most rural females live in or near poverty, and they cannot afford to retire. As rural older women get older and suffer health problems, their economic situation further deteriorates.

FACTORS RELATED TO POVERTY

Poverty is associated with other characteristics, such as age (Barusch, 1994), educational attainment (Rogers, 1998), marital status and living arrangement (Glasgow & Brown, 1998; Rogers, 1999), and health (McLaughlin & Jensen, 1994). When these factors are considered together, it is apparent that rural female elders are facing more severe financial problems than urban female elderly. In their study of 3,029 elderly, Chung et al. (2005) reported the results of a nationwide survey on living status and the welfare needs of Korean elderly in 2004. It showed income distribution and the average income of the elderly by general characteristics such as gender, age, education level, marital status, and living arrangement (Table 4). Although the data did not directly compare the income and other demographic characteristics by place of residence and gender, it suggested that gender, age, educational attainment, marital sta-

TABLE 3. Status of Financial Support by Residence and Sex (Unit: %)

	Urban			Rural		
	Total	Male	Female	Total	Male	Female
Self-support	26.1	40.5	17.3	41.9	58.7	31.4
Received partial-support	49.6	42.3	54.0	39.4	29.8	45.5
Received full-support	24.3	17.2	28.6	18.6	11.4	23.1

Adapted from: Korean National Statistical Office (2001): 2000 population and housing census report

tus and living arrangement are important factors affecting income of the older people.

LONGEVITY

Longevity alone brings increased risk of poverty (Barusch, 1994). Older women do outnumber older men, and this gender imbalance increases with advancing age. In rural areas as well as urban areas, women are disproportionately represented among the oldest-old, making up 75.8 percent of the population over 85 years of age in 2000 (Table 5).

Average yearly income for rural families was 29,001,000 won in 2004 (Table 6). As the age of the head of household increases, the median income decreases. The rural elderly over the age of seventy lived with less than forty percent (39%) of income of age between thirty and thirty-nine. As Table 6 suggests, economic well-being declines with advancing age. Because women live longer than men on average, their economic status is quite vulnerable at later ages. Gender and longevity combine to increase women's risk of poverty dramatically. This illustrates the notion of "cumulative disadvantage" introduced by Crystal and Shea (1990), since the disadvantage associated with being a woman appears first in young adulthood and then increases with age.

EDUCATIONAL ATTAINMENT

Along with low incomes, the rural female elderly lack education (Rogers, 1998). Educational level makes striking difference in the income of older people. Lower educational attainment has an adverse effect on eco-

TABLE 4. Income Distribution of the Elderly by General Characteristic (Unit: %)

	>200,000 won	200,000~ 400,000 won	400,000~ 600,000 won	600,000+ won	N	Average income (won)
Total	33.3	32.0	12.1	22.7	3,029	486,000
Region						
Urban	32.4	32.0	11.8	23.8	2,051	529,000
Rural	35.1	32.0	12.7	20.3	977	397,000
Gender						
Male	19.3	23.9	13.3	43.5	1,171	783,000
Female	42.1	37.1	11.3	9.5	1,858	299,000
Age						
65-69	28.6	25.1	12.6	33.8	1,215	641,000
70-74	31.2	37.0	11.9	19.9	901	432,000
75+	41.7	36.2	11.6	10.5	911	337,000
Education						
Can't read	43.0	38.5	11.7	6.7	537	257,000
Read	42.3	37.8	10.7	9.2	608	302,000
1-6 years	31.3	33.2	14.8	20.6	1,098	412,000
7-12 years	26.4	23.4	10.5	39.8	611	718,000
Over college	8.6	13.8	6.9	70.7	174	1,501,000
Marital Status						
Married	33.1	25.6	11.4	29.9	1,711	587,000
Widowed	33.5	40.2	13.0	13.3	1,318	356,000
Living Arrangement						
Live Alone	13.3	54.1	17.2	15.4	669	420,000
Live/Spouse	31.4	26.4	12.8	29.5	1,082	615,000
Live/children	48.2	23.7	8.2	19.9	1,100	412,000
Etc.	27.5	33.7	12.9	25.8	178	424,000

Adapted from: Chung et al. (2005): 2004 nationwide survey on living status and the welfare needs of Korean elderly.
*$1 is equivalent to 1,020won

nomic well-being (Barusch, 1994). Elderly who attained college gradua-tion have 5 times more income than elders who cannot read. Educational differences by sex and place of residence are even more striking (Table 7). Rural areas have a larger share of less-educated older women residents. While 48.3% of older women in urban areas have no education experi-ence, 71% had none in rural areas. The share of older women with more

TABLE 5. Percentage of Elders by Residence and Age Distribution

		65-74	75-84	85+
Total	Male	41.1	33.9	23.1
	Female	58.9	66.1	76.9
Urban	Male	41.1	32.3	22.2
	Female	58.9	67.8	77.8
Rural	Male	41.0	36.2	24.2
	Female	59.0	64.8	75.8

Adapted from: Korean National Statistical Office (2001): 2000 population and housing census report.

TABLE 6. Yearly Income for Rural Families by Age of Family Head (Unit: 1,000 won)

Age	Average	30-39	40-49	50-59	60-69	70+
Income	29,001	47,637	38,446	36,111	27,410	18,603

Adapted from: Korean National Statistical Office (2004): 2004 Agriculture Basic Statistics.

TABLE 7. Percentage of Elderly by Education Level, Place of Residence, and Sex

	Urban			Rural		
	Total	Male	Female	Total	Male	Female
No education	35.6	14.7	48.3	57.0	34.8	71.0
1~6 years	34.6	31.0	36.8	32.7	43.7	25.7
7-9 years	10.8	17.2	7.0	4.8	9.4	1.9
10-12 years	11.0	19.0	6.1	3.7	7.9	1.1
13 years and over	8.0	18.1	1.8	1.8	4.2	0.2

Adapted from: Korean National Statistical Office (2001): 2000 population and housing census report.

than 10-12 years of education in urban areas is 7.9% but in rural areas the percentage of older women who have more than 10-12 years of education is only 1.3%. Many female rural elders have less education than their urban counterparts. The less-educated older women residents in rural areas are particularly vulnerable to adverse economic circumstances.

MARITAL STATUS AND LIVING ARRANGEMENT

The family status of males and females differs sharply based on the sex ratio and marital status. About half of rural elders were married, with males at 86.9% and females at 35.0% (Table 8). Males are twice as likely to be married as females, while females are much more likely to be widowed. As a result, a large and growing number of widowed females live alone in rural Korea. The romantic image of the rural elderly passing their later years away in an idyllic country setting, surrounded by beautiful vistas and the extended family, has been abandoned as more realistic data have been gathered.

Seven out of every ten women aged 65 and over, or about 68.2%, are without a spouse, whereas, in contrast, four out of every five men (85.7%) in this age category are married and live with their wives. In large part, this picture reflects higher rates of widowhood among women, whose life expectancy at age 65 is 8 years longer than men's and whose tendency to marry men older than themselves, coupled with lower rates of remarriage, increases their chances of living alone. Thus, living in poverty for the current cohorts of rural elderly women is partially the result of changes in family status. This is because today's elderly women were unlikely to work outside of the home during their younger years; consequently, they depend heavily on their spouses' incomes and pension for their own support. Marital dissolution, including the onset of widowhood, is likely to disrupt the spouse-related income stream and trigger a woman's transition into poverty (Glasgow & Brown, 1998). While rural elders are more

TABLE 8. Percentage of Elders by Marital Status and Place of Residence

Residence	Age	Married		Widowed/divorced		Never married	
		Male	Female	Male	Female	Male	Female
Urban	Total	84.9	29.2	14.8	70.5	0.2	0.3
	65-74	89.0	38.5	10.8	61.1	0.1	0.3
	75-84	75.7	13.3	24.2	86.5	0.2	0.2
	85+	50.8	3.7	49.0	96.2	0.1	0.1
Rural	Total	86.9	35.0	12.9	64.9	0.2	0.1
	65-74	90.7	45.7	9.1	54.2	0.2	0.2
	75-84	80.2	17.9	19.7	82.0	0.1	0.1
	85+	57.1	4.5	42.7	95.4	0.2	0.1

Adapted from: Korean National Statistical Office (2001): 2000 population and housing census report.

likely to be married than their urban counterparts, cross-sectional data indicate that once they experience marital disruption, rural elderly women living alone have higher poverty rates than those living in urban areas (Glasgow, 1988; McLaughlin & Holden, 1993). This suggests that the deleterious effect of widowhood may be greater among rural elders.

Because marital status and living arrangements are linked, the patterns of living arrangements mirror those of marital status. The living arrangements of the elderly have an important bearing on their poverty status and overall well-being. Those living alone are more likely to lack social support networks, to report themselves in poorer health, and to experience poverty (Rogers, 1999). Widowhood increases with advancing age, as does the likelihood of living alone. The older and frailer women, a large majority of them widows, live alone. While 6.8% of elderly males live alone in rural areas, over 4 times as many female elderly (29.7%) live alone (Table 9). A much greater proportion of older men were living in a family setting than were older women. For the majority of these men this family included a spouse, but significantly fewer women were living in families that included a spouse. Older persons living alone are considerably more likely to be poor than are older married couples (Rogers, 1999). As suggested in Table 4, the average income of elderly people who live with a spouse (615,000 won) was one third higher than elderly persons who live alone (420,000 won).

TABLE 9. Percent of Living Arrangement of Elders by Sex and Place of Residence

Residence	Living arrangement	Total	Male	Female
Urban	Live with Spouse	26.9	41.9	17.7
	Live with Children	4.9	1.9	6.7
	Live with Spouse & Children	35.5	35.7	35.4
	Live Alone	13.5	5.4	18.4
	Etc.	19.3	15.2	21.8
Rural	Live with Spouse	42.8	61.2	31.1
	Live with Children	2.7	0.8	3.9
	Live with Spouse & Children	19.9	20.3	19.6
	Live Alone	20.8	6.8	29.7
	Etc.	13.8	10.9	15.6

Adapted from: Korean National Statistical Office (2001): 2000 population and housing census report.

HEALTH

Income has a clear impact on the physical health of older adults. Lower income is also associated with poorer self-rated health. This is probably because those with limited incomes suffer poorer nutritional status and limited access to preventive care (Barusch, 1994). Rural elders are more likely to have characteristics associated with poorer health because they are more likely to be less educated and financially worse off than the urban elderly, and lower socioeconomic status is strongly associated with poor health.

After comprehensive review of the literature on rural/urban health differences, Ecosometrics (1981) stated that no matter what measurement of health status is used, the results are always the same: the rural elderly are in relatively poor health. Rural disadvantage of health status have also reported by Nelson (1980), Palmore (1983), Han (2002), and Chung et al. (2005). Acute health conditions are more commonly experienced by rural elderly primarily because of underdeveloped health care systems that do not detect and treat conditions effectively before they become serious. Among rural elderly, female elderly report more serious health problems. While 84.4 % of the male elderly reported they have chronic illness, 95% of female elderly reported they suffer from chronic illness (Chung et al., 2005). As indicated in Table 10, 57.6% of female elderly people perceived their health as poor compared to 37.3% of male elderly (Korean National Statistical office, 2004). Although few studies have specifically examined the health status of rural women, limited evidence suggests that rural elderly female suffer more health problems than their male counterparts (Kim, 2002; Han 2002). Han (2002) also reported that 57.5% of rural female elderly in her study assessed their subjective health as poor while 39.7% of male elderly perceived themselves to be in poor health.

TABLE 10. Percent of Self-Reported Health Status of the Elderly by Sex and Age

	Very Healthy	Healthy	Fair	Poor	Very Poor
Total	2.4	17.5	31.1	38.2	10.9
Male	4.0	24.3	34.3	28.5	8.8
Female	1.2	12.6	28.7	45.2	12.4

Adapted from: Korean National Statistical Office (2004): 2004 Social Indicators in Korea.

In old age, gender differences in morbidity translate into higher incidence of acute illness among men and greater chronic illness among women. Women over 65 thus experience more injuries, bed disability, and restricted activity days than their male counterparts, with these sex differences becoming most dramatic in the 75 and over age group (Minkler & Stone, 1985). Those elderly with significant health problems not only must deal with the physical and mental discomfort associated with their maladies, but they also may require costly health care. Lack of the financial resources is the most serious difficulty facing older people. Forty-one percent of rural elderly female and 36.3% of rural male elderly reported medical expenses next to living expenses to be the second largest economic burden on them (Han, 2002). This result is consistent with the findings from Chung et al. (2005) and elderly statistics released by Korean Statistical Office (2005). Rural female elderly not only suffer physical illness but also face economic hardship accompanied by health problems. According to W. R. Lassey and M. L Lassey (1985),

> Poor rural older people suffer from what might be referred to as the 'poverty-illness syndrome'–that is, they are poor, which . . . limits their access to medical services while subjecting them to many of the risk factors associated with the higher incidence of chronic disease. Because of their chronic disease, they are often unable to improve their incomes. Geographic and social isolation limit their ability to escape from either poverty or health. (p. 86)

Health status is an important determinant of the elder's behavior and life style and is also strongly related to life satisfaction among aged (George & Bearon, 1980). It is clear that health status is among the most prominent concerns of older people as they evaluate their quality of life. Thus, the health status of the elderly raises significant issues not only for the elderly but for the health care system as well (Krout, 1986).

As Rogers (1999) has noted, problems of poor health in rural communities are exacerbated by structural barriers to accessing health care services, including physicians, hospitals and other health facilities that tend to be concentrated in urbanized areas. Table 11 shows that health services are less available and accessible to rural persons. The number of general hospitals, dental hospitals and oriental hospitals is less than 8% of those in urban areas. Rural elders are more likely than urban elders to have to travel greater distances taking longer times to reach their usual source of care.

TABLE 11. Number of Hospitals by Place of Residence

Type of Hospital	Urban (number)	Rural (number)	Share of urban (%)
General Hospital	265	18	6.8
Hospital	546	184	33.7
Long-term Care Hospital	45	23	51.1
Dental Hospital	97	2	2.1
Oriental Hospital	141	10	7.1
Psychiatric Hospital	72	16	22.2

Adapted from: Ministry of Health and Welfare (2004): 2004 Yearbook of Health & Welfare Statistics.

CONCLUSIONS AND POLICY IMPLICATIONS

This study has examined the economic status of the rural female elderly and demographic factors related to the poverty. Data from previous studies and Korean national census indicate that rural female elderly have lower incomes than their male counterparts in rural areas. The causes of poverty among rural female elderly are complex, reflecting the interaction of individual choice and social conditions (Barusch, 1994). However, it is reasonable to attribute poverty among women in old age in rural areas to societal failings throughout their lives. For today's aged, the communal wrongs of earlier years continue to dictate income status. For the rural female elderly, poverty, illness, social and geographic isolation are all related to each other. The overall picture, then, is of a sizeable number of rural elderly who are at great risk– the older widowed female with low education, low income, living alone. Being old, female, and living alone in a rural area represents a particular kind of "multiple jeopardy."

Although rural elderly women represent the fastest growing and the single poorest segment of Korean society, discussions of the feminization of poverty for the most part have tended to neglect this critical population group. As the examination of the status of the rural elderly female has unfolded, it has become evident that little if any effort has been made at the national level to develop a viable policy to address the unique problems of the rural female elderly (Ambrosius, 1979).

Factors contributing to lower National Pension benefits and higher poverty among elderly women include lower lifetime earnings, the breakdown of the nuclear family, fewer years spent in the labor force, relatively long life expectancy, lower likelihood of receiving pension income, and lower financial net worth (Rupp, Strand, & Davies, 2003). In addition, elderly women are less likely to be married than elderly men and more likely to be widowed. The death of a husband is followed by a decline in living standards and substantial reductions in wealth. To improve the economic status of rural female elderly, policymakers need to consider several policy options related to National Pension. First, Supplemental Special Old-Age Pension should be developed to include all of the rural elderly who could not enroll in the National Pension due to the age limitation. Han (2002) investigated respondents' perspectives on what programs or policies would help rural women in their situation. Thirty-two percent of respondents answered income support policy for the elderly population and sixteen percent indicated a need for general welfare policies for the elderly people.

In addition, social workers in rural areas believed that the income support policy is the most important and urgent policy needed to help rural elderly people (Mo, 2002). Compulsory coverage of Old-Age Pension was extended to farmers, fishermen, and all residents in rural areas in July 1995. Also, for those aged from 50 to less than 65 who cannot meet the requirement for Old-Age Pension because of their old age, the Special Old-Age Pension program was created in 1995 and furthered in 1999.

However, Special Old-Age Pension fails to raise the rural elderly out of poverty due to nonparticipation. Only 13.5% of the rural elderly were receiving Special Old-Age Pension as of 2002. Since the maximum age of the Special Old-Age Pension was less than 65 when it started in 1995, elderly who were over 65 were ineligible. Yoo (2002) reported that 41% of the elderly respondents in his study answered that the reason they did not enroll the Special Old-Age Pension was the age limitation. Furthermore, many married women chose exemption, forfeiting the right to their own National Pension. Considerable numbers of female elders live without a pension in their own right. Moreover, most of them live even without widow's pension which is called *Survivors Pension*. Therefore, special policy which includes all of the rural elderly who could not enroll the pension due to the age limitation needs to be developed.

Second, effective advertisement about the pension is necessary particularly for rural elderly people. The lack of advertisement about the pension precluded participation. Mo (2002) reported that 28% of female rural elderly people reported they never heard of Farmer-Fisherman pension, and 51% reported they heard about it but do not know what it was. (Only 6% of the female elderly knew the contents of the Farmer-Fisherman pension well.) Most of rural female elderly have lower educational attainment, making it harder for them to understand government policies and programs. Therefore, outreach, through door-to-door canvassing, extensive public announcements or other means, is one effort that could familiarize people to services and benefits available to them (Rim, 2004). In addition, information and referral/assistance programs need to assist older persons, their families, and community agencies who need information but do not know where to turn. Nationwide toll-free numbers could assist with linking older persons with appropriate services and resources available in the community to individuals 60 and over.

Third, it is necessary to make widow(er) benefits more generous to reflect the need for a higher percentage of pre-widowhood income to maintain the same standard of living. Under the current law, the payment rate for Survivor Pension ranges from only 40% to 60% based on insured period of former insured person at the time of his/her death– 40% for less than 10 years, 50% for period from 10 to less than 20 years, and 60% for more than 20 years. Since women outlive men, females are the primary beneficiaries of the Survivor's Pension. However, the official poverty threshold assumes that a one-person household needs 80 percent of the income of a two-person household to have an equal standard of living (Ansick & Weaver, 2001). Therefore, increasing Survivor pension benefits to 80 percent would help poor female elderly move out of poverty.

Along with considering policy options related to National Pension policy, providing a training program for new farming technology for the rural elderly is another way to improve their income (Kim, 2003). Until now, farming education was provided to young and middle age farmers. Since 43.1% of the managers of the farm household are over 65 (Korean National Statistical Office, 2004), educating elders with recent farming technology will maximize their profit from farming.

However, the most fundamental step to alleviate the risk of poverty of older women in rural areas involves rejuvenating the nation's agriculture economy and developing a regionally balanced national economy. Rural economies underwent a dramatic transformation during the working lives of today's elders. Local economic conditions will continue to affect the life of the elderly and range of services available to older persons. Poverty among rural female elderly can be addressed by stimulating the rural economy thus improving their quality of life (Han, 2002).

Those living in the rural community find limited relief in health care services. Governmental programs systematically discriminate against the rural elderly. Perhaps the most obvious reason for the smaller number of services found in rural areas is lack of funds. However, it is not simply lack of money that restricts the availability of services for the elderly in rural areas. A "person power" shortage is found in rural areas. A major policy issue associated with the increasing number of elderly is the allocation of public resources. The elderly require a disproportionate level of services and account for a disproportionate share of the public budget (Siegel, 1993). Residential differences in physical limitations as well as access to and availability of services need to be considered in planning for services in particular communities.

It is clear that more research is needed to determine the nature and degree of economic status differences of the rural versus urban elderly by gender. Both national level research and community level research are necessary to obtain more regionally specific data. With so many limitations, it is no wonder that a single model of service delivery will not fit all communities. Each community, with its differences in population, economic resources, geographic characteristics, and political policies must therefore have programs and services that fit its specific locale. Urban models can be transferred to a rural setting, but several adaptations must occur (Bull, 1998).

There still remains a general lack of knowledge on the part of national officials about nationwide older rural populations. There is an urgent need to bridge this information gap with reliable data that go beyond the nationwide aggregate level. Continuing education of elected officials is needed at all levels of government. Unfortunately, many officials at the national level, especially in the large bureaucratic agencies (Seoul-oriented or city-oriented) are apt to write regulations that fit only urban programs, so that new and existing programs often cannot be adapted to provide the greater variety needed in rural areas. Based on research about the needs and life status of the region, community based policy should be developed. The regionally focused research implies the complementary goal of regionally designed and implemented policies and programs to consider special circumstances of various regional sections. Residential differences in physical limitations as well as access to and availability of services need to be considered in planning for services in particular communities.

This study could not show the direct income comparison between rural female elderly and their urban counterparts. In many governmental data bases and research outcomes in Korea, there was no classification based on age, gender, and place of residence. Governmental officials and researchers should become aware that gender and place of residence are important factors that can affect the well-being of the older population. This shortcoming limits our understanding of the ways rural women interpret their world, the factors that affect their quality of life, and similarities and differences between older rural women and other older women. Although the Korean government has enacted the Welfare Act for Older Persons in 1981 and has implemented various policies to provide benefits to the elderly, little attention has been paid to the gender differences and particular needs of older women, particularly older women in rural areas. It is necessary to pay attention to the particular characteristics and needs of rural female elderly, and ageing policy and gender policy need to converge.

Elderly policies should be gender specific and gender sensitive. Gender sensitive policies are generally preventive, offering the promise of security to later generations of women. Policy makers and practitioners need to develop the programs and policies that may better serve the needs of older women and thus may work to promote needed social policies in both the private and the public sector. Such policies should attempt to put an end to gender inequalities in pay and pension benefits, recognize and deal justly with such factors as the sexual division of labor, including caregiving, and strive to meet the needs of women of all ages, including, importantly, the rural female elderly (Minkler & Stone, 1985). Efforts to improve the financial status of older women must start with younger women, enabling them to lay the foundation for economic security in old age (Barusch, 1994). The growing number of elderly women in rural Korea points to the importance of initiating a new discourse on the needs and abilities of older women and women of all ages, their preferred styles of empowerment, and the implication for social work practice to improve the quality of life of the rural elderly female.

REFERENCES

Ambrosius (1979). *In search of a national policy on the rural older person: An analysis of the 1978 Amendments to the Older American Act.* Council on Ageing, University of Kentucky, Lexington, Kentucky.

Auerbach, A. J. (1976). The elderly in rural areas: Differences in urban areas and implications for practice. In L. Ginsberg (Ed.), *Social Work in Rural Communities* (pp. 99-108). New York: Council on Social Work Education.

Barusch, A. S. (1994). *Older women in poverty: Private lives and public policies.* New York: Springer Publishing Co.

Bengtson, U. L., Olander, E. B., & Haddad, A. A. (1976). The generation gap and ageing family members: Toward a conceptualized model. In J. F. Gubrium (Ed.) *Time, roles, and self in old age* (pp. 237-263). New York: Human Science Press.

Bull, C. N. (1998). Ageing in rural communities. *National Forum, 78,* 38-41.

Cape, E. (1987). Ageing women in rural settings. In V. W. Marshall (2nd ed.), *Ageing in Canada* (pp. 84-99). Markham, Ontario: Fitzhenry & Whiteside.

Chung, K. H., Suk, J. E., Do, S. E., Kim C. H., Lee, Y. K., & Kim, H. K. (2005). 2004 Nationwide survey on living status and the welfare needs of the elderly. Korea Institute for Health and Social Affairs.

Crystal, S., & Shea, D. (1990). Cumulative advantage, cumulative disadvantage, and inequality among elderly people. *The Gerontologist, 30,* 437-443.

Ecosometrics. 1981. *Review of reported differences between the rural and urban elderly: Status, needs, services, and service costs.* (Contract No. 150-80-6-065). Washington, D.C.: Administration on Ageing.

George, L., & Bearon, L. (1980). *Quality of life in older persons: Meaning and measurement.* Boston, MA: Human Sciences Press.

Glasgow, N. & Brown, D. (1998). Older, rural, and poor. In R. T. Coward & J. A. Krout (Eds.), *Ageing in rural settings* (pp 187-207). New York: Springer Publishing Company.

Glasgow, N. (1993). Poverty among rural elders: Trends, context and directions for policy. *Journal of Applied Gerontology, 12,* 302-319.

Haghes, B. (1990). Quality of Life. In S. M. Peace (Ed.), *Researching Social Gerontology* (pp 46-58). Canada: Sage.

Han, K. H. (2002). *The living status of rural elderly female.* Paper presented at the 9th Women's Policy Forum, Korean Women's Developmental Institute.

Harris, C. S. (1978). *Fact book on ageing, a profile of America's older population.* Washington, DC: National Council on Ageing.

Kim, I. K., & Choe, E. H. (1992). Support exchange patterns of the elderly in the Republic of Korea. *Asia-Pacific Population Journal, 7,* 89-104.

Kim, E. K. (2002). The effects of family relations on life satisfaction of the rural elderly in Korea. *Journal of Asian Regional Association for Home Economics, 9* (2), 66-71.

Kim, E. K. (2002). Issues and policies of the rural female elderly. *Journal of Korean Society of the Welfare for the Aged, 16,* 175-191.

Kim, P. K. (1981). The low income rural elderly: Under-served victims of public inequity. In P. K. Kim & C. Wilson (Eds.), *Toward Mental Health of the Rural Elderly* (pp. 289-316), Washington D.C.: University Press of America.

Korean National Statistical Office (2001). *2000 population and housing census report.*

Korean National Statistical Office (2004). *2004 Agriculture Basic Statistics.*

Korean National Statistical Office (2004). *2004 Social Indicators in Korea.*

Krout, J. A. (1986). *The aged in rural America.* Westport, CT: Greenwood Press.

Krout, J. A., & Coward, R. T. (1998). Ageing in rural environments. In J. A. Krout & R. T. Coward (Eds.), *Ageing in Rural Settings: Life Circumstances & Distinctive Features* (pp. 3-14). New York, NY: Springer Publishing Company.

Lassey, W. R. & Lassey, M. L. (1985). The physical health status of the rural elderly. In R. T. Coward & G. R. Lee (Eds.) *The elderly in rural society* (pp. 83-104). New York: Springer.

McLaughlin, D. K., & Jensen, L. (1993). Poverty among older Americans: The plight of nonmetropolitan elder. *Journal of Gerontology: Social Sciences, 48,* S44-54.

McLaughlin, D. K., & Jensen, L. (1994). *Poverty dynamics among U.S. elders: Implications of occupation, gender, and residence.* Paper presented at the 1994 Meeting of the Population Association of America.

McLaughlin, D. K., & Holden, K. (1993). Nonmetropolitan elderly women: A portrait of economic vulnerability. *Journal of Applied Gerontology. 12*, 320-334.

Ministry of Health and Welfare (2004). *2004 Yearbook of Health & Welfare.*

Minker, M., & Stone, R. (1985). The feminization of poverty and older women. *The Gerontologist, 25*, 351-357.

Mo, S. H. (2002). *The welfare status and problems of rural female elderly.* Paper presented at the 9th Women's Policy Forum, Korean Women's Developmental Institute.

Nelson, G. (1980). Social services to the urban and rural aged: The experiences of area agencies on ageing. *The Gerontologist, 20*, 200-207.

New York State Senate (1980). *Old age and ruralism: A case of Double Jeopardy, Report on the Rural Elderly.* Albany, NY: New York State Senate.

Palmore, E. (1983). Health care needs of the rural elderly. *International Journal of Ageing and Human Development, 18*, 39-45.

Pearce, D. (1978). The feminization of poverty: Women, work and welfare. *Urban and Social Change Review, 74*, 11-19.

Rim, C. S. (2004). Future issues and agendas for the ageing society. *Journal of Welfare for the Aged, 11*, 125-144.

Rogers, C. C. (1998). Poverty of older women across rural-urban continuum. *Rural Developmental Perspectives, 13*, 2-9.

Rogers, C. C. (1999). *Changes in the older population and implication for rural areas.* Washington, DC: U.S. Department of Agriculture.

Rupp, K., Strand, A., & Davies, P. (2003). Poverty among elderly women: Assessing SSI options to strengthen Social Security reform. *Journal of Gerontology: Social Seicnces, 58*, S359-S368.

Vourlekis, B. S. & Leukefeld, C. (1989). *Making our case.* Silver Spring, MD: NASW Press.

Yoo, S. H. (2002). *The policy issues of rural female elderly.* Paper presented at the 9th Women's Policy Forum, Korean Women's Developmental Institute.

doi:10.1300/J137v14n01_07

Chapter 8

The Role of African-American Pastors in Mental Health Care

Kimberly Farris

SUMMARY. This chapter uses a biopsychosocial and spiritual model to examine the help-seeking behavior of African-American individuals with mental illness. It addresses questions related to African-Americans undertutilization of formal mental health services and how spriutal factors contribute to their secking help from African-American pastors. doi:10.1300/J137v14n01_08 *[Article copies available for a fee from The Haworth Document Delivery Service: 1-800-HAWORTH. E-mail address: <docdelivery@haworthpress.com> Website: <http://www.HaworthPress.com> © 2006 by The Haworth Press, Inc. All rights reserved.]*

KEYWORDS. African-American pastors and support systems, spirituality, mental illness

INTRODUCTION

The National Survey of Black Americans conducted by Taylor and Chatters (2003) examined mental health and help-seeking among Afri-

[Haworth co-indexing entry note]: "The Role of African-American Pastors in Mental Health Care." Farris, Kimberly. Co-published simultaneously in *Journal of Human Behavior in the Social Environment* (The Haworth Press, Inc.) Vol. 14, No. 1/2, 2006, pp. 159-182; and: *Contemporary Issues of Care* (ed: Roberta R. Greene) The Haworth Press, Inc., 2006, pp. 159-182. Single or multiple copies of this article are available for a fee from The Haworth Document Delivery Service [1-800-HAWORTH, 9:00 a.m. - 5:00 p.m. (EST). E-mail address: docdelivery@haworthpress.com].

can-Americans. Their findings showed that when the need for treatment is defined by the presence of psychopathology, African-Americans underutilize mental health services. Rather, African-Americans tend to seek help through their social networks which include the Black church and African-American pastors. Therefore, African-American pastors play a key role in meeting the needs of African-American individuals, families, and communities, including caregivers and consumers. This chapter uses a biopsychosocial and spiritual model to examine the help-seeking behavior of African-American individuals with mental illness. It addresses questions related to African-Americans underutilization of formal mental health services and how spiritual factors contribute to their seeking help from African-American pastors.

MENTAL HEALTH STATISTICS

In 2003, the National Survey on Drug Use and Health (NSDUH) reported that an estimated 19.6 million adults, ages 18 or older, had a serious mental illness representing 9.2 percent of all adults. This rate is higher than the rate of 8.3 percent in 2002. The NSDUH (2003) also reported that 8.4 percent of individuals with a serious mental illness were African-American adults, ages 18 or older. In 2001, the Surgeon General's supplement report, *Culture, Race, and Ethnicity*, showed that approximately 12% (33.9 million individuals) of the United States population identified themselves as African-American.

Previous studies examining the prevalence of serious mental illness in African-Americans, including the National Comorbidity Study (NCS) and Epidemiologic Catchment Area (ECA) study showed that while there are existing variations for some disorders, the frequency of serious mental illness in African-Americans was almost comparable to that of Whites, with the exceptions of schizophrenia and phobias. The findings of the NCS show that even without controlling for demographic and socioeconomic differences, African-Americans had a lower lifetime prevalence of mental illness than Whites.

However, this finding is subject to challenge due to the overrepresentation of African-Americans in high need populations, including psychiatric hospitals, prisons, the inner city, and poor rural areas that were not surveyed by researchers for accessibility reasons. The inclusion of the mentally ill among these high need populations could increase the rates of mental illness among African-Americans. The NCS also revealed that African-Americans with serious mental illnesses are significantly less likely than Whites to seek treatment for mental health related problems

(Neighbors, Musick, & Williams, 1998). This revelation leads to the question whether some African-Americans in need of help recognize or know what the symptoms of mental illness are. The studies' findings demonstrate the existence of disparities for individuals of color, the limited knowledge about mental illness and culture, and the greater level of burden potentially faced by individuals of color due to unmet needs (Davis, 2001).

SERVICE USE BY AFRICAN-AMERICANS

Barriers

The literature provides some understanding of the barriers members of specific groups encounter in regards to service delivery systems. Snowden, Collinge, and Runkle (1982) maintain that

> the question of why potential clients do not become actual clients is considerably more complicated than is often recognized. Behind any potential episode of professional help is a background of perceptions, judgments, and actions, all moving the person toward or away from contact with services. (p. 281)

Historically, African-Americans have been among those populations that underutilize mental health services. Research findings generally show that African-Americans are less likely than Whites to seek help from private practice therapists, mental health centers, and physicians, but are more likely than Whites to use emergency room services (Snowden, 1999). The Surgeon General's Report on Mental Health (2001) also discussed service use patterns among African-Americans. The Report indicated that African-Americans who are mentally ill choose to use other sources of support, including family, friends, the church, and pastors, in times of distress.

Snowden (1999), who examined racial differences in use of mental health services, indicated that an under-representation of mental health care services by African-Americans may be accounted for by clinical and socio-demographic differences as well as the inadequate sampling of difficult-to-reach populations. Underutilization may also be due to distrust of the mental health service system, lack of available community mental health resources, misdiagnosis of psychiatric symptoms, stigma, and low levels of knowledge in understanding the etiology of mental illness (Neighbors & Jackson, 1984; Pickett-Schneck, 2002).

Cultural Differences

Cultural differences may also play a major role in the underutilization of mental health services (Biegel, Johnsen, & Shafran, 1997; Pickett-Schneck, 2002). It has been suggested (Hunt, 1996) that variations in experiences often indicate differences in history, culture, and generalized experiences, with the result that African-Americans tend to identify more with each other as a group than Whites or other disadvantaged groups (Gurin, Miller, & Gurin, 1980). The strong group identification has the potential to encourage African-Americans to view social issues in terms of problems facing fellow African-Americans even if they do not experience the problem themselves (Hunt, 1996). As a result, African-Americans' beliefs about mental illness may be strongly influenced by circumstances faced as a group and by the inferences of various explanations of mental illness for public debates about race (Schnittker, Freese, & Powell, 2000).

Pastoral Help

Reasons for African-American individuals seeking mental health care from their pastors may be found in the study by Schnittker, Freese, and Powell (2000). Their research suggested that African-Americans may be more likely than Whites to believe that mental illness is a result of God's will because of the reports of stronger religious beliefs and higher levels of religious participation (Taylor & Chatters, 1991; Taylor et al., 1996; Taylor, Levin, & Chatters, 2003). Evidence also shows that Blacks use prayer more or consult religious leaders for assistance with personal and psychological problems (Milstein, Guarnaccia, & Midlarsky, 1995; Taylor & Chatters, 1991; Taylor, Chatters, & Levin, 2003). In addition, African-Americans may be more likely than Whites to attribute mental illness to bad character, with some research showing that African-Americans more commonly believe that disorders including schizophrenia and depression are due to lack of willpower (Hall & Tucker, 1985).

BIOPSYCHOSOCIAL AND SPIRITUAL ASPECTS OF MENTAL ILLNESS

A person's belief about the causes or etiology of mental illness is a determinant of where people seek help and a necessary component of client assessment. That is, does he or she perceive mental illness as having biological, psychological, social or spiritual roots? Personal conceptions may include biological causes, such as genetic inheritance or chemical imbalance or environmental factors, such as family background and social stressors. Still others may think about mental illness in terms of individual responsibility or divine judgment (Schnittker, Freese, & Powell, 2000). By contrast, sociologists studying etiological beliefs of mental illness examine various contributing explanations such as economic inequality, gender and race differences, education, homelessness, or environmental issues as they attempt to understand how individuals construct the beliefs about the world they live in, attitudes towards others, their definition and framing of social problems, endorsement of public policies, and their own behavior (Brown, 1992; Feagin, 1975; Furnham, 1988; Kluegal & Smith, 1986; Lee, Jones, & Lewis, 1990). Therefore, a bio-psycho-social-spiritual model, an extension of the traditional social work bio-psycho-social model, is used here to allow for an understanding how mental health professionals and the African-American community differently embrace the causes of mental illness (Schnittker, Freese, & Powell, 2000).

Within the field of social work, the goal of the psychosocial approach is to determine a psychosocial assessment of a client including history and developmental processes (Jordan & Franklin, 2003; Figure 1). Cumella (2002) has amplified how health professions have adopted biopsychosocial models to conceptualize and treat physical and mental illness. She notes that a biopsychosocial and spiritual model acknowledges that mental illness occurs through an interactive process involving: (1) genetic and biomedical factors, (2) psychological, emotional, behavioral, and cognitive factors, and (3) social and family factors (Cumella, 2002). It is further noted that each area may generate a susceptibility to, or protect against, the development of specific mental illnesses. It is among the complex bio-psycho-social interactions that mental illness occurs, progresses, heals, or fails to develop at all (Cumella, 2002). Moreover, because spiritual beliefs are assumed to influence thoughts and choices and are many times formed within a social context such as the family or church, conventional sources have begun to recognize spirituality as an important characteristic of individual psychology and social/family functioning. Thus, spirituality is viewed as a crucial part of the "psycho-social" part of the model, addressing all dimensions of mental health and illness.

FIGURE 1. Bio-Psycho-Social Framework for Assessment

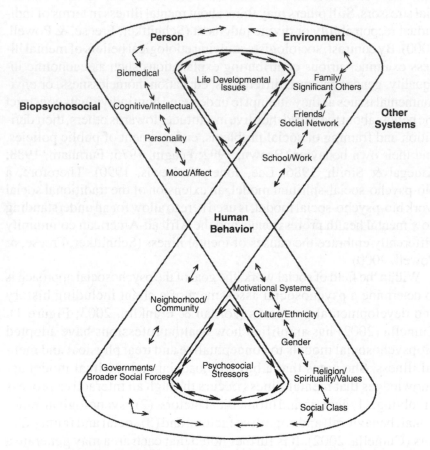

Jordan, C. & Franklin, C. (2003). *Clinical Assessment for Social Workers: Quantitative and Qualitative Methods.* (2nd ed.). Chicago: Lyceum Books, Inc. Reprinted by permission of Lyceum Books, Inc.

HELP-SEEKING BEHAVIORS AND AFRICAN-AMERICANS

Formal and Informal Services

Once persons recognize and accept the need for help with a mental illness, they may find assistance from various sources. That is, they may choose to utilize services from health and mental health care, and other formal organizations or they may choose informal sources of care. Help-seeking may be thought of as "any communication about a problem or troublesome event that is directed toward obtaining support, advice, or assistance in times of distress" (Gourash, 1978). For example, according to Poole and Salgado de Snyder (2002), "people usually first try to remedy a symptom through self-care. They attribute the symptom to a physical or psychological problem, evaluate the severity of their pain and suffering, and apply their own knowledge of healing remedies" (p. 51). Veroff et al. (1981) called this process an individual's readiness for self-referral involving three decision points: (1) defining the problem in mental health versus potential terms; (2) seeking help versus not seeking help; and (3) choosing other alternative potential sources of help.

Pathways to Help

Help seeking behaviors may also be understood as help seeking *pathways*, or the "structured patterns of interaction with social networks, informal helping systems, and formal sources of care" (Poole & Salgado de Snyder, 2002). Lewis (1980) suggests that understanding how clients seek help should take on a system perspective. He gives as an example the practice of Native Americans who have a long history of using natural helping systems. According to Lewis (1980), it is important for practitioners to remember that when a Native American needs help, he or she prefers to go first to the immediate family. If the problem is not resolved, he or she will go to members of his or her social network, next to the spiritual or religious leader, and then to the tribal council. If all else fails, only then will he or she go to a formal agency. Therefore, help seeking behavior may encompass the use of professional services as a discrete act or as a process grounded in both personal attitudes and social experiences (Snowden et al., 1982).

Social Networks

The use of social networks in help seeking assumes that "the whole process of seeking help involves a network of potential consultants, from the intimate and informal confines of the nuclear family through successively more select, distant, and authoritative laymen, until the professional is reached" (Rogler & Cortes, 1993, p. 377). Social networks usually consist of biological and extended family members, friends, and others that have an established relationship with the individual or family. When individuals are in need of help, the social network, in many cases, provide counsel, emotional support and financial assistance, share personal experiences with comparable issues, and suggest ways to stabilize and improve their situation. In many cases, individuals are also connected to help outside of the network (Poole & Salgado de Snyder, 2002).

For practitioners to understand the role of social networks, it is also important to identify individuals and services that are included in the network and the importance of their role. For some, particularly African-Americans, their social network typically includes individuals and settings that are considered informal sources of support, specifically the church and informal helpers, which include church leaders, more specifically pastors or priests.

RELIGION, RELIGIOUS PARTICIPATION, AND MENTAL HEALTH CARE

Many African-Americans use other networks including the church as a source of help for mental health issues. Therefore, it is essential to understand the role of religion and religious participation by African-Americans. Religion has been defined in terms of "the search for significance in ways related to the sacred" (Pargament, 1997, p. 32) and its association with an institutional base (Fallot, 1998). Furthermore, "religiousness . . . can refer to adherence to the beliefs and practices of an organized church or religious institution" (Shafranske & Maloney, 1990, p. 72).

In looking at the relationship between religion and African-Americans, Taylor, Chatters, and Levin (2004) underscore that

> religion and religious institutions of African-Americans have had a profound impact on individuals and broader black communities. This influence is documented in the historical experiences of blacks within American society, as well as the role of religion and black churches in the development of independent black institutions and communities. (p.13)

The authors also note that discussions regarding the form and purposes of religion and religious involvement among African-Americans must be viewed through an understanding of the historical origins of traditions as well as the social, cultural, economic, and political experiences that assisted in defining the individual and collective religious expression for this group (Taylor, Chatters, & Levin, 2004).

Previous literature has argued that theological orientations and religious practices of African-Americans originated from the distinctive social, political, and historical circumstances characterizing their position within American society (Frazier, 1974; Lincoln & Mamiya, 1990; Taylor, Chatters, & Levin, 2004). However, because black religious expression also transpired within the context of an antagonistic larger society, the aims and purposes of religious belief and expression were distinctively adapted toward addressing life circumstances that were harmful to the well-being of African-Americans (Taylor, Chatters, & Levin, 2004). Also, as pointed out by Lincoln and Mamiya (1990), the religious traditions of African-Americans have historically reflected the significant issues of emancipation, individual and community enfranchisement, civil and human rights, and social and economic justice.

Religion and Mental Health

In examining the impact of religion on serious mental illness, Koenig, Larson, and Weaver (1998) mentioned the fact that for many years, the area of religion was considered by some mental health professionals and researchers to be a strong contributor to mental illness. Therefore, positive roles that religion may have played in the treatment of mental illness were overlooked. The authors also noted the belief of incompatibility between religion and science led most researchers to ignore the relationship between religion and mental illness (Koenig, Larson, & Weaver, 1998; Larson & Milano, 1997).

Levin and Chatters (1998) noted that numerous epidemiologic and clinical studies have recognized the influence of religious affiliation and religious involvement on physical and mental health outcomes. Although it has been an ambiguous area of research, various authors also noted that over 200 published studies investigated religious differences in numerous health outcomes and examined the effects of dimensions of religiosity on health status indicators and measures of disease states (Levin & Chatters, 1998; Levin & Schiller, 1987).

Research has shown positive effects of religion on various mental health outcomes (Jang & Johnson, 2004, 2003; Johnson, Thompson, & Webb, 2002; Koenig, McCullough, & Larson, 2000; Levin, Markides, & Ray, 1996; Regnerus, 2003; Ross, 1990; Sherkat & Ellison, 1999; Williams et al., 1991). A great amount of the research ascribes the beneficial effects of religious involvement to numerous factors that religion promotes, including social integration and support, psychological resources, coping behaviors and resources, and various positive emotions and healthy beliefs (Jang & Johnson, 2004). Religion and spirituality have been seen as related to positive mental health outcomes, contributing to self-understanding and recovery experiences of many individuals with mental illness. Understanding the importance of religions with particular cultures is important to culturally competent services and to an empowerment-focus (Fallot, 1998).

Religious involvement may also have a beneficial effect due to the perceptions of support, relationship with God, as well as guidance from God during stressful times (Pargament & Brant, 1998). On the other hand, research regarding mental health and religious effects has shown that individuals who are actively involved in religion or are religiously committed are less distressed than those who are nominally religious or not religious at all (Jang & Johnson, 2004; Mirowsky & Ross, 1989; Sherkat & Ellison, 1999).

Furthermore, religion appears to exert disease prevention and health promotion influences for African-Americans (Taylor, Chatters, & Levin, 2004). Taylor, Chatters, and Levin (2004) note that religion reveals its influence in two ways: (1) a *protective factor* serving to protect subsequent mental illness and psychological distress, and (2) a *moderating factor* serving to ease the impact of harmful impact of life stress and physical challenges on subsequent mental health and well-being. Moreover, research has demonstrated that higher levels of spiritually-based coping are associated with higher levels of psychological adjustment to various stressors. Three helpful forms of religious coping include: (1) spiritual support and collaborative religious coping, (2) congregational support, and (3) benevolent religious reframing (Pargament & Brant, 1998).

Mental health researchers have found that social patterns of distress offer evidence of the social origin of individuals' psychological well-being (Aneshensel, 1992; Jang & Johnson, 2004; Mirowsky & Ross, 1986, 1989; Pearlin, 1989). The social patterns show that individuals who live in disadvantaged positions in the social structure are more likely to face distressful situations than more advantaged individuals, including factors such as racism, economic disadvantage, and inadequate residential neighborhoods (Jang & Johnson, 2004; Mirowsky & Ross, 1989; Schulz et al., 2000).

Finally, the effectiveness of the interventions provided by clergy is continuously in question. Koenig, Larson, and Weaver (1998) note that it is unlikely that the use of religious therapies alone is sufficient in managing individuals with serious mental illness; however, it is their belief that religious therapies can be used to complement traditional therapies fairly well as shown through a study completed by Propst and others (1992). In their study on medical inpatients, the authors found that cognitive symptoms on depression, including hopelessness, depressed mood, and so on, were less prevalent among individuals who maintained a heavy dependence on religious belief and activity in coping, while the more biological or somatic symptoms of depression, including weight loss, fatigue, insomnia, and so on, were not associated with religious coping (Propst et al., 1992).

As pointed out by Koenig, Larson, and Weaver (1998), these findings suggest that religious treatments are mostly beneficial for individuals with milder forms of depression, whereas severe depression requiring more specialized psychiatric treatment and antidepressant drug therapy. They also note that combination treatment addressing psychological issues and conflicts (the mind), religious concerns (the spirit), and biological causes for mental illness (the body), may hold potential for the best results, although there has been little scientific research completed on such hypotheses. Koenig, Larson, and Weaver (1998) acknowledge that religious commitment has often been an overlooked factor in mental health research, concluding "it would be in mental health professionals'—and their patients'—best interest to begin to examine this overlooked factor in improving patient coping as well as treatment and care outcomes" (ibid., p. 92).

SPIRITUALITY AND MENTAL HEALTH CARE

Just as the subject of religion and religious participation has raised concerns in the field of mental health, spirituality, along with the ability to differentiate between religion and spirituality, has done the same. Spirituality has been defined as "the sense of the sacred and divine" (Martin & Martin, 2002, p. 1). Spirituality provides Black people with the strength to continue in the face of threats to their existence, self-worth, and dignity when oppressive forces attempt to take away their humility, hope, even when there appear to be none. Feelings of joy were also confronted by hardship, frustration, and pain.

Thus, spirituality can be seen as embedded in the Black helping tradition, "the largely independent struggle of Black people to collectively promote their survival and advancement from one generation to the next" (ibid., p. 11). That is, when faced with demoralizing situations, spirituality provided Black people with encouragement, a will to live, and a determination to make their life worth living. Martin and Martin (2002) also discuss the historical expressions of Black spirituality which include singing, dancing, moaning, mourning, affirming, worshipping, contemplating, reflecting, shouting, praying, preaching, and testifying, including lifting the spirit or finding that divine spark.

Within the Black helping tradition, spirituality tends to surpass religiosity expressed through a deep concern for and commitment to the collective well-being. Specifically, spirituality in the Black helping tradition:

- promoted a sense of community and social support
- enhanced communal and racial self-development
- established social myths to counter racial mythomania (lies or distortions)
- laid the foundation for creating a Black strengths perspective
- helped Black people to develop the ability to mourn
- served as a major source of inspiration and hope (Martin & Martin, 2002, p. 5)

To Black ministers, who were viewed as chief helping professionals in early African-American history, inspiration was considered the most important tool of their work. Early black social workers also viewed inspiration as crucial to evading the growth of alienation, defeatism, bitterness, and despair among Black people (ibid.).

MENTAL HEALTH CARE
AND THE ROLE OF THE BLACK CHURCH

The role of the church in the lives of African-American families as an informal source of support has been examined for many years. As noted by Taylor and Chatters (1988), historically, religion and the Black church maintain great importance in the lives of African-Americans. This has been the case due to the high level of responsiveness of Black churches to the needs of the community, whereas access to formal social institutions has always been limited. Martin and Martin (2002) state that even when the Black church was under White control, the church primarily served three functions: (1) a social center, (2) a source of social therapy and social support, and (3) a form of social control.

Lincoln and Mamiya (1990) provide a conceptual framework for understanding features of Black churches and religious involvement, specifically, the pivotal role of the church in communities and the diverse functions and objectives it fulfills. The authors highlight particular characteristics of African-American culture, within the larger American context, that have developed into a tradition in which religious and secular concerns are only partly differentiated (Lincoln & Mamiya, 1990). The mission within Black religious traditions have been historically defined as one of transforming the social and political conditions that influence the lives of African-Americans as a whole, whether the involvement includes direct political action, civic projects, health ministries, or educational activities. The result is the inability to fully differentiate between religious pursuits from secular concerns (Taylor, Chatters, & Levin, 2003).

Evidence of this is seen through the Black church being viewed as instrumental in developing Black self-help traditions, such as mutual aid societies, and in the provision of institutional foundations for educational, civic, and commercial activities within the African-American communities (Taylor, Chatters, & Levin, 2003). The historic and ethnographic research on the type of Black religious involvement validates its multidimensional quality (Cone, 1985). Therefore, Black churches are often noted for their role in social welfare, political, and civic and community functions (Frazier, 1974; Taylor, Chatters, & Levin, 2003; Taylor, Thornton, & Chatters, 1987). Taylor, Chatters, and Levin (2003) note the evident diversity of roles within Black churches, and Black religious involvement by and large, suggesting numerous means by which spiritual, emotional, social, and political strivings of African-Americans may be attained.

Traditionally, many African-American families have depended on the Black church to provide both religious and spiritual guidance as well as emotional, financial, and social support. Empirical findings suggest that religion has a special eminence in the lives of many African-Americans, with the Black church assuming a particularly prominent role. Approximately 9 of 10 African-Americans consider the church as fulfilling multifaceted roles in African-American communities, and as having an encouraging influence on their lives (Taylor, Ellison, Chatters, Levin, & Lincoln, 2000; Taylor, Thornton, & Chatters, 1987).

The multifaceted role of the black church is reflected in the variety of community outreach programs that may provide services such as:

- assistance with basic needs (such as food and clothing distribution, home care)
- income maintenance programs (such as financial services and low-income housing)
- counseling and intervention for community members (such as family counseling, parenting/sexuality seminars, and at-risk programs for youth)
- education and awareness programs (such as child care, life skills, and academic tutoring)
- health-related activities (such as HIV/AIDS care, substance abuse counseling, recreational and fellowship activities for individuals and families) (Taylor, Chatters, & Levin, 2003).

McRae, Carey, and Anderson-Scott (1998) maintain that the church operates as a social network where individuals are able to obtain assistance in handling the problems they face in day-to-day living, discover that they are not the only ones living their particular experiences, and are able to develop a feeling of acceptance within their social milieu. The positive experience gained from the church encourages hope and faith so that one can successfully resolve problems of daily living.

Lincoln and Mamiya (1990) observe that Black churches are closely associated with Black family life and, because of the church's teachings, belief systems, and rituals, these institutions overlap in terms of the relationships they structure. Significantly, the authors note, Black churches constitute a "quasi" family environment, such as the church family, in which fellow congregants are thought of in terms of kinship and honorific titles are given to respected church elders. The concept of church family and kin symbolizes the special "family-like" quality of the relationships where rights and responsibilities of kinship are bestowed on fellow church members (Lincoln & Mamiya, 1990). This includes the development of lasting social and personal relationships and exchanges of informal social support (Chatters, Taylor, Lincoln, & Schroepfer, 2002).

Finally, and most important here, several studies have also discussed the extensive provision of support by African-American churches to address the emotional and instrumental needs of the congregants as well as improve their well-being through a variety of services (Taylor & Chatters, 1988; Caldwell et al., 1994; McRae et al., 1998). Ellison (1994) notes that religious involvement may reduce psychological distress, increasing health in four ways: (1) shaping behavioral patterns and lifestyles, (2) generating social resources, (3) enhancing psychological resources, including self-esteem and personal mastery, and (4) providing specific coping resources.

THE AFRICAN-AMERICAN PASTOR AS GATEKEEPER

Within the Black church, the African-American pastor is acknowledged as a pivotal figure whose guidance and direction are vital in order for parishioners to understand the types of programs organized in the church as well as the relationship of the church with the broader community. African-American pastors assume various roles in relation to programs and interventions that are church-based, particularly as mediators of health-related behavioral and social changes. Programs and interventions offered include, but are not limited to, health-care screenings, mentorship programs, programs for the disadvantaged including food pantries and temporary shelters, and community economic development programs.

In relation to formal mental health services, pastors often serve as "gatekeepers" and referral sources. The concept of a gatekeeper is defined by Poole and Salgado de Snyder (2002) as an individual who guides or connects people to promising sources of help. They identify gatekeepers as "family, friends, neighbors, ministers, priests, shopkeepers, beauticians, barbers, bartenders, and folk healers" who serve as links to those in need of formal helping services in the community (p. 52).

Mental health researchers have often suggested that African-American pastors be utilized as gatekeepers, collaborators, and referral sources to formal mental health services (Neighbors, 2003; Neighbors & Jackson, 1984; Neighbors, Musick, & Williams, 1998; Pickett-Schneck, 2002; Taylor et al., 2000). However, as Neighbors (2003) points out, the idea of pastors operating only as gatekeepers or referral agents must be thought through more carefully. Viewing African-American pastors only as gatekeepers or referral agents assumes that they are facing conditions they are not qualified to address (Neighbors, 2003). However, this view is not uniformly true. Neighbors (2003) acknowledges that it is not clear who is more qualified to treat issues faced by African-Americans, pastors or formal mental health systems. Because individuals with a range of religious concerns as well as mental health problems seek help from their pastors, religious leaders must be able to differentiate between problems they can solely respond to and those which warrant consultation from mental health professionals (Milstein, Midlarsky, Link, Rauc, & Bruce, 2000).

Clergy counsel individuals on a wide variety of issues, including alcoholism and other forms of substance abuse, depression, marital and family conflict, teen pregnancy, unemployment, and legal problems (Taylor, Chatters, & Levin, 2004). The authors point out that, "in fact, the type and severity of psychiatric problems that clergy encounter in counseling do not differ significantly from those seen by mental health practitioners. However, given the heterogeneity of this group, the counseling and referral practices of individual clergy diverge considerably" (ibid., pp. 7-53).

It is also noted that level of education of pastors is an important predictor of level of knowledge of mental health issues (Taylor, Chatters, & Levin, 2004). The literature has shown that pastors who have received post-graduate education receive minimal training in counseling individuals experiencing basic daily life problems (e.g., marital and family conflict) and are completely unfamiliar with the area of psychopathology and symptoms of severe mental illness (Bentz, 1970; Gottlieb & Olfson, 1987; Virkler, 1979; Taylor, Chatters, & Levin, 2004).

Additionally, the literature has discussed the possibility of pastors underestimating the severity of psychotic symptoms, compared to other mental health practitioners, and may be least likely to recognize suicide lethality (Domino & Sevain, 1985-1986; Larson, 1968). The religious and ministerial training received by pastors may lead them to interpret mental or emotional problems in religious terms or interpret clinical symptoms, such as hallucinatory behaviors as evidence of religious conflict (Taylor, Chatters, & Levin, 2004). At the same time, more pastors are currently being trained as pastoral counselors or receiving other graduate training in clinical counseling, becoming more successful in responding to the counseling needs of their congregants. In addition, "the quality of mental health services provided by pastors is determined, in part, by their ability to identify serious mental health problems and their willingness to refer people to professional mental health practitioners" (Taylor et al., 2000, p. 76).

It is apparent that there will be a difference in the type of services that pastors are able to provide based upon the type and level of training that they have received. It is obvious that parallels exist in the support that individuals and families can receive from formal support groups as well as informal support systems such as the church. Examining the potential benefit of collaboration between these two systems has been a potentially overlooked solution in increasing the participation of African-American individuals and families. Community-based partnerships acknowledge that the church occupies a high level of trust and respect within the African-American community, tapping into longstanding traditions of communal assistance and self-sufficiency to improve the health of members of the participating communities (Taylor et al., 2000).

Social workers can apply the same principle in connecting individuals and families from their informal support systems to formal support groups with the church as the link and the pastor as the gatekeeper. Neighbors et al. (1998) contend that "more than any other influence on the help-seeking behaviors of African-Americans, pastors hold the most potential for opening a wider pathway between the Black community and specialty mental health care" (p. 774).

IMPLICATIONS FOR SOCIAL WORK PRACTICE

Expanding the Role of African-American Pastors

Regardless of attempts to make mental health services more culturally relevant, most African-Americans do not seek help through professional services. When individuals are confronted by serious personal problems, they can choose from a variety of professional helpers, including psychiatrists, clinical psychologists, social workers, physicians, lawyers, marriage counselors, and vocational guidance counselors (Taylor, Chatters, & Levin, 2004). However, research has shown that individuals choose pastors as their helper and that they play a significant role in addressing a variety of personal problems and concerns (Taylor et al., 2000).

Pastors are consulted for life problems and concerns that are considered to be consistent with their traditional ministerial roles and training, including comforting the bereaved and advising individuals who are physically ill (Taylor, Chatters, & Levin, 2004). They also counsel individuals for concerns including marital and family issues and serious mental health problems (Chalfant et al., 1990; Veroff et al., 1981).

The tendency to seek assistance from pastors may be related to several factors, including treatment expense, access, and experience with and knowledge of this type of help. Insurance coverage, co-payments, or other bureaucratic actions for a consultation are not required by pastors (Taylor, Chatters, & Levin, 2004). Additionally, individuals seeking help from a pastor usually do so within the perspective of a meaningful personal relationship with him where trust has already been established. Lastly, individuals may be more apt to seek out pastors for help in dealing with personal issues because of the common philosophy shared with regard to helping others, shared worldviews about the sort of problems, and traditional and accepted ways of coping with difficult experiences in life that are expressly religious (ibid.).

Neighbors (2003) recognizes several significant points concerning the relationship between African-American pastors and African-American individuals and families. He urges that, "first, the field of mental health and mental health professionals must understand that African-American pastors are strongly rooted within African-American communities in a way that mental health professionals will never be. Second, pastors are considered as accessible as other sources of informal support, including family and friends. Third, pastors maintain a level of respect and responsibility that places them in a special category within the lives of African-Americans. Finally, pastors play a key role in meeting the needs of African-American families, including caregivers and potential consumers."

FUTURE DIRECTIONS FOR SOCIAL WORK

The issues presented including using pastors as gatekeepers or sole service providers, gaps in collaborative efforts, and effectively meeting the needs of the African-American community opens the door to the debate regarding the adequate preparation of social work students to collaborate with mutually helping social networks and the inclusion of spirituality in the social work curriculum. However, the overarching theme is the importance of understanding culture and social workers maintaining the ability to provide services that are culturally relevant to their population through identifying innovative ways to reach the community. In order to effectively meet clients' needs, culture must be acknowledged as an important variable; thus, the discussion of evaluating the preparation of social work students in working with mutually helping social networks and incorporating spirituality into the curriculum are important.

There have been suggestions made for modes of implementation of collaboration from social work literature. Chalfant et al. (1990) suggest that attempts be made to work out a bi-directional referral system between mental health professionals and clergy. In order to make this system beneficial, the authors recommend an intensive community mental health care orientation for pastors, practitioners of family medicine, psychiatrists/psychologists, and psychiatric social workers. By creating this type of system, the referral process between pastors and mental health professionals becomes a two way street. This, in turn would allow individuals in need to continue doing what they already do. They can go to different sources depending on their perception of need in order to obtain guidance from the sources most suited to their particular needs by way of a referral system between pastors and mental health professionals.

In addition, Taylor, Ellison et al. (2000) proposed that use of a liaison between service agencies and pastors would open a line of communication between formal and informal systems, providing a pathway of access to individuals and families, and present legitimacy of the relationship between the two groups. The authors suggest that service providers and formal support groups should provide in-service training programs for clergy and other church leaders, providing pastors with the ability to address referral issues. In turn, pastors could train service providers and formal support group leaders on religious beliefs and practices that may influence experiences of personal and family problems. Collaborative efforts between the groups would be useful in addressing issues of individuals and families, including serious and persistent issues of concern, such as caregiving, that call into question an individual's basic conviction about life and the meaning of their role in their family member's life (Taylor, Ellison et al., 2000).

It is noted that collaboration requires commitment and a cooperative effort on the part of service delivery systems, policy makers, and pastors in order to make a difference. In order for the collaboration to reach its potential, the church with the pastor being recognized as the key individual must put aside possible feelings of disinclination to form a partnership. This is due, in part, to the longstanding history of mistrust of the formal institutions based on previous patterns of both discrimination and prejudice by helping professionals in their dealings with African-American communities (Neighbors, 2003). Furthermore, individuals in the helping profession must reflect upon their own personal views and biases regarding religion and religious institutions, and their willingness to work in a collaborative effort with the Black church and the pastor (Taylor, Ellison et al., 2000).

CONCLUSION

With the needs of many African-American caregivers and consumers remaining unmet, acknowledging the significance and the role of the pastor is congruent with literature presented and recommendations from the President's New Freedom Commission on Mental Health (2003). Social work practitioners are in the best position to collaborate with mutually helping social networks, such as the Black church, increasing comfort and providing support to pastors, families, and consumers, and guiding to formal mental health services as needed. Inclusion of pastors in bi-directional collaborations and training for social work students would assist practitioners in teaching consumers and families ways to navigate the system, address cultural issues; therefore improving quality of care with culturally relevant services in order to reach those not readily served.

Policymakers must continuously assist in the development of comprehensive federal and state plans along with creating early screening programs. Policymakers must recognize the need for comprehensive plans in order to provide effective services that are easily navigated and utilize flexible funding streams in order to loosen restrictions on how and for whom funds are used. Development of early screening programs lead to promotion of assessments and referrals as common practice rather than as the last resort. Provision of federal funding should be used to address important issues of accessibility and accountability, remove policy barriers, encourage choice and self-determination of consumers and families along with involving them in planning, evaluating treatment processes, and support services.

Research is especially important in the development and advancement of the knowledge base of understudied areas, populations, effective treatments, and service delivery strategies. Also, evidence-based practice reflects the range of effective treatments and services.

The issues of collaboration of social workers with mutually helping social networks and inclusion of spirituality in the social work curriculum are important. In order for these issues to be placed on the table for serious consideration, there must be a buy-in from all groups including pastors, social work students, practitioners, educators, and the community. The Black church has long been a source of support for African-American families and communities faced with day-to-day struggles, with the pastor being one of the most influential and easily recognized leaders and support systems.

REFERENCES

Aneshensel, C. (1992). Social distress: Theory and research. *Annual Review of Sociology*, 18, 15-38.

Bentz, W. (1970). The clergyman's role in community mental health. *Journal of Religion and Health*, 9, 7-15.

Biegel, D., Johnsen, J., & Shafran, R. (1997). Overcoming barriers faced by African-American families with a family member with mental illness. *Family Relations*, 46, 163-178.

Brown, P. (1992). Popular epidemiology and toxic waste contamination: Lay and professional ways of knowing. *Journal of Health and Social Behavior*, 33, 267-281.

Caldwell, C., Greene, A., & Billingsley, A. (1994). Family support programs in black churches: A new look at old functions. In S. L. Kagan, & B. Weissbourd (Eds.). *Putting Families First: America's Support Movement and the Challenge of Change.* (pp.137-160). San Francisco: Jossey-Bass.

Chalfant, H., Heller, P., Roberts, A., Briones, D., Aguirre-Hochbaum, S., & Farr, W. (1990). The clergy as a resource for those encountering psychological distress. *Review of Religious Research,* 31, 305-313.

Cone, J. (1985). Black theology in American religion. *Journal of the American Academy of Religion*, 53, 755-771.

Cumella, E. (2002). Bio-psycho-social-spiritual: Completing the model. *The Remuda Review: The Christian Journal of Eating Disorders*, 1, 1-5.

Davis, K. (2001). The Intersection of Fee for Service, Managed Health Care, and Cultural Competence. In N. Veeder and W. Peebles-Wilkins (Eds.). *Managed Care Services: Policies, Programs, and Research*. (pp. 50-73). New York: Oxford University Press.

Domino, G., & Servain, B. (1985-1986). Recognition of suicide lethality and attitudes toward suicide in mental health professionals. *Omega: Journal of Death and Dying*, 16, 3010-3018.

Ellison, C. (1994). Religion, the life-stress paradigm, and the study of depression. In J. Levin (Ed.), *Religion in aging and health: Theoretical foundations and methodological frontiers* (pp. 78-121). Thousand Oaks, CA: Sage.

Fallot, R. (1998). The place for spirituality and religion in mental health. In R. Fallot (Ed.). *Spirituality and Religion in Recovery from Mental Illness, New Directions for Mental Health Services, no. 80* (pp. 3-12). San Francisco: Jossey-Bass.

Feagin, J. (1975). *Subordinating the Poor: Welfare and American Beliefs*. New Jersey: Prentice-Hall.

Frazier, E. (1974). *The Negro church in America*. New York: Schocken.

Furnham, A. (1988). *Lay Theories: Everyday Understanding of Problems in the Social Sciences*. Pergamon.

Gottlieb, J., & Olfson, M. (1987). Current referral practices of mental health care providers. *Hospital and Community Psychiatry*, 38, 1171-1181.

Gourash, N. (1978). Help seeking: A review of the literature. *American Journal of Community Psychology*, 6, 413-424.

Gurin, G., Miller, A., & Gurin, G. (1980). Stratum identification and consciousness. *Social Psychology Quarterly*, 43, 30-47.

Hall, L., & Tucker, C. (1985). Relationships between ethnicity, conceptions of mental illness, and attitudes associated with seeking psychological help. *Psychological Reports*, 57, 907-916.

Hunt, M. (1996). The individual, society, or both? A comparison of Black, Latino, and White beliefs about the causes of poverty. *Social Forces*, 75, 293-322.

Jang, S., & Johnson, B. (2004). Explaining religious effects on distress among African-Americans. *Journal of the Scientific Study of Religion*, 43, 239-260.

Johnson, B., Thompson, R., & Webb, D. (2002). *Objective hope-Assessing the effectiveness of faith-based organizations: A review of the literature*. CRRUCS report. Philadelphia: University of Pennsylvania.

Jordan, C., & Franklin, C. (2003). *Clinical Assessment for Social Workers: Quantitative and Qualitative Methods*. (2nd ed.). Chicago: Lyceum Books, Inc.

Kluegal, J., & Smith, E. (1986). *Beliefs about Inequality*. Aldine de Gruyter.

Koenig, H., Larson, D., & Weaver, A. (1998). Research on religion and serious mental illness. In R. Fallot (Ed.). *Spirituality and Religion in Recovery from Mental Illness: New Directions for Mental Health Services*. (pp. 81-95). San Francisco: Jossey-Bass.

Koenig, H., McCullough, M., & Larson, D. (2000). *Handbook of religion and health*. New York: Oxford University Press.

Larson, R. (1968). The clergyman's role in the therapeutic process: Disagreement between clergymen and psychiatrists. *Psychiatry*, 31, 250-260.

Larson, D., & Milano, M. (1997). Making the case for spiritual interventions in clinical practice. *Mind/Body Medicine*, 2, 20-30.

Lee, B., Jones, S., & Lewis, D. (1990). Public beliefs about the causes of homelessness. *Social Forces,* 69, 253-265.

Levin, J., & Chatters, L. (1998b). Research on religion and mental health: An overview of empirical findings and theoretical issues. In H. Koenig (Ed.), *Handbook on religion and mental health* (pp. 33-50). San Diego: Academic Press.

Levin, J., Markides, K., & Ray, L. (1996). Religious attendance and psychological well-being in Mexican Americans: A panel analysis of three-generations data. *Gerontologist*, 36, 454-463.

Levin, J., & Schiller, P. (1987). Is there a religious factor in health? *Journal of Religion and Health*, 26, 9-36.

Lincoln, C., & Mayima, L. (1990). *The Black church in the African-American experience*. Durham, NC: Duke University Press.

McRae, M., Carey, P., & Anderson-Scott, R. (1998). Black churches as therapeutic systems: A group process perspective. *Health Education & Behavior*, 25, 778-789.

McKee, D., & Chappel, J. (1992). Spirituality and medical practice. *Journal of Family Practice*, 35, 201, 205-208.

Macrae, C., Bodenhausen, G., Milne, A., & Jetten, J. (1994). Out of mind but back in sight: Stereotypes on the rebound. *Journal of Personality and Social Psychology*, 67, 808-817.

Martin, E., & Martin, J. (2002). *Spirituality and the Black helping tradition in social work.* Washington, DC: NASW Press.

Milstein, G., Guarnaccia, P., & Midlarsky, E. (1995). Ethnic differences in the interpretation of mental illness: Perspectives of caregivers. *Research in Community and Mental Health*, 8, 155-178.

Mirowsky, J., & Ross, C. (1986). Social patterns of distress. *Annual Review of Sociology*, 12, 23-45.

Mirowsky, J., & Ross, C. (1989). *Social causes of psychological distress*. New York: Aldine de Gruyter.

Neighbors, H. (2003, November). The African-American minister as a source of help for serious personal problems: Bridge or barrier to mental health care? Paper presented at the meeting of the Central Texas African-American Families Support Conference, Austin, TX.

Neighbors, H., & Jackson, J. (1984). The use of formal and informal help: Four patterns of illness behavior in the black community. *American Journal of Community Psychology*, 12, 629-644.

Neighbors, H., Musick, M., & Williams, D. (1998). The African-American minister as a source of help for serious personal crises: Bridge or barrier to mental health care? *Health Education & Behavior*, 25, 759-777.

New Freedom Commission on Mental Health, *Achieving the Promise: Transforming Mental Health Care in America. Final Report*. DHHS Pub. No. SMA-03-3832. Rockville, MD: 2003.

Pargament, K. (1997). *The Psychology of Religion and Coping: Theory, Research, and ractice*. New York: Guilford Press.

Pargament, K., & Brant, C. (1998). Religion and coping. In H. Koenig (Ed.), *Handbook of religion and mental health* (pp. 111-128). San Diego: Academic Press.

Pearlin, L. (1989). The sociological study of stress. *Journal of Health and Social Behavior*, 30, 241-256.

Pickett-Schneck, S. (2002). Church-based support groups for African-American families coping with mental illness: Outreach and outcomes. *Psychiatric Rehabilitation Journal*, 26, 173-180.

Poole, D., & Salgado de Snyder, V. (2002). Pathways to health and mental health care: Guidelines for culturally competent practice. In A. Roberts, & G. Gilbert (Eds.) *Social Workers' Desk Reference* (pp. 51-56.). New York: Oxford.

Propst, L., Ostrom, R., Watkins, P., Dean, T., & Mashburn, D. (1992). Comparative efficacy of religious and nonreligious cognitive-behavior therapy for the treatment of clinical depression in religious individuals. *Journal of Consulting and Clinical Psychology*, 60, 94-103.

Regnerus, M. (2003). Religion and positive adolescent outcomes: A review of research and theory. *Review of Religious Research*, 44, 394-413.

Rogler, L., & Cortes, D. (1993). Help-seeking pathways: A unifying concept in mental health care. *American Journal of Psychiatry*, 150, 554-561.

Ross, C. (1990). Religion and psychological distress. *Journal of the Scientific Study of Religion*, 29, 236-245.

Schnittker, J., Freese, J., & Powell, B. (2000). Nature, nurture, neither, nor: Black-White differences in beliefs about the causes and appropriate treatment of mental illness. *Social Forces*, 78, 1101-1130.

Schulz, A., Williams, D., Israel, B., Becker, A., Parker, C., James, S., & Jackson, J. (2000). Unfair treatment, neighborhood effects, and mental health in the Detroit metropolitan area. *Journal of Health and Social Behavior*, 41, 314-332.

Shafranske, E., & Malony, H. (1990). Clinical psychologists' religious and spiritual orientations and their practice of psychotherapy. *Psychotherapy*, 27, 72-78.

Sherkat, D., & Ellison, C. (1999). Recent developments and current controversies in the sociology of religion. *Annual Review of Sociology*, 25, 363-394.

Snowden, L. (1999). African-American service use for mental health problems. *Journal of Community Psychology*, 27, 303-313.

Snowden, L., & Cheung, F. (1990). Use of inpatient mental health services by members of ethnic minority groups. *American Psychologist*, 45, 347-355.

Snowden, L., Collinge, W., & Runkle, M. (1982). Help seeking and underservice. In L. R. Snowden (Ed.). *Reaching the Underserved: Mental Health Needs of Neglected Populations* (pp. 281-298). Beverly Hills: Sage.

Taylor, R., & Chatters, L. (1988). Church members as a source of informal social support. *Review of Religious Research*, 30, 193-203.

Taylor, R., & Chatters, L. (1991). Religious life. In J. Jackson (Ed.), *Life in Black America* (pp. 105-123). Thousand Oaks, CA: Sage.

Taylor, R., & Chatters, L. (2003). National survey of black Americans. In R. Taylor, & Chatters, L. (Eds.). *Religion in the lives of African-Americans*. Thousand Oaks, CA: Sage.

Taylor, R., Chatters, L., Jayakody, R., & Levin, J. (1996). Black and White differences in religious participation: A multisample comparison. *Journal for the Scientific Study of Religion*, 35, 403-410.

Taylor, R., Chatters, L., & Levin, J. (2004). Religion in the lives of African-Americans: Social, Psychological, and Health Perspectives. Thousand Oaks, CA: Sage.

Taylor, R., Ellison, C., Chatters, L., Levin, J., & Lincoln, K. (2000). Mental health services in faith communities: The role of clergy in black churches. *Social Work*, 45,
73-87.

Veroff, J., Douvan, E., & Kulka, R. (1981). *The inner American: A self portrait from
1957 to 1976*. New York: Basic Books.

Virkler, H. (1979). Counseling demands, procedures, and preparation of parish ministers: A descriptive study. *Journal of Psychology & Theology*, 7, 271-280.

Williams, D., Larson, D., Buckler, R., Heckmann, R., & Pyle, C. (1991). Religion and
psychological distress in a community sample. *Social Science and Medicine*, 11,
1257-1262.

doi:10.1300/J137v14n01_08

Chapter 9

Self-Care Practices and Hispanic Women with Diabetes

Olivia Lopez

SUMMARY. Diabetes is a major public health problem in the United States, and a dangerous disease that can lead to serious long term complications. Left uncontrolled, diabetes can lead to blindness, heart failure, kidney failure, and low extremity amputations. This challenge is further magnified by the fact that Hispanics already constitute the largest minority group in the U.S., which suggests the potential of diabetes to reach epidemic proportions. This chapter explores the role of culture and self-care practices among Hispanic women with diabetes. doi:10.1300/J137v14n01_09 *[Article copies available for a fee from The Haworth Document Delivery Service: 1-800-HAWORTH. E-mail address: <docdelivery@haworthpress.com> Website: <http://www.HaworthPress.com> © 2006 by The Haworth Press, Inc. All rights reserved.]*

KEYWORDS. Hispanic women, diabetes, self-care

[Haworth co-indexing entry note]: "Self-Care Practices and Hispanic Women with Diabetes." Lopez, Olivia. Co-published simultaneously in *Journal of Human Behavior in the Social Environment* (The Haworth Press, Inc.) Vol. 14, No. 1/2, 2006, pp. 183-200; and: *Contemporary Issues of Care* (ed: Roberta R. Greene) The Haworth Press, Inc., 2006, pp. 183-200. Single or multiple copies of this article are available for a fee from The Haworth Document Delivery Service [1-800-HAWORTH, 9:00 a.m. - 5:00 p.m. (EST). E-mail address: docdelivery@haworthpress.com].

doi:10.1300/J137v14n01_09 *183*

INTRODUCTION

Diabetes is a major public health problem in the United States, and a dangerous disease that can lead to serious long term complications. Left uncontrolled, diabetes can lead to blindness, heart failure, kidney failure, and low extremity amputations (Hunt, Arar & Larame, 1998). Diabetes is associated with severe morbidity and premature death and affects U.S. Hispanics disproportionately (Center for Disease Control, 2003). Mexican Americans suffer from increased prevalence, a greater number of risk factors, and more severe complications.

This challenge is further magnified by the fact that Hispanics already constitute the largest minority group in the U.S., which suggests the potential of diabetes to reach epidemic proportions. By the year 2050, Hispanics will number 97 million and constitute almost 25 percent of the U.S. population (Census Data, 2000).

The Mexican American elderly represent a large and ethnically-diverse part of the Mexican American population. It is estimated that by the year 2050 Mexican American elders will likely represent 16% of adults age 65 or older (Coon, Rubert, Solano, Mausback, Kraemer, Arguelles, Haley, Thompson & Gallagher-Thompson, 2004). With this estimated population growth among Mexican Americans elders it is also likely that we will see a marked increase in the number of families taking on the caregiving role. For example, Neary and Mahoney (2005) report that one-third of middle-aged U.S. Latinos care for elders, and Phillips, Torrez de Ardon, Komminenich et al. (2000) report that most caregivers are women.

BIOLOGICAL ASPECTS OF DIABETES

Older Mexican Americans are among the highest-risk groups for diabetes and its complications. These complications include retinopathy (a diabetic eye disease that is the leading cause of blindness in the United States), nephropathy (kidney disease), and peripheral vascular disease (nerve damage affecting the legs and feet) (Wu, Haan, Dang, Ghosh, Gonzalez & Herman, 2003). Such diabetes complications have an impact on functional limitations and disability, particularly visual impairment, which is the leading cause of functional disability and diminished quality of life (DiNuzzo, Black, Lichtenstein & Markides, 2001).

Spanish-speaking Hispanics older than 60 years report greater limitations for activities of daily living (ADLs) and instrumental activities of daily living (IADLs). Commonly used to assess the disability in basic life activities among the population that is greater than 65 years of age, ADLs measure the activities for personal care, such as walking across the room, bathing, grooming, dressing, eating, transfer from bed to chair and toileting, and IADLs measure the person's ability to use the telephone, driving a car, shopping, preparation of own meals, housework (light/ heavy), taking medication, management of finances, and walking up and down stairs (Wu et al., 2003; DiNuzzo et al., 2001). Limitations with both ADLs and IADLs increase with age and are associated with higher levels of disability. For example, Hispanic elderly who are 85 and older are at ten times the risk of becoming blind compared to those aged 65 to 70 (DiNuzzo et al., 2001).

PSYCHOLOGICAL RESPONSE TO DIABETES

Older Hispanic diabetics suffer increased rates of cognitive impairment than other non-Hispanic populations (Reyes-Ortiz, Kuo, Di-Nuzzo, Ray, Raji & Markides, 2005; Wu et al., 2003), and older Hispanics with near vision impairment have been found to have low cognitive functioning. Cognitive impairment increases rapidly with age and low education levels (Wu et al., 2003). Often, cognitive impairment can lead to dementia in the elderly population, especially the elderly Hispanic population.

Near vision tasks are similar to adult daily living skills and include crafts, recreation activities, eating, personal care and hygiene, work tasks and reading. Reyes-Ortiz et al. (2005) have suggested that near vision affects cognitive functioning by decreasing the level of participation in stimulating activities that can lead to reduced brain stimulation. Higher levels of cognitive decline have been associated with the incidence of diabetic complications, which, as has been mentioned earlier, is common among elderly Hispanics. These complications include hypertension, stroke, heart attack, kidney disease, diabetic retinopathy (diabetic eye disease) and amputation (Wu et al., 2003). This, in turn, may lead to higher dementia among elderly Hispanics and affect the caregiving experience. For example, cognitive incapacity among elderly Hispanics has been perceived by spouses as burdensome, whereas children providing care have perceived cognitive incapacity as less burdensome (Phillips, Tores de Ardon, Komnenich, Killeen & Rusinak, 2000).

SOCIOCULTURAL ASPECTS OF DIABETES

Cultural Beliefs and Illness

Cultural norms, values, and beliefs help create shared collective knowledge about disease within a group (Christman & Kleinman, 1983). Beliefs about diabetes are related to how individuals respond to disease and can provide explanations about illness perceptions. Mercado-Martinez and Ramos-Herrera (2002) conducted a qualitative study in Guadalajara, Mexico to examine laypersons' perceptions of diabetes causality. Results indicate that participants described diabetes in a variety of ways. The most common cause of diabetes cited was the combination of economic, social, and relational factors that produce fright. A fright was described as an accident, fear of amputation, and death. Results also indicate gender differences in beliefs of diabetes causality. Women emphasized psychosocial factors and domestic problems as the origin of diabetes, whereas men emphasized employment and rage as the origin of diabetes.

The meaning of diabetes is highlighted in another study conducted by Luyas (1991). This study reported a two-pronged meaning for (a) diabetes, and (b) sugar diabetes. Diabetes referred to amputations, loss of eyesight, and dialysis. Sugar diabetes referred to how sugar accumulated in the blood and was described as eating too much sugar during childhood. Participants did not have a clear understanding of how foods are processed in the body and did not understand that starches such as tortillas, bread, and potatoes convert to glucose in the blood. Many participants attempted to "dilute" their blood sugar by drinking sour juices or adding extra salt to counteract the sweet. Finally, eating "diet food" such as fruits and vegetables was identified as a treatment strategy for controlling high blood sugar levels. By and large, participants included family problems as part of the etiology of diabetes.

Building on this causal theme, Hunt, Valenzuela and Pugh (1998) conducted a qualitative study in South Texas with Mexican-Americans with type II diabetes. This study focused on causal stories and treatment behaviors. Open-ended interviews were conducted with 49 participants and addressed concepts of experiences managing diabetes and self-care behaviors. Results indicate that the primary cause of diabetes was attributed to heredity and diet by 93% of participants followed by 43% of participants who attributed lifestyle as a cause and 33% who attributed emotional trauma as a cause and finally 20% attributed physical disorder/trauma as a cause of diabetes. In addition, 45% of participants cited events as causes of diabetes. Causes of diabetes were grouped into two categories: (a) behaviors, and (b) events. Behaviors refer to things the patient has done or failed to do. Events refer to things that happened to the participant. Results also indicate that participants who reported behaviors (diet, lifestyle) as having caused diabetes were more likely to be involved in their diabetes treatment than those reporting events as having caused diabetes. However, participants who were active in their diabetes treatment were no more likely to have good glucose control than those that did not participate in their treatment. Finally, results indicate that the core of participant's causal understanding of diabetes is based in personally relevant events and behaviors rather than emphasizing biomedical-based constructs.

In a similar vein, a qualitative study conducted by Weller, Baer, Pachter, Trotter, Glazer, de Alba Garcia, and Klein (1999) explored beliefs about diabetes and assesses the heterogeneity in beliefs across groups among Latinos in four communities: Hartford, Connecticut; Edinburg, Texas; Guadalajara, Mexico; and rural Guatemala. Participants in this study were primarily women with different levels of acculturation, education, and location of residence (urban/rural). A structured questionnaire was given to 130 participants and focused on the causes, symptoms, and treatment of diabetes. Results indicate that all sites shared a core description of causality. Participants believed diabetes was caused by heredity, genetics, lack of insulin, uncontrolled sugar levels, eating too much sugar, and poor diet. The Mexican and Guatemalan sample identified *Susto* as the cause of diabetes. However, diabetic symptoms were found to be generally in agreement with biomedical diabetic symptom definitions. Participants in this study believed diabetes was best treated by a physician and that oral medication was helpful in processing blood sugar. Results of this study found no differences in beliefs by age or gender. Results also indicate that beliefs about diabetes were consistent with biomedical beliefs. Finally, beliefs about diabetes did not differ by having diabetes, knowing someone with diabetes, or having a family member with diabetes.

Not only are personal beliefs about diabetes causality a factor in participation in diabetes treatment, home remedies have also been reported to influence diabetes treatment. Home remedies for type II diabetes was the focus of a qualitative study conducted by Poss, Jezewski and Stuart (2003) in El Paso, Texas. In this study, 22 Mexican-American participants were interviewed using an open-ended format to elicit participants' beliefs about the appropriate treatment for diabetes. Results indicate participants in this study combine traditional herbal remedies with western medicine. The most common remedies purchased in Mexico are Diabetil Tea, Diabe Cure, and Te Malabar (Malabar tea). The most common home remedies used by participants were *nopal* (cactus), and *sabila* (aloe vera). Results also indicate that most participants had an elementary understanding of how diabetic medication worked on the body, and some had advanced understanding about how diabetic medication assists the pancreas to produce more insulin. However, most participants did not inform their physicians that they were taking herbal home remedies because they feared being scolded.

Similar to Poss et al. (2003) Hunt, Arar and Akana (2000) conducted a qualitative study of low income Mexican-Americans focusing on the use alternative treatment for diabetes and prayer. Forty-three participants from San Antonio and Laredo, Texas, were interviewed using an interview guide of standardized questions. Results indicated that 84% of participants reported they had heard of using herbs as a possible treatment for diabetes; however, most participants reported minimal use of herbs. The most common herbs cited by participants were *nopal* (cactus), *sabila* (aloe vera), and *nispero* (loquat or Chinese plumb). Only 9% of participants reported current use of herbs, and a majority of participants were skeptical about the value of using herbs for treatment of diabetes. Results also indicate religion as a factor in treating diabetes. Seventy-seven percent of participants reported they thought prayer helped their diabetes by reducing stress. Participants viewed medical treatment as a mechanism through which God could heal them of diabetes. Participants in this study did not report competition between alternative and conventional treatment. Finally, results indicate that participants may give priority to biomedical treatment strategies over alternative strategies.

The results from these various studies highlight the influential nature cultural factors play in health care decisions. Moreover, these results suggest that integration of cultural beliefs and practices into standard medical practices can assist Mexican-Americans to achieve and maintain safe blood glucose levels.

A CONTRAST:
BELIEFS AMONG NON-HISPANIC WHITES
AND OTHER POPULATIONS

A review of the literature yielded three studies among non-Hispanic whites that focused on perceptions of type II diabetes. One study focused on Taiwanese perceptions about illness and treatment. Another study focused on disease models among Latinos and European Americans. The last study assessed perceptions on Black Americans and white Americans with type II diabetes. This section will provide a detailed review of each study.

A qualitative study conducted by Lai, Lew-Ting and Chiet (2004) focused on perceptions about illness and treatment strategies among Taiwanese participants with type II diabetes. Authors interviewed 22 participants (10 women/12 men) using an in-depth interview format. The themes emerging from this study include (a) dietary management, (b) exercise practice, and (c) pharmaceutical treatment.

Participants in this study agreed diet and exercise were important factors in controlling type II diabetes; however, diet modifications were limited to a reduction of sweets and carbohydrates, and did not include fruits and vegetables. Exercise was considered helpful in managing diabetes, although participants more strongly believed that vigorous exercise consumed blood glucose and eliminated pharmaceutical toxins through sweat. It is important to note that in Chinese culture the notion of exercise has to do with "survive and move," which means if you want to survive you have to keep moving. Participants also believed that an increase in water consumption would dilute blood glucose, which would be eliminated from the body through urine. Participants in this study were ambivalent about medication. Participants held a positive attitude towards medication, while others were more concerned with side effects, such as kidney damage. For example, participants reported not taking their medications on days when they did not consume sweets. Results from this study indicate that participants integrate both biomedical practices and cultural beliefs into their perceptions of type II diabetes, although it is important to note that participants were more in favor of cultural practices.

While Lai, Lew-Ting and Chiet (2004) focused on illness perception and treatment strategy among participants in Taiwan, Chelsa, Skaff, Baratz, Mullan and Fisher (2000) focused on the differences in personal disease models among Latinos and European Americans (EA). Disease models were defined as participants' working knowledge about diabetes, based on contact with providers, diabetes educators, and disease management experience. In this qualitative study, 76 Latinos and 116 EA were interviewed using open-ended interviews. Participant responses were examined separately and comparisons across ethnic groups were made. Participants were asked questions about perceived cause of diabetes, nature, seriousness course, future course of diabetes and impact on daily life. Results indicate that both Latino and European Americans recognized heredity, weight loss, diet, and stress as causes of diabetes. Results also indicate a three-pronged categorization of disease models: (a) experiential, (b) biomedical, and (c) psychosocial.

An *experiential* disease model refers to descriptions of diabetes in terms of symptoms, such as tender feet, fatigue, or increased irritability; however, the prominent description for diabetes is that one had too much sugar. A *biological* disease model refers to both elementary and sophisticated descriptions of diabetes as having high blood sugar, a pancreatic malfunction, insufficient insulin, or insulin resistance. A *psychosocial* disease model includes biological, psychosocial, and social descriptions of diabetes. For example, participants described how job stress or interactions with family and friends might affect the disease process.

In addition, results also indicate variations of disease descriptions by ethnicity. Latinos used an experiential model to describe type II diabetes, while European Americans used a biomedical model. Significant differences in life changes were noted. Latinos reported changes in fatigue and mood, whereas European Americans reported changes in exercise and spontaneity. In terms of cause, seriousness and treatment efficacy both groups gave similar assessments for these categories. Both Latino and European Americans had future concerns about physical decline; however, Latinos were more concerned with financial worries and concerns that their children would inherit the disease. The effect of diabetes on the daily lives of Latinos and explanatory models differed. Latinos reported troubling symptoms of diabetes, while European Americans reported changes in self-care activities. Concluding, the authors note that Latinos and European Americans do not differ in their assessment of causality, seriousness, or treatment efficacy, rather they differ in how they understand the disease process and experience its impact on their daily lives. The authors suggest that taking a broad look at personal models of diabetic patients is critical for the design of research and interventions for diverse populations.

Continuing with differing perceptions of diabetes, Ford, Havstad, Brooks and Tilley (2002) examined the perceptions of diabetes among African-Americans and white Americans in an urban health care system in the Midwest using a quantitative research methodology. Forty-five participants with type II diabetes were randomly stratified by race and socioeconomic status (SES). Perceptions were measured using scales from an illness meaning questionnaire assessing impact, loss, and stress associated with type II diabetes. Salient themes include: (a) perceptions of diabetes, and (b) involves assessing measurement instruments within racial subgroups. No differences in SES were found between Black Americans and white Americans. A majority of Black Americans perceived diabetes as disfiguring, which was defined as amputations, loss of vision, loss of sexuality and loss of youth. Black Americans cited familial experience as evidence. In contrast, white Americans affirmed that diabetes was not disfiguring. Reliability coefficients in the combined groups, measured by Cronbach's alpha, were well above 0.68 for the Impact, Loss, Stress and Perceptions of Physician Efficacy scales. However, the Loss scale did not fit the white American subgroup, and the Stress and Perceptions of Physician Efficacy scales did not fit the African American subgroup. The authors conclude that perceptions of diabetes may vary by race, even when controlling for SES. Moreover, the authors state that overall measures of reliability may mask the instability of scales within specific study groups. In sum, the literature suggests that variation in understanding the diabetes disease process may exist among different cultural groups.

EXPLANATORY MODELS WITHIN A CULTURAL CONTEXT

Explanatory models are ideas and beliefs about an illness that help persons to understand and make sense of an illness within a cultural context (Poss, Jezewski & Stuart, 2003). They are tied to a specific cultural system of knowledge, norms, and values. Explanatory models are constructed through interaction with the sociocultural environment, although much of their content is based on a common sense understanding of body functions (McSweeney, Amey & Coward, 1998). The primary characteristic of explanatory models is that they stress understanding an illness experience from the subjective culturally-based view of the client (McSweeney, 1990). Explanatory models may contain explanations for (a) etiology, (b) onset of symptoms, (c) pathophysiology, (d) course of sickness (severity and type of sick role), and (e) treatment (Kleinman, 1978). Explanatory models are held by both patients and health practitioners, with each group having its own version. Moreover, explanatory models of patients and health practitioners are in conflict (Kleinman, 1978). For example, patients view illness as a psychosocial experience and focus on the meaning of the perceived illness. Glucose control is based on feeling better and factors such as medical insurance, socioeconomic status, and the effect on the family. On the other hand, health practitioners view disease as a malfunctioning of the biological process. Glucose control is based on blood glucose levels as less than 140 mg/dL, medication, diet, exercise, and regular appointments with a primary care physician, nutritionist, and endocrinologist (Hunt, Arar & Larme, 1998).

Kleinman (1980) makes clear distinctions between the concepts of *disease* and *illness*. *Disease* refers to the process of interpretation that occurs when patients visit health practitioners of one kind or another. *Disease* is conceptualized as the practitioner's construction of the patient's illness using the terminology and conceptual framework of the western medical health system (Poss, & Jezewski, 2002). According to Kleinman (1978, 1980, 1986), practitioners reconstruct the patient's meaningful experience of illness according to how their particular profession's theoretical orientations classifies the symptoms and illness experience.

On the other hand, *illness* is first conceptualized in lay society, where the sick person and family draw from paradigms of everyday practical knowledge and culturally approved management strategies that have been transmitted through personal and familial experience and membership in a cultural system. *Illness* signifies the experience of disease (or perceived disease) and the societal reaction to the disease. *Illness* is a way the sick person, his/her family, and social network perceive, label, explain, valuate, and respond to illness. Kleinman maintains that patients seek not only symptom relief, but also personally and socially meaningful explanations and psychosocial treatments for illness. Kleinman (1980) points out that patients often do not volunteer their explanatory models to health care professionals and may be hesitant to divulge them due to lack of trust or fear of being devalued and shamed. For this reason explanatory models are better elicited by conducting research in the participant's home or in places of comfort.

Illness Meaning

Kleinman (1986) outlines seven types of illness meanings derived from the patient and local culture: (1) overt meanings of symptoms such as pain, deformity, disfigurement, and disability; (2) illness as suffering, involving religious or moral idioms of distress in the patient's culture; (3) meanings involving culturally marked salience of particular symptoms in particular societies; (4) meanings of illness embodied and absorbed through personal and social significance, taking into consideration the psychological and social distresses that are likely to amplify symptoms; (5) meanings related to the practitioner's construction of illness within the framework of biomedicine focusing on social use and functions of illness for a particular person in a particular situation at a particular time; (6) meaning through the creation of retrospective narratives that function to relate illness to life history of illness and to make sense of sickness; and (7) meaning derived from the selective illness accounts audited by clinicians and researchers according to their particular interests.

STUDIES USING EXPLANATORY MODELS

Thus far, this literature review has analyzed research studies that focused on beliefs about diabetes, causality and its relationship to treatment behaviors and traditional and home remedies as treatment for diabetes, as well as perceptions of diabetes among non-Hispanics and other populations. Explanatory models are holistic and bring together beliefs about illness, treatment, and causality. Explanatory models are ideas and beliefs about an illness that help persons to understand and make sense of an illness within a cultural context (Poss, Jezewski & Stuart, 2003). The following review will analyze studies based on explanatory models of illness and type II diabetes. Virtually all studies using explanatory models have been on Mexican Americans or Latino populations.

Jezweski and Poss (2002) conducted a qualitative study with the purpose of developing a culturally specific explanatory model of diabetes among Mexican Americans living along the U.S.-Mexico border. Twenty-two participants (18 women/4 men) from El Paso, Texas were interviewed using an open-ended interview format. Results indicate that Mexican American's perceptions of diabetes using four constructs: (a) cause, (b) symptoms, (c) treatment, and (d) social significance. A majority of participants described *susto* as the cause of diabetes and believed *susto was* unavoidable. Participants identified and interpreted their symptoms within the western biomedical view of type II diabetes; although participants were unsure about the symptoms of hyperglycemia and hypoglycemia. Participants integrated both biomedical and traditional treatments into their explanatory model of type II diabetes based on diabetes education classes. Diet regulation was believed to be important in diabetes treatment, yet participants reported substantial confusion regarding diet. Many participants believed that eating any amount of fat was acceptable as long as it was not lard. Others believed they could eat candy and limit carbohydrates. Participants also believed they could eat everything as long as it was in small portions. The home remedy most commonly used to treat type II diabetes was *nopal* (cactus), and it was prepared as a tea and a meal. Most participants discussed diabetes with their families and reported family members offering support and reminders about taking care of themselves, although several participants reported feeling ashamed of having diabetes and as a result did not confide in family members or seek advice or social support.

Building on characterizing explanatory models among Mexican Americans, Coronado, Thompson, Tejeda and Godina (2004) conducted a qualitative study in a rural agricultural area of Washington state. Forty-two men and women participated in focus groups and data from these groups was used to characterize perceptions about beliefs, causes, and treatment strategies among Mexican Americans. Participants defined diabetes as a serious, life-threatening illness that "kills you little by little." Others compared diabetes to HIV or cancer. Symptoms were in accordance with medically recognized symptoms of diabetes. Participants identified genetic and environmental risk factors as causes of diabetes, which are also in accordance with medically recognized causes. Others viewed *susto* (fright) as the cause of diabetes. Participants commonly cited diet, exercise, and oral medication as treatment for diabetes. Others cited the combination of traditional treatment and western medical strategies as effective treatment. Traditional remedies commonly used were *nopal* (cactus), sabila (aloe vera), *espina de pochete* (silk cotton tree), *chaya* (tree spinach), *arnica* (arnica), and *agua de violeta* (violet water). Findings from this study support the notion that the biomedical system and folk beliefs influence beliefs about diabetes, and the authors suggest that intervention programs should acknowledge and reinforce aspects of both biomedical and folk beliefs to improve adherence to health recommendations.

Guided by Kleinman's model, Luyas (1991) studied low income, Mexican American women's explanatory model of type II diabetes, and examined how the explanatory model of these women compares with the bio-medical model. The author examined labels and meaning of diabetes, ways of knowing one is sick, attributions to the cause of diabetes, and ways of treating diabetes. Participants reported a two-pronged meaning for (a) diabetes, and (b) sugar diabetes. Diabetes referred to amputations, loss of eyesight, and dialysis. Sugar diabetes referred to how sugar accumulated in the blood and was described as eating too much sugar during childhood. Symptoms were the primary method of knowing one was sick. The cause of diabetes was attributed to the cumulative effects of problems and life circumstances experienced since childhood. Finally, eating "diet food" such as fruits and vegetables were identified as a treatment strategy for controlling high blood sugar levels. However, participants stated they often could not afford such foods and instead used fillers such as rice to bulk rationed beef and pork. By and large, participants included family problems as part of the etiology of diabetes. The author argues for the integration of this domain in treatment planning.

Advancing the concept of explanatory models, Alcozer (2000) conducted a secondary data analysis based on her original study on the perceptions and meanings of type II diabetes among Mexican American women. In the original study twenty women were interviewed using an open-ended interview format. Unlike several studies in this review, participants in this study were high school and college graduates, had higher acculturation levels, and average annual earnings of $16,000 to $30,000. Perceptions and meanings of type II diabetes were categorized as defining, getting, having, describing, or taking care of diabetes. Results indicated a two-pronged definition of diabetes: (a) borderline or glucose intolerant, and (b) diabetes. Participants reported that borderline or glucose intolerant meant having sugar in their urine and this was not considered to be negative. Participants reported that diabetes meant less sugar in the blood, dialysis, and insulin. Participants were fearful of diabetes due to complications that happen. In discussing etiology of diabetes participants also reported a two-pronged definition in getting diabetes: (a) heredity was considered as a major cause of diabetes given family history, and (b) eating too many sweets was thought to stress the body's glucose storing system. Participants reported a two-pronged definition of having diabetes: (a) it was described as having high sugar, and (b) as a confusing and silent illness. Participants described a diabetic state as having periods of high glucose. Participants reported that glucose is excreted in the urine as a way for the body to maintain a normal glucose levels. Diabetes was considered a confusing and silent illness because participants did not feel ill. How participants describe diabetes was less clear as they linked the definitions of borderline and diabetes to the symptoms of illness. Participants mentioned insulin as complications of diabetes, such as blindness, amputations, and kidney failure. Participants reported very little variation between treatment of diabetes and their definitions of borderline and diabetes. They reported diabetes was to be treated with oral medication or insulin. Participants described the meaning of diabetes as a life threat, complications and a shortened life. As is the case in many of the studies analyzed in this review, the biomedical model of diabetes was incongruent to participants' explanatory models, which the author states explains the prevalent confusion regarding care and information received from health care providers.

FAMILY CAREGIVING DYNAMICS AND DIABETES

Although Mexican Americans constitute the fastest growing segment of the elderly population, little is known about their approach to caregiving for their elderly (Joilcoeur & Madden, 2002). The elderly are respected among Mexican American culture and families, and it is largely considered the responsibility of children, primarily daughters, to provide care (Mintzer, Rubert & Herman, 1994; Joilcouer & Madden, 2002). There are, however, natural support systems within the Mexican American communities that can be helpful during the caretaking experience. Natural support systems include family, friendship groups, and local informal caregivers (Delgado & Humm-Delgado, 1982). The extended family, folk healers, religious institutions, and community clubs have been cited as important components in the natural support systems of Mexican Americans (Delgado & Humm-Delgado, 1982; Joilcouer & Madden, 2002).

Within the Mexican American culture, family is considered the primary social support during a crisis. The definition of extended family includes blood relatives and adopted relatives. Adopted relatives are known as "compadres" who are close friends that have proven themselves trustworthy and committed to participation in important family matters (Delgado & Humm-Delgado, 1982). Folk healers are considered consultants within this culture. Often folk healers are trusted community members and considered wise in their advice and decisions regarding illness and treatment. Religion is also a key support among many Mexican Americans. The belief that God can cure illness and prayer can give strength and alleviate symptoms is a common theme among this group. Community clubs are considered places that fulfill a culture-specific role within the community. For example, a Mexican bakery and botanical shop provide culturally related items needed by families and community members as well as serving as a meeting place for community members. Extended family, healers, religion, and community understand the culture and can provide emotional support, advocacy, financial assistance, day care, and respite.

Caregivers

Mexican American caregivers are primarily daughters, although spouses and members of the immediate family also provide care (Mintzer, Rubert & Herman, 1994). Mexican American caregivers have unique cultural norms and patterns related to care giving (Talamentes, Lawler & Espino, 1995). That is, caregiving is filtered through the belief systems, perceptions, and cultural practices, specific cultural groups (Mintzer, Rubert & Herman, 1994). Cultural beliefs and practices can influence how the caregivers feel about caregiving responsibilities, understanding dementia, and how the person receiving care feels about the care she/he is receiving (Neary & Mahoney, 2005). These personal beliefs are used by caregivers to recognize, interpret, and respond to a particular illness. The organization of such beliefs comprises an explanatory model of illness and serves to mediate the caregiving role and their interaction with the person for whom they are caring.

PROFESSIONALS AND EXPLANATORY MODELS

Explanatory models are characterized by vagueness, multiple meanings, frequent changes, and lack of sharp boundaries. They are unconsciously formed, tend to change over time, and are influenced by environment, ethnicity, individual interpretation, familial illness experience, exposure to western medical practices, and tacit knowledge (Luyas, 1991; McSweeney, 1990). Explanatory models of individuals may very well differ from those of the family or social and community networks. As such, the ongoing experience with a specific illness, particularly a chronic illness, new knowledge, or a significant health event may modify them (McSweeney, Alan & Mayo, 1997). The capacity to take on additional illness meanings indicate that health care professionals of all types can influence explanatory models by teaching meaningful health information to patients, family members, and peer groups.

The holistic nature and diversity of explanatory models acknowledge physiological, affective, cognitive, and the phenomenological process of the individual's illness experience (Tijerina, 2000). Perhaps more important is the model's emphasis on ethno-cultural context as the foundation of the illness experience (McSweeney, Allan & Mayo, 1997). Establishing the explanatory models of diabetes among Mexican American women is a useful framework for practitioners to collect and analyze data that can ultimately provide theoretical models for understanding the meaning of type II diabetes among Mexican American women.

Most importantly, such theoretical models can be used to negotiate meaningful and culturally appropriate treatment strategies. The holistic nature of this framework will provide a deeper, richer understanding of the perceptions and meanings of caregiving among Mexican American women and diabetes. This information can help explain how Mexican

American caregiver women construct explanatory models of illness and helps practitioners gain an understanding of the intersection between their explanatory models of illness and standard medical practices. Moreover, understanding the structures and function of explanatory models contributes to the theoretical construction under which practitioners and bio-medicine are guided. The merging of differing disciplines, such as the social work profession and medical profession, provides an opportunity for the revision or shifting of the paradigm of the current theoretical medical models guiding health delivery by systematically analyzing the relevant effects of sociocultural determinants on sickness and care (Kleinman, 1980).

For many decades, it has been widely recognized by agencies providing services to farmworkers that this population requires special attention from the health community (Luna, 2003; Villarejo, 2003), social services, and the social work profession. Their needs require a holistic approach. A holistic approach can be defined as the incorporation of cultural beliefs, values and experiences, and the inclusion of family, extended family and community networks that are involved in the health care decision making process. For example, Holland and Courtney (1998) report that many Mexican Americans do not think of their cultural health beliefs and practices as "folk" medicine. These authors suggest that rather than asking patients if they use folk medicine, practitioners can ask how *susto* or *mal de ojo* (evil eye) is treated, questions demonstrating cultural understanding and creating a positive partnership between patients and practitioners. Similarly, client goals and needs should suggest appropriate interventions that incorporate such systems (Hepworth, Rooney & Larsen, 1997).

The incorporation of a holistic system of care is consistent with social work values in which treatment begins "where the patient is" and the development of meaningful treatment strategies is based on client needs. Social workers have the potential to improve the quality of the lives of farmworking women with type II diabetes through well-established roles as educators, advocate, counselor, therapist, community developer, and resource broker (DeCoster, 2001).

In sum, cultural beliefs about diabetes likely play a major role in determining how farmworking women feel about illness and health (Anderson, Wiggins, Rajwani, Holbrook, Blue and Ng, 1995) and influence how these women understand illness, symptoms, and causes. Thus, the failure to recognize ethno-specific illnesses on the part of health and social service professionals can result in farmworkers failing to recognize early symptoms of diabetes or from effectively using current conventional forms of intervention.

REFERENCES

Anderson, J.M., Wiggins, R., Rajwani, A., Holbrook, C., Blue, C. & Ng, M. (1995). Living with a chronic illness: Chinese-Canadian and Euro-Canadian women with Diabetes–exploring factors that influence management. *Social Science Medicine*, 41 (2), 181-195.

Centers for Disease Control. Retrieved February 2, 2003, from http://www.cdc.gov

Delgado, M. & Delgado, D. (1982, January). Natural support systems as sources of strength in Hispanic communities. *Social Work*, 83-89.

DiNuzzo, A.R., Black, S.A., Lichtenstein, M. J. & Markides, K.S. (2001). Prevalence of functional blindness, visual impairment, and related functional deficits among elderly Mexican Americans. *Journal of Gerontology*, 56A(9), M548-M551.

Hepworth, D.H., Rooney, R.H. & Larson, J.A. (1997). Direct Social Work Practice: Theory and Skills (5th ed.). Pacific Grove: Brooks/Cole Publishing.

Holland, L., & Courtney, R. (1998). Increasing cultural competence with the Latino community. *Journal of Community Health Nursing*, 15(1), 45-53.

Hunt, L.M., Arar, N.H. & Akana, L.L. (2002). Herbs, prayer, and insulin: Use of medical and alternative treatment by a group of Mexican-American diabetic patients. *Journal of Family Practice*, 49 (3), 216-223.

Hunt, L..M., Arar, N.II. & Larme, A.C. (1998). Contrasting patient and practitioner Perspectives in type II diabetes management. *Western Journal of Nursing Research*, 1, 656-676.

Hunt, L.M., Valenzuela, M.A., & Pugh, J.A. (1998). Porque me toco a me? Mexican American diabetes patient's causal stories and their relationship to treatment behaviors. *Social Science Medicine*, 46(8), 959-969.

Jezewski, M.A. & Poss, J. (2002). Mexican-Americans' explanatory model of type II Diabetes. *Western Journal of Nursing Research*, 24 (8), 840-859.

Kleinman, A. (1979). Concepts and a model for the comparison of medical systems as cultural systems. *Social Science and Medicine*, 23, 85-93.

Kleinmen, A. (1980). Patients and Healers in the Context of Culture: An Exploration of the Borderland Between Anthropology, *Medicine and Psychiatry*, 77-107.

Lai, W.A., Lew-Ting, C-Y, & Chiet, W.-C. (2004). How diabetic patients think about and manage their illness in Taiwan. *Diabetes Medicine*, 22, 286-292.

McSweeney, J.C. (1990). Making behavior changes after a myocardial infarction: A naturalistic study. Published Dissertation: University of Texas at Austin.

McSweeney, J.C., Allan J. D., & Mayo, K. (1997). Exploring the use of explanatory models in nursing research and practice. *Image Journal of Nursing Scholarship*, 29 (3), 243-248.

Poss, J.E. (2001). Developing a new model for cross-cultural research: Synthesizing the Health Belief Model and Theory of Reasoned Action. *Advanced Nursing Science*, 23 (4), 1-15.

Poss, J., Jezewski, M.A. (2002).The role and meaning of susto in Mexican-American's explanatory model of type II diabetes. *Medical Anthropology Quarterly*, 16(3), 360-377.

Poss, J.E., Jesewski, M.A. & Gonzalez-Stuart, A. (2003). Home remedies for type II diabetes used by Mexican-Americans in El Paso, Texas. *Clinical Nursing Research*, 12 (4), 304-323.

Reyes-Ortiz, C.A., Kuo, K.Y., DiNuzzo, A.R., Ray, L.A., Raji, M.A. & Markides, K.S. (2005). Near vision impairment predicts cognitive decline: Data from the Hispanic established populations for epidemiologic studies of the elderly. *Journal of American Geriatric Society*, 53(4), 681-686.

Tijerina, M. (2000). Mexican-American's perspective on end stage renal disease and the hemodialysis regimen: Psychosocial influences on compliance with treatment recommendations. Doctoral Dissertation.

Vilarejo, D. (2003). The health of U.S. hired farm workers. *Annual Review Public Health*, 24, 175-193.

Wu, J.H., Haan, M.N., Dang, J., Ghosh, D., Gonzalez H. M. & Herman, W.H. (2003). Diabetes as a predictor of change in functional status among older Mexican Americans. *Diabetes Care*, 26(2), 314-319.

Wu, J. H., Haan, M.N., Liang, J., Ghosh, D., Gonzalez, H. M. & Herman, W.H. (2003). Impact of diabetes on cognitive function among older Lationos: A population based cohort study. *Journal of Clinical Epidemiology*, 56, 686-693.

doi:10.1300/J137v14n01_09

Chapter 10

Care Needs of Older Adults Following a Traumatic or Disastrous Event

Roberta R. Greene
Sandra A. Graham

SUMMARY. This chapter addresses biopsychosocial and spiritual needs of older adults following a traumatic or disastrous event. It assumes that most older adults have established a pattern of positive adaptation over the life course as they encountered acute stress or chronic adversities. The importance of social supports and mutual aid is also described. doi:10.1300/J137v14n01_10 *[Article copies available for a fee from The Haworth Document Delivery Service: 1-800-HAWORTH. E-mail address: <docdelivery@ haworthpress.com> Website: <http://www.HaworthPress.com> © 2006 by The Haworth Press, Inc. All rights reserved.]*

KEYWORDS. Trauma, care needs, older adults, survivorship

This article addresses the biopsychosocial and spiritual needs of older adults following a traumatic or disastrous event. Combining the Functional Age Model (FAM) and a resilience-enhancing point of view (REM; outlined in Chapter 1), survivorship is explored from a strengths

[Haworth co-indexing entry note]: "Care Needs of Older Adults Following a Traumatic or Disastrous Event." Greene, Roberta R., and Sandra A. Graham. Co-published simultaneously in *Journal of Human Behavior in the Social Environment* (The Haworth Press, Inc.) Vol. 14, No. 1/2, 2006, pp. 201-219; and: *Contemporary Issues of Care* (ed: Roberta R. Greene) The Haworth Press, Inc., 2006, pp. 201-219. Single or multiple copies of this article are available for a fee from The Haworth Document Delivery Service [1-800-HAWORTH, 9:00 a.m. - 5:00 p.m. (EST). E-mail address: docdelivery@haworthpress.com].

perspective, assuming that most older adults have established a pattern of positive adaptation over the life course as they encountered acute stress or chronic adversities (Masten, 1994). The importance of social supports and mutual aid is also described. Composite cases illustrating various aspects of disaster work obtained from Federal Emergency Management Agency (FEMA) and American Red Cross (ARC) workers are provided.

INTRODUCTION: POSTTRAUMATIC STRESS AND RESILIENCE

When establishing the care needs of older adults following disastrous or critical events, practitioners need an assessment and intervention plan. Usually this plan involves integrating several models of care, in this case, the functional-age model of intergenerational therapy (FAM) and the resilience-enhancing model (REM). Both models share several assumptions including the need to address the biopsychosocial and spiritual functioning of the individual, the significance of examining the family as a developmental system, and the importance of involving ecological systems in care planning.

Risk

When initiating a plan of care, practitioners must first consider whether an individual is at high risk of negative side effects following the threat of the disaster. *Risk* is a statistical concept referring to "any influences that increase the probability of onset, digression to a more serious state, or maintenance of a problem condition" (Kirby & Fraser, 1997, pp. 10-11). Risk factors are those characteristics thought to present a group of people with a higher probability of an undesirable outcome, such as in the case of a disaster, experiencing PTSD following an emergency situation.

Research on how older adults respond to disaster has revealed four primary factors that may place older adults at risk: (1) older adults are less likely to evacuate their homes/property after warnings have been posted; (2) they live in homes that are more structurally unsound and prone to damage in disasters; (3) they experience greater psychological and emotional trauma than younger people as a result of losses associated with the disaster; and (4) they are less likely to receive assistance than younger survivors (Sanders, Bowie, & Bowie, 2003, p. 25). In addition, the physical, emotional, and social losses taken together may bring about the feeling that the environment in which they lived can no longer be trusted.

Because many older adults and those living on fixed incomes are more likely to reside in poorly maintained homes, they are at increased risk for injury or loss in a disaster such as a flood, tornado or hurricane. Residential structures in a state of deferred maintenance become particularly vulnerable to severe weather conditions.

It is common that many older adults refuse help and relocation services that would protect them from dangerous conditions resulting from a disaster event. During a flooding disaster in central Texas in 1998, FEMA disaster workers assisted thousands of survivors in obtaining safe, sanitary and secure housing. In many cases this meant temporarily relocating from their disaster-stricken homes. The Smith Family, five members two of whom were disabled, refused to move to a safer location. From conversations with the mother, it was evident that they were afraid to leave behind their belongings and their pets. American Red Cross (ARC) shelters do not have room to accommodate families' belongings and pets. They decided to recover whatever was usable from their home, take their pets, and move temporarily into a tent they set up away from their flooded home. Neighbors eventually persuaded them to move into an ARC shelter and make arrangements for someone else to care for the pets.

Disasters and Posttraumatic Stress

A *disaster*–an ecological phenomenon that occurs suddenly and is of sufficient magnitude to require external assistance (WHO, 1980)–is an occurrence of such severity and magnitude that it normally results in death, injuries, and property damage and cannot be managed through routine procedures (FEMA, 1983). A disaster requires the immediate, coordinated response of multiple government agencies, the private sector, and trained professionals to meet people's needs. A resilience point of view to the aftermath of trauma does not negate the fact that a disaster can be a frightening and out-of-the-ordinary experience. Nor does it deny that trauma can bring about extreme stress and uncertainty, with a few people experiencing severe aftereffects referred to as *posttraumatic stress disorder* (PTSD).

In fact, it is conservatively estimated that 10 percent of disasters survivors suffer adverse psychological effects akin to PTSD (National Institute of Mental Health, 1990). Posttraumatic stress involves a constellation of conscious and unconscious behaviors and emotions related to coping with the stressors immediately after a catastrophe as well as those associated with memories of the stressor (Figley, 1985). Symptoms may include intense fear, helplessness, horror, and psychic numbing (American Psychiatric Association, 1994). To make a judgment about whether a person is experiencing PTSD, practitioners must consider the type and severity of trauma experienced, preexisting psychiatric, family, and behavioral problems, as well as a person's subjective reaction to the critical event. Such reactions as sleep disturbance or loss of concentration should not be ignored, especially if they persist. The nature of a person's current social supports and societal attitudes such as racism or ageism may also contribute to higher levels of stress (Lightfoot, 1997). In addition, assessment judgments should consider whether the new stressors have triggered past trauma (Salerno & Nagy, 2002).

> Disaster workers need to be alert to the fact that older adults may appear to be unable to negotiate their surroundings and systems that previously were easily accomplished and accessible. In such situations, disaster recovery workers immediately refer the older adult to mental health counselors who are often at ARC shelters and within local community outreach posts such as storefronts, schools, churches, and fire stations. Social workers often serve as the mental health counselors. Other agencies such as the local Area Agency on Aging (AAA) and senior citizen centers will be contacted to activate support services and resources for the elderly.

Protective Factors

Although the risks to older adults following critical events must be evaluated, the social worker must also assess strengths and resiliency at all systems levels and initiate interventions that encourage and support survivorship. Contrary to popular belief, current research has documented that although some people experience disasters in negative ways, many people successfully regain their equilibrium (Kaniasty & Norius, 1999). This knowledge has led to the study of protective factors, involving a conceptual shift and change in the models of inquiry that direct the researcher's attention from risk factors to the process of how people successfully negotiate risk (Jessor, 1993; Rutter,1987). *Protective factors* generally refer to the circumstances that moderate, interrupt, or even prevent the effects of risk and enhance adaptation (Masten, 1994), and are therefore critical to take into account when care planning.

For example, there is evidence that older adults who have undergone stressful historical events, such as WWII, the Holocaust, or the Depression, may have greater resilience in the aftermath of more recent stressful events (Staudinger et al., 1999; Staudinger, Marsiske, & Baltes, 1995). That is, they have been able to maintain their psychological well-being even though they have experienced great disruptions in their lives (Brennan, Horowitz, & Reinhardt, 2003). Such adaptation is due to protective factors that have contributed to a resilient self, such as supportive social ties developed over the life course (Greene, 2002).

That is, when social workers approach older adults following a traumatic event, they should consider the following assumptions: Older adults who have remained resilient across the life span have social competence, a capacity to be flexible, empathetic, and to communicate effectively. Older adults are also relatively able to problem-solve, to plan, to seek help, and to think critically and reflectively. They can continue to benefit from contacts with their social ties (Greene, 2002; Rowe & Kahn, 1998).

> During Hurricane Andrew, a disaster worker recounts the scene in which an older man who was walking around the neighborhood strewn with debris helping other people by consoling them, reminding them of their ability to cope and offering words of hope. . . . *I've been through this before, and remember, you have too! We will make it again.*

Resilience

Positive assumptions about recovery following adverse events stem from the belief that people have an innate self-righting mechanism known as *resilience* (Garmezy, 1993), a term often used interchangeably with *positive coping, adaptation,* and *persistence* (Winfield, 1994). Resilience has also come to describe a person having a good track record of successful adaptation in the face of stress or disruptive change (Werner & Smith, 1992). In addition, the term has come to mean sustaining competence under pressure (Masten, 1994). *Resilience* is, then, "a universal capacity which allows a person, group, or community to prevent, minimize or overcome the damaging effects of adversity" (Grotberg, 1995, p. 2).

In short, when professionals first meet an older adult following an adverse event, they must be alert to symptoms that reflect severe stress or a loss in function. However, practitioners must also have a belief in the older adult's capacities. Namely, emotional upset should be dealt with while attempting to put a healing process into place.

When disaster workers first speak with survivors, they can contribute to healing as they:

- set a positive tone
- listen to their story
- find positive aspects of their experiences
- remind them of past successes with adversity
- indicate that help is on the way
- give encouragement

After the initial "normalizing" contact–a time when people are assured they are safe and basic needs are met–survivors may then be referred to mental health workers who will conduct needs assessments and make recommendations for follow-up. This requires that the practitioner be able to understand the interplay of a person's biopsychosocial spiritual functioning and how these factors influence and are influenced by the various social systems in which people live.

BIOPSYCHOSOCIAL AND SPIRITUAL ASSESSMENT FACTORS

Risk and resilience theory, an evolving human behavior and social work practice approach, may be understood as a biopsychosocial and spiritual phenomenon (Figure 1). As such it can serve as a basis for assessment and intervention (Greene, 2002). *Biological factors* to be assessed following a critical event are related to functional capacity and include health, physical capacity, or vital life limiting organ systems; *psychological factors* encompass an individual's affect state or mood, cognitive or mental status, and their behavioral dimensions; and *sociocultural aspects* to consider involve the cultural, political, and economic aspects of life events (Greene, 2000). *Spiritual factors* may include a person's relationship with his or her faith/religious community and or an inner system of beliefs.

Biological Functioning

One important biological risk factor to keep in mind is that older adults are less likely to have an acute sense of smell, touch, vision, and hearing. Therefore, interviews need to be adjusted accordingly (Table 1). Any older

FIGURE 1. The Resiliency Model

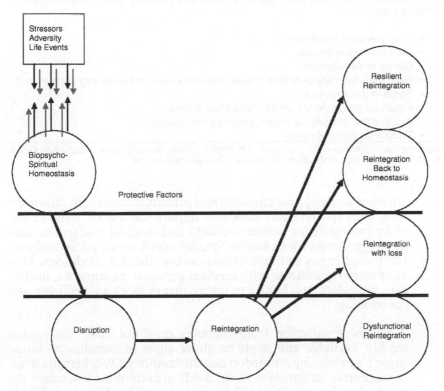

Richardson, G. E. (2002). Metatheory of resilience and resiliency. *Journal of Clinical Psychology,* *58*(3), 307-321. Reprinted with permission of John Wiley & Sons, Inc.

adults may be frail and have diminished functional capacities which may include strength and mobility. In addition, older adults may respond more slowly to ongoing disaster events. The survivor may have a history of tiredness, loss of interest and appetite, weight loss, or inability to sleep.

However, a resilience perspective also suggests that people have a "biological imperative for growth and development that unfolds naturally" that may be tapped by the practitioner (Bernard, 1995, p. 1). Therefore, although development is shaped by a person's genetic and biological substrate, social workers can promote resilient behaviors following an emergency.

TABLE 1. Tips for Talking to the Hearing Impaired

Are there ways to talk more effectively to someone with a hearing loss of which I should become more aware?

- Don't talk from another room.
- Face the person directly.
- Get his or her attention
- Recognize that hard-of-hearing people understand less well when they are tired or ill
- Speak in a normal tone.
- Keep your hands away from your face when talking.
- Avoid eating, chewing, or smoking during a conversation.
- Reduce background noises.

Adapted from: Schneider, R.L., & Kropf, N.P. (1987) (1992). Gerontological social work: Knowledge, service settings, and special populations. Chicago: Nelson Hall.

Disaster workers give attention and priority treatment to those persons with special conditions that require the use of assistive devices (wheelchairs, walkers, canes) and medical equipment such as oxygen tanks for example. Special needs create additional mobility challenges and restrictions during disaster conditions. Disaster works coordinate with medical personal, pharmacies, healthcare providers, and family to insure that devices are available and functioning.

A survivor suffering from diabetes may not have medication readily available and begin to show signs of unbalanced blood sugar by exhibiting confusion and unsteadiness. Workers must obtain accurate information about medical conditions to explain the reason for this condition. Thus, attention to medication refills is one of the first items for professionals to address.

Psychological Functioning

Psychological characteristics associated with resilience include a higher sense of self-esteem and self-efficacy (Werner, 1989), as well as hope, optimism, and self-understanding (Seligman, 1990). Therefore, assessment must take into account how effectively an older individual seems to be mastering his or her environment. Psychological risk factors to take into account during assessment of an older adult following a disaster include obtaining knowledge of prior life attitudes and mental health conditions.

Professionals should understand that an estimated 15 to 25 percent of the nation's older adults have symptoms of mental illness that may be exacerbated by living through a disastrous event (Estes, 1995). Perhaps, the first symptom a professional will notice is confusion. It is important to assess whether confusion is caused by underlying prior conditions. These prior-existing conditions may include depression, one of the most common psychiatric conditions among older adults, involving a range of feelings from mild indifference to complete demoralization. Care in assessment should be given as dementia should not be mistaken with delirium, a sudden and temporary change in mental functioning that may be connected with the disaster (Greene, 2000). Consequently, getting a medical history from a family member is sometimes necessary.

At the same time, the social worker needs to assess an older adult's ability to counteract stress and maintain a sense of continuity. Continuity theory suggests that older adults exhibit "considerable consistency over time in their patterns of thinking, activity profiles, and social relationships" (Atchley, 1995, p. 227). Therefore, learning how a person has positively dealt with change and successfully made difficult life transitions can help the social worker assist the client following a critical event. That is, the practitioner will want to assess the client's coping level (Table 2).

> Disaster workers develop a heightened awareness to signs of excessive stress, and look for survivors exhibiting behaviors such as uncontrollable crying, excessive talking, extreme expressions of anger, unmanageable anxiety, and withdrawal, apathy and silence. These are indications of poor coping strategies and identify those people who need more attention and services. This form of triage is common during disaster work.

Social Functioning

Positive social functioning following an adverse event is related to resiliency and how a person's has made role transitions across his or her life time. Various events across the life course may be *normative*, referring to events that most people experience over their lifetime or *nonnormative*, encompassing situations that are not expected to occur and are experienced by an entire cohort such as the Great Depression, the Nazi Holocaust, or September 11th. In the words of a senior,

> Senior citizens today are a sturdy, reliable generation. We've proven time and again our ability to survive everything from the Great Depression to world wars and the threat of nuclear holocaust. We've lived through droughts, floods, and all sorts of other natural disasters. We've given birth, supported our families, and stood by our loved ones through personal and financial losses. We are proud, tough, and resilient. ("Voices of Wisdom: Seniors Cope with Disaster" Videotape Project Cope, 1992)

TABLE 2. Person-in-Environment System Coping Index

- Outstanding coping skills: The client's ability to solve problems, to act independently, and to use ego strength, insight, and intellectual ability to cope with difficult situations is exceptional.
- Above-average coping skills: The client's ability to solve problems, to act independently, and to use ego strength, insight, and intellectual ability to cope with difficult situations is more than would be expected in the average person.
- Adequate coping skills: The client is able to solve problems, can act independently, and has adequate ego strength, insight, and intellectual ability.
- Somewhat adequate coping skills: The client has fair problem solving ability, but has major difficulties in solving the presenting problems, acting independently, and using ego strength, insight, and intellectual ability.
- Inadequate coping skills: The client has some ability to solve problems but it is insufficient to solve the presenting problems; the client shows poor ability to act independently; and the client has minimal ego strength, insight, and intellectual ability.
- No coping skills: The client shows little or no ability to solve problems, lacks the capacity to act independently, and has insufficient ego strength, insight, and intellectual ability.

Adapted from: Karls & Wandrei (1994). Person-in-Environment System. Washington, DC: NASW Press, (p. 33).

It is the unexpected, extreme nature of a disastrous event, then, that can either trigger a resilient response or renew prior trauma. The emotional state of discomfort may occur with two types of situations: (1) unusual single occurrences, such as a hurricane; and (2) ongoing sustained violence or intimidation, such as elder abuse. This is the distinction the professionals need to make.

> Many older adults have lived through traumatic events, including wars, the Great Depression, and losses of loved ones. New stressful events, such as the terrorist attacks on the United States, often trigger memories of past traumatic experiences and new symptoms of loss, stress, and grief. Feelings of anxiety, helplessness, hyper arousal, and depression are common, as are recurrent thoughts about the new images and events. (Lantz & Buchalter, 2001, p. 35)

Furthermore, positive attachments to others are known to foster resilience (Garmezy, 1991). Studies of people's response to disasters such as floods or hurricanes suggest that there is a high level of mutual helping, involving assistance to and from people. Understanding community altruism and promoting a heightened sense of internal solidarity may lessen a threat and be less psychologically injurious (Janoff-Bulman, 1992).

Research suggests that following disasters communities may establish their own therapeutic milieu involving solidarity, togetherness, and reciprocity. Because disruptions in social networks can negatively affect psychological distress, it is important for professionals and lay leaders to immediately mobilize social support to enhance resiliency. In addition, people feel reconnected to others and are better able to transform their lives (Blundo & Greene, 2007).

Cultural Influences

Because cultural norms can influence help-seeking behavior, it is another factor that affects how people respond to disasters. *Culture* is the shared heritage of a group including language, customs, traditions, and rituals as well as a set of learned beliefs. Culture may be characterized by national origin, length of origin in the United States, age, gender, sexual orientation, education level or socioeconomic status, creating "one medium through which people develop the resilience that is needed to overcome adversity" (Athey & Moody-Williams, 2003, p. 23).

Disaster workers may be unfamiliar with coping strategies that stem from particular cultures. For example, in some cultures hurricane parties are natural events that accompany the natural disaster. Festive gatherings can include music, dancing, and laughter, drinking and eating, and recovery parades. The opportunity to recover and heal together within familiar cultural surroundings contributes to the hope of regaining some form of normalcy.

Spiritual Functioning

Spiritual belief systems can contribute to help maintain a resilient self, fostering a person's ability to transcend the immediate situation and to discover meaning in seemingly meaningless events. Practitioners will want to tap this propensity to growth in the healing process. Survivors may spontaneously mention their faith belief about how they have survived the disaster. Others may want to talk with clergy available at the site.

Clergy are valuable resources during disaster recovery and serve effectively as members of the disaster recover teams. In this way interested disaster survivors are assured to have opportunities for spiritual comfort. Clergy remain important members of the relief team along with medical personnel and safety workers. In addition, houses of worship often serve as shelter sites for survivors and a place for the recovery team to receive respite.

INTERVENTION

Individual

Most importantly, professionals should understand that recovery is a process. Highly structured regimens and the commonly held assumptions about fixed stages of recovery are now coming under scrutiny in terms of efficacy and effectiveness (Brody, 2004). Research has generally indicated that preplanned sessions or established treatments show no greater benefit than the more spontaneous discussions among those who went through the disaster (Greenberg, 1995). Therefore, professionals are leaning to a form of triage, assessing who might need emergency mental services and those who might benefit from mutual aid groups and the mobilization of informal supports (Greene, 2002).

However, some older adults will experience a decline in their sense of control following disasters (Wolinsky et al., 2003). At the same time, it is important for professionals not to mistake the fact that survivors may be stunned following a disaster with the myth that older adults can not help themselves. In reality, many older adult survivors may be able to care for themselves or even to care for others (Oriol, 1999).

Recovery begins with relief assistance that provides people with practical necessities (Greene & Livingston, 2002). This assistance usually involves being able to once again handle the basics of daily living and return to normal routines. The focus on resilience and survivorship has shifted the focus of intervention strategies to how a person heals from loss and is able to reconstruct a sense of perspective (Chung, 2003). For example, it is often normal for denial and shock during early phases after the disaster. Such denial may help survivors postpone or even alleviate more painful emotions (Oriol, 1999). Because a disaster usually makes no immediate sense or is essentially senseless, practitioners who work with survivors from a resilience perspective often use a narrative or storytelling approach (Table 3). It is much less threatening for professionals to talk about their services as "assistance" or "talking" (ibid.). Responding in an active, genuine, and concerned manner allows for recovery to get further under way. Listening to a survivor's story, or a simple account of what has happened, allows for the grieving process (Greene & Armenta, 2007), permits the survivor to externalize the problem (Abel & Abel, 2001), and encourages the formation of a coherent sense of self (Smyer & Qualls, 1999). The professional can also learn how to tap survivors' generative or growth producing processes (Saleebey, 1996). Survivors may realize that they are not alone and that their reactions to such a horrendous event are "normal."

TABLE 3. Narrative and Solution-Focused Assumptions and Interventions

Narrative

1. People are proactive and self-organizing.

2. People's behavior is shaped by the meaning they give to events.

3. As people create meaning in interaction with others, they develop a life story.

4. A person's life story contains information about how they have met life's critical events. The story gives life coherence and continuity.

5. If a story is problem-saturated, the client can be helped to reauthor it and discover alternative solutions.

6. Practitioners aim to broaden the client's view of reality and find alternative ways to overcome an impasse.

Solution-Focused

1. The focus of therapy is to create future solution.

2. Practitioners explore what the client hopes to achieve by going step by step to find positive solutions.

3. Client-social worker conversation helps the client gain control by imagining a positive self-chosen direction.

4. Practitioners help clients explore alternative ways of gradually achieving success.

Adapted from: Greene, R. R. (2007). *Social Work Practice: A Risk and Resilience Perspective* (with CD-ROM). Belmont, CA: Wadsworth.

Systems

Resilience is not limited to individuals but is also a large-scale social phenomena (Grotberg,1995). Therefore, intervention plans should be ecologically-based, involving pertinent social systems. Most importantly, survivors need to come to the realization that what is *individual trauma*, or a blow to their personal well-being, is also a *collective trauma*, or a blow to the fabric of social life (Oriel, 1999). Thus, resilience is "a nested context for social competence" (Walsh, 1998, p. 12). Practitioners work with small-scale *microsystems*, such as families and peer groups; the connection between systems, known as *mesosystems*, such as the family and health care systems; *exosystems*, the connections between systems that do not directly involve the person, such as insurance companies; and *macrosystems*, or overarching large-scale systems, such as legal, political, and value systems.

Because of the magnitude of many disasters, they may require a public health response involving individual and community interventions encompassing clinical, research, and community organization skills (Galambos, 2005). The objectives of a public health response, as delineated by Noji (2000), include:

1. assessing the needs of disaster-affected populations;
2. matching available resources to those needs;
3. preventing further adverse health affects; implementing disease control strategies for well-defined problems; and
4. evaluating the effectiveness of disaster relief programs, and improving contingency plans for various types of future disasters (p. 21).

Family

One of the first steps for a disaster worker is to reunite families. If this is possible, the professional can focus on a family's natural resources, patterns of functioning, and capabilities that enable them to meet and even thrive in the face of crisis. From this viewpoint, the focus is upon the family's behavior as a group and its ability to positively approach life challenges. Wherever possible, the professional builds on a family's assets, endurance, and survival skills to confront negative stressors (Germain, 1994; Wolin & Wolin, 1995). The professional will also want to know if a family has had a trauma affecting several generations such as refugee status (Graziano, 2003).

Support Systems

Social supports are "those interpersonal transactions involving mutual aid and affirmation" (Gitterman & Shulman, 1986). Being a part of a social support network has a stress-buffering effect on individual well-being (Tracy & Whittaker, 1990). For example, Tyler's (2000) research found that older adult survivors of the Midwest flood in the early 1990s who had secure social supports exhibited less depression than those with weaker support systems. Social support network characteristics may vary by size and composition, frequency of contact, length of relationships, and perceived availability. The four largest sources of social support are households, relatives, friends, and formal service providers (Greene, 2005). Family and kin have been shown to be the best source of support following disasters, providing an opportunity to reconnect with daily life.

PHASES OF RECOVERY

The National Institute of Mental Health (1983) has delineated seven phases that individuals and communities tend to follow when moving towards recovery. These stages are not linear, but may overlap or blend together.

1. *Warning or Threat Phase.* A time of advance notification about an adverse event such as a hurricane or flood. Elderly citizens are less likely to want to relocate following a warning.
2. *Impact Phase.* A time when the adverse event occurs and the destruction becomes apparent. Survivors' reactions may include disbelief, confusion, and anxiety.
3. *Rescue or Heroic Phase.* A time when professionals move into rescue operations and work together to save lives and property. Survivors may be keenly aware of separation from the family's emotional support, and their usual sources of food, clothing, or medicines.
4. *Remedy or Honeymoon Phase.* A time when survivors tend to be optimistic and work together as a community. Because this phase involves cultural perceptions of healing, this is a particular time to be cognizant of culturally sensitive interventions.
5. *Inventory Phase.* A time of when disaster survivors are more interested in discussing their thoughts but not necessarily exploring their feelings (CMHS, 1994). There may be high levels of experiencing grief and loss. Survivors may want to discuss property loss such as homes and treasured possessions.
6. *Disillusionment Phase.* A time when survivors recognize the reality of their loss and the limits of outside help. They may experience feelings of anger and helplessness. Professionals may want to acknowledge these concerns as well as begin to reconstruct the meaning of events.
7. *Reconstruction or Recovery Phase.* A time that may last up to a year in which survivors integrate the changes in personal and community life. Professionals may want to assist through rituals and ceremonies that move people towards the healing process.

CULTURALLY COMPETENT CARE PLANS

The culture of the survivors "provides the lens through which community members see their recovery" (Athey & Moody-Williams, 2003, p. 20). A professional should understand what constitutes a friendly gesture or if a touch is appropriate. Professionals who aspire to culturally competent interventions following adverse events need an understanding of the historical, social, and political events that affect the survivors' physical and mental health.

According to Cross (1989), professionals should understand cultural competence as an ongoing developmental process requiring a long-term commitment over time to work effectively across cultures. Practice requires the professional to gain a set of values, behaviors, attitudes, and practice strategies that honor and respect individuals, families, and communities receiving services. Cultural competence is not easily achieved and may be thought of as a professional and systems-wide process involving six levels of achievement:

1. *Cultural Destructiveness*, involving behaviors that are damaging to a culture such as denying equal services to people of color.
2. *Cultural Incapacity*, referring to a paternalistic posture toward "lesser" groups such as maintaining stereotypes.
3. *Cultural Blindness*, involving an indifference to difference such as believing all people are the same.
4. *Cultural Pre-Competence*, moving toward some self-awareness that services need to improve.
5. *Cultural Competence,* requiring self assessment to achieve a higher comfort level when working across cultures.
6. *Cultural Proficiency*, involving professionals and agencies who hold diversity of culture in high esteem.

PLANNING AHEAD FOR MENTAL HEALTH RECOVERY

During Hurricane Andrew, rescue workers learned that proactive planning is a key to success, especially if relocation is needed (Silverman & Weston, 1995). Planning ahead involves knowing community demographics, identifying and understanding various cultural groups, determining the community's socioeconomic considerations, identifying mental health resources as well as gaps, determining government roles and responsibilities, assuring nongovernmental organizations' roles in disaster, and developing community partnerships (Athey & Moody-Williams, 2003). Involving disaster advocates, senior citizen centers, adult day service centers, and nursing home staff is essential. An eldercare locator service may be initiated (Oriol, 1999).

REFERENCES

Abels, P. & Abels, S. L. (2001). *Understanding narrative therapy.* New York: Springer Publishing.
Atchley, R. (1995). Continuity theory. In G. L. Maddox et al. (Eds.). *Encyclopedia of Aging, Activity and Aging* (2nd edition, pp. 5-16). Newbury Park, CA: Sage.
Athey, J. & Moody-Williams, J. (2003). *Developing cultural competence in disaster mental health programs: Guiding principles and recommendations.* Rockville, MD: U. S. Department of Health and Human Services Substance Abuse and Mental

Health Services Administration Center for Mental Health Services, DHHS Publication No. SMA 3828.

Blundo, R. & Greene, R. R. (2007). Survivorship in the face of traumatic events and disasters: Implications for social work practice. In R. R. Greene (Ed.), *Social work practice: A risk and resilience perspective* (pp. 160-173). Monterey, CA: Thompson Brooks/Cole.

Brennan, M., Horowitz, A., & Reinhardt, J. P. (2003). The September 11th attacks and depressive symptomatology among older adults with vision loss. *Journal of Gerontological Social Work, 40,*(4), 55-72.

Brody, J. (2004). Often, time beats therapy for treating grief. *The New York Times,* Tuesday, January 27, p. D7.

Bronfenbrenner, U., Moen, P., & Garbarino, J. (1984). Family and community. In R. Parke (Ed.), *Review of child development research* (Vol. 7, pp. 283-328). Chicago: University of Chicago Press.

Carter, B., & McGoldrick, M. (1999). *The expanded family life cycle: Individual, family, and social perspectives.* Boston: Allyn & Bacon.

Chung, I. (2003). The impact of the 9/11 attacks on the elderly in NYC Chinatown: Implications for culturally relevant services. *Journal of Gerontological Social Work, 40,*(4), 37-54.

Conrad, A. P. (1999). Professional tools for religiously and spiritually sensitive social work practice. In R. R. Greene (Ed.), *Human behavior theory and social work practice* (2nd ed., pp. 63-72). New York: Aldine de Gruyter.

Cross, T. L. (1989). Towards a culturally competent system of care. Vol. I: A monograph of effective services for children who are severely emotionally disturbed. Washington, DC: Georgetown University Child Development Center.

Estes, C. L. (1995). Mental health services for the elderly: Key policy elements. In M. Gatz (Ed.), *Emerging issues in mental health and aging.* Washington, DC: American Psychological Association.

Federal Emergency Management Agency (1983). Preparing for Disaster: A Conference on Emergency Planning for Disabled and Elderly Persons. Washington, DC: Author.

Figley, C. (1985). Introduction. In C. Figley (Ed.), *Trauma and its wake: The study and treatment of post-traumatic stress disorders.* New York: Brunner/Mazel.

Galambos, C. (2005). Natural disasters: Health and mental health considerations. *Health & Social Work, 30*(2), 83-85.

Germain, C. B. (1994). Human behavior in the social environment. In F. G. Reamer (Ed.), *The foundations of social work knowledge* (pp. 88-121). New York: Columbia University Press.

Gitterman, A., & Shulman, L. (1986). *Mutual aid groups and the life cycle.* Itasca, IL: F. E. Peacock.

Graziano, R. (2003). Trauma and aging. *Journal of Gerontological Social Work, 40,*(4), 3-22.

Greene, R. R. (2005). The changing family of later years and social work practice. In L. Kaye (Ed.). *Productive Aging* (pp. 1-7-122). Washington, DC: NASW Press.

Greene, R. R. (2002). *Resiliency theory: An integrated framework for practice, research, and policy.* Washington, DC: NASW Press.

Greene, R. R. (2000) *Social work with the aged and their families*. (2nd edition). Hawthorne, New York: Aldine de Gruyter.

Greene, R. R. (1999). *Human behavior theory and social work practice* (2nd edition). New York: Aldine de Gruyter.

Greene, R. R. & Armenta, K. (2007). The REM: Phase II–Practice strategies. In R. R. Greene (Ed.), *Social work practice: A risk and resilience perspective* (pp. 67-87). Monterey, CA: Thompson Brooks/Cole.

Grotberg, E. H. (1995, September 27-30). *The international resilience project: Research, application, and policy.* Paper presented at the Symposio Internacional Stress Violencia, Lisbon, Portugal.

Lantz, M. S., & Buchalter, E. N. (2001). Posttraumatic stress: Helping older adults cope with tragedy. (12), 35-36.

Lightfoot, O. (1997). Biopsychosocial trauma and the urban elderly. *Journal of Geriatric Society, 30*(1), 175-192.

Masten, A. (1994). Resilience in individual development: Successful adaptation despite risk and adversity. In M. C. Wang & E. W. Gordon (Eds.), *Educational resilience in inner-city America: Challenges and prospects* (pp. 3-25). Hillsdale, NJ: Lawrence Erlbaum.

National Institute of Mental Health (1983). *Training manual for human service workers in major disasters*. (Pub. No. ADM 83-538). Washington, DC: Department of Health and Human Services.

Noji, E. K. (2000). The public health consequences of disasters. *Prehospital and Disaster Medicine, 15*(4), 85-105.

North, C. S. & Pfefferbaum, B. (2002). Research on the mental health effects of terrorism. *Journal of the American Medical Association* (JAMA), *288*, (5), 633-636.

Oriol, W. (1999). Psychosocial issues for older adults in disasters. Substance Abuse and Mental Health Services Administration Center for Mental Health Services. DHHS Publication No. ESDRB SMA 99-3323. Washington, DC: http://www.mentalhealth.org

Project COPE (1992). *Voices of wisdom videotape and brochure*. Ventura County, CA.

Saleebey, D. (1996). The strengths perspective in social work practice: Extensions and cautions. *Social Work, 41*(3), 296-305.

Salerno, J. A. & Nagy, C. (2002). Terrorism and aging. *Journal of Gerontology: Medical Sciences, 57A* (9),M552-M554.

Sanders, S., Bowie, S. L., & Bowie, Y. D. (2003). Lessons learned on forced relocation of older adults: The impact of Hurricane Andrew on health, mental health, and social supports of public housing residents. *Journal of Gerontological Social Work, 40*,(4), 23-36.

Schneider, R. L. & Kropf, N. P. (1987) (1992). Gerontological social work: Knowledge, service settings, and special populations. Chicago: Nelson Hall.

Silverman, M. A. & Weston, M. (1995). Lessons learned from Hurricane Andrew: Recommendations for care of the elderly in long term care facilities. *Southern Medical Journal, 88*, 603-609.

Smyer, M. A., & Qualls, S. H. (1999). *Aging and mental health*. Malden, MA: Blackwell Publishers.

Staudinger, U. M., Freund, A. M., Linden, M. & Maas, I. (1999). Self, personality, and life regulations: Facets of psychological resilience in old age. In P. B. Baltes & K. U. Mayer (Eds.), *The Berlin aging study* (pp. 302-328). Cambridge, U.K: Cambridge University Press.

Staudinger, U. M., Marsiske, M., & Baltes, P. B. (1995). Resilience and reserve capacity in later adulthood: Potential and limits in development across the life span. In D. Ciccetti & D. Cohen (Eds.), *Developmental psychopathology: Risk, disorder, and adaptation* (Vol. II, pp. 801-847). New York: John Wiley and Sons.

Tyler, K.A. (2000). The effects of an acute stressor on depressive symptoms among older adults. *Research on Aging, 22,* 143-165.

Tracy, E. M., & Whittaker, J. K. (1990). The social network map: Assessing social support in clinical practice. *Families in Society, 71,* 461-470.

Rowe, J. W., & Kahn, R. L. (1998). *Successful aging.* New York: Pantheon Books.

Walsh, F. (1998). *Strengthening family resilience.* New York: Guilford Press.

Willis, S. L. (1996a). Everyday cognitive competence in elderly persons: Conceptual issues and empirical findings. *Gerontologist, 36,* 595-601.

Wolin, S., & Wolin, S. (1995). Resilience among youth growing up in substance abusing families. *Pediatric Clinics of North America, 42,* 415-429.

Wolinsky, F., Wyrwich, K. W., Kroenke, K., Babu, A. N., & Tierney, W. (2003). 9-11, personal stress, mental health, and sense of control among older adults. *Journal of Gerontology, 58B,* 146-150.

doi:10.1300/J137v14n01_10

Chapter 11

Caregivers of Children with Cancer

Barbara L. Jones

SUMMARY. When a child is diagnosed with cancer, families experience a devastating life event with immediate and long-term impact on quality of life, actvities of daily living, family dynamics, self identity, parental role, and sense of meaning in the world. However, despite the trauma, more recent studies are highlighting the resilience and functioning of families facing cancer in childhood. This chapter explores these family dynamics. doi:10.1300/J137v14n01_11 *[Article copies available for a fee from The Haworth Document Delivery Service: 1-800-HAWORTH. E-mail address: <docdelivery@haworthpress.com> Website: <http://www.HaworthPress.com> © 2006 by The Haworth Press, Inc. All rights reserved.]*

KEYWORDS. Childhood cancer, family dynamics, resilience

INTRODUCTION:
CANCER IN CHILDHOOD AND IMPACT ON THE FAMILY

When a child is diagnosed with cancer, families experience a devastating life event with immediate and long-term impact on quality of life, ac-

[Haworth co-indexing entry note]: "Caregivers of Children with Cancer." Jones, Barbara L. Co-published simultaneously in *Journal of Human Behavior in the Social Environment* (The Haworth Press, Inc.) Vol. 14, No. 1/2, 2006, pp. 221-239; and: *Contemporary Issues of Care* (ed: Roberta R. Greene) The Haworth Press, Inc., 2006, pp. 221-239. Single or multiple copies of this article are available for a fee from The Haworth Document Delivery Service [1-800-HAWORTH, 9:00 a.m. - 5:00 p.m. (EST). E-mail address: docdelivery@haworthpress.com].

doi:10.1300/J137v14n01_11

tivities of daily living, family dynamics, self identity, parental role, and sense of meaning in the world (Van Dongen-Melman et al., 1998, Bowman et al., 2003; Young et al., 2002). Siblings of children with cancer also undergo extreme shifts in identity and well-being, often resulting in significant emotional and behavioral problems (Sahler et al., 1994; Davies, 1999). Previous work in this area has looked at maladaptive responses and adverse outcomes to families with a child with cancer. These negative outcomes can include post-traumatic stress disorder, anxiety, depression, financial distress, marital discord, social and behavioral problems, and prolonged and complicated mourning (Bowman et al., 2003; Hoekstra-Weebers et al., 1999, 2001; Kazak et al., 1998; Manne et al., 2000).

However, despite the trauma and disruption that families experience upon diagnosis and throughout treatment of a child with cancer, more recent studies are highlighting the resilience and functioning of families facing cancer in childhood (Svavarsdottir, 2004; Young et al., 2002). Changing the focus from one of pathology to one of resilience allows practitioners to engage in the work of understanding the complexity of caregiving for this population (Greene, 2002; Young et al., 2002). Caregiving roles and tasks of providing care to children with cancer may have a mediating effect on the traumatic impact of the diagnosis and the care (Young, 2002; Moore & Beckwitt, 2004; Bowman, 2003). The resilience of these families in the midst of personal crisis is an area for further exploration. This chapter will highlight the caregiving experiences of families of children with cancer and focus on a model of understanding and enhancing family resilience (Greene, 2002; McCubbin & McCubbin, 1996; Walsh, 1998).

PREVALENCE OF CHILDHOOD CANCER

Each year more than 12,000 children under the age of twenty in the United States receive a diagnosis of cancer (National Institutes of Health, 1999). Childhood cancer survival rates have steadily increased in the United States over the past 20 years (National Cancer Institute, 2004). With current treatments, more than 70% of children diagnosed with cancer are expected to become long-term survivors (National Cancer Institute, 2004). However, the end of cancer treatment does not finish the need for care and support from the effects of the cancer. Survivors diagnosed as children may experience learning difficulties, social stigma, trouble with peer relations, depression, anxiety, post-traumatic stress disorder, difficulty integrating their cancer experience into their current life, difficulty transitioning to adult healthcare, and infertility (Hewitt et al., 2004; National Cancer Institute, 2004). Therefore, caregiving needs may continue for families of survivors well beyond the actual course of treatment.

Despite the rarity of diagnosis and the advances in treatment, cancer is still the leading cause of death from disease in children under fifteen (National Cancer Institute, 2002). More than 2,000 children each year die from cancer-related causes (SEER, 2004, National Institutes of Health, 1999) leaving their families with significant loss and many unanswered questions (Cincotta, 2004). The death of a child has been shown to be a predictor of complicated mourning in surviving family members (Rando, 1993). Families may erroneously feel that they have failed as a parent because they were unable to protect their child from their death (Cincotta, 2004). Consequently, the role of caregiving takes on even more importance as the family approaches end-of-life care and the death of the child.

THE CHALLENGES TO FAMILIES IN HEALTHCARE

Families entering today's healthcare system are often overwhelmed and confused by the volume of technical information and the pace at which it is delivered to them. While confronting their own deep fears about their child's health, families find themselves trying to respond to the requests being made of them by healthcare professionals. Cultural issues in healthcare are paramount as many practitioners are unable to respond with the cultural humility and sensitivity needed to allow families to receive care that is congruent with their beliefs (Tervalon & Murray-Garcia, 1998) Additionally, the United States healthcare system has a culture of its own that families must learn to understand, interpret, and ultimately comply with if they are to receive the treatment they wish for their child. As one family put it,

> Sometimes, a place can be so overpowering and overwhelming that it asserts a culture of its own. A hospital can be such a place. Its culture is mysterious and imposing to families, but the families acknowledge and respect this institutional culture. The family bends over backwards, really, to conform to this culture because they know that doing so will benefit their child . . . getting good care for Leah required us to be easy to work with.

> Regardless of their ethnicity, the circumstances that keep families in a hospital force them (us, once upon a time) to adopt this culture. . . while they are inside the hospital, the strange new culture they adopt to make do and get by is more important than the culture they may identify themselves with when they are "outside." (Insook, 2004)

Families of young children who are diagnosed with cancer carry all of the same burdens of other families with young children. They have responsibilities for work, care of their well children, relationships, paying bills, care for their home, and perhaps even other caregiving roles they were already fulfilling such as caring for a parent or sibling. However, the healthcare system does not slow for families to adjust to the new caregiving responsibilities that can sometimes place families in a quandary about whose needs will get met and whose will not.

Finally, when a child is diagnosed with a life-threatening condition, the family is placed in a position of extreme vulnerability that only exacerbates the power differential in modern healthcare between patient and provider. In a recent study of pediatric palliative care service provision in hospitals, parents reported experiencing distress as a result of selected staff interactions and a feeling that their child's pain was not adequately assessed or managed (Contro et al., 2002).

> One of the most striking findings was how a single event could cause parents profound and lasting emotional distress. Parents recounted incidents that included insensitive delivery of bad news, feeling dismissed or patronized, perceived disregard for parents' judgment regarding the care of their child, and poor communication of important information. Such an event haunted them and complicated their grief even years later. (ibid., 2002)

PARENTS AND FAMILIES AS CAREGIVERS

Parenting is itself a caregiving role replete with responsibilities for the safety, health, development, and well-being of the child. However, when a child is diagnosed with a life-threatening condition, the caregiving responsibilities multiply exponentially. Parents are often not prepared for the extent of the shift in their role from parent to parent of a child with cancer (Young et al., 2002). Upon diagnosis, parents begin a process of "becoming" the parent of a child with cancer (ibid.). This identity and role shift may actually start before diagnosis as the parent seeks to understand some set of curious medical symptoms and to obtain adequate medical assistance (ibid, Moore & Beckwitt, 2004). Because of the rarity of childhood cancer, diagnosis is not easy and parents can experience many delays and misdiagnoses as they desperately try to discover what is happening to their child. This period of uncertainty can cause the parents to feel that their knowledge of their child is discounted by professionals (Young et al., 2002). This transition to the role of "parent of a child with cancer" is not easy and can set up barriers between the familial caregivers and professional caregivers that must later be mediated.

From the moment of a diagnosis of cancer, the entire family system is immediately changed and coping strategies and previously agreed-upon roles are challenged. The sense of disbelief upon diagnosis is extreme when the patient is a child; the emotional impact on the family cannot be overstated. The understanding of a cancer diagnosis is both medically and socially constructed with the threat of death as a real and present danger. However, current healthcare practices expect a great deal of self-care and dependent care from children and their parents even before the shock of the diagnosis has dissipated (Moore & Beckwitt, 2004). Immediately, the child and family receive voluminous and complicated medical information directly related to their expected caregiving responsibilities and ultimately their child's health. Families are expected to take on difficult medical and emotional caregiving responsibilities for their child as a course of treatment. These responsibilities can include frequent medical appointments and hospital stays, home-based high tech medical care, and psychological support of the child and siblings (Jones, 2006; Cincotta, 2004). Caregivers face extensive emotional, social, spiritual, and often financial burdens as they attempt to learn the rigorous treatment regimens while maintaining some sense of normalcy for the child and family. Despite these tremendous burdens, the medical urgency of the situation demands that an empirically-based oncology protocol for care be followed. These protocols always involve family responsibility for care.

In the United States, most of the 250 children's hospitals are members of the Children's Oncology Group, the national research organization that brings together the nation's pediatric oncology physicians, nurses, psychologists, and social workers to develop protocols of pediatric oncology care to cure cancer, reduce suffering, and manage symptoms. Most pediatric oncology protocols place immediate caregiving responsibilities on the family in order to succeed. Depending upon the type of malignancy, the protocol may involve learning complicated treatment regimens, staying in the hospital for a series of days, weeks, or months, adhering to a frequent schedule of outpatient hospital visits, learning to administer medicines, responding to the often severe side effects of treatment, and being ready to return to the hospital emergently as the situation demands. These responsibilities come, like in many other caregiving situations, at a time of profound crisis and in the midst of all of the other responsibilities of modern families. What is unique about caregiving when the patient is a child is that the parents are already caregivers but the new responsibilities far surpass those expected of families whose children are not sick. The parents usually face multiple caregiving responsibilities–for the child with cancer, for their other children, and perhaps for their parents.

Siblings, too, can be expected to assume caregiving responsibilities sometimes related to the identified patient or to the tasks that the parents must forego to meet the demands of treatment. It is not uncommon for siblings to report having to care for themselves in ways that were previously done for them due to their parents' sudden preoccupation with the identified patient (Davies, 1999). Suddenly, the burden of care for everyone is quite different and takes on dire importance. The system of caregivers can extend well beyond the parents and siblings to include grandparents, aunts, uncles, cousins, family friends, classmates and other children, community members and members of the hospital staff. All of this shared caregiving can both mitigate and potentially complicate the caregiving responsibilities. It can be difficult for those who "care" about the family to know how to lessen the burden of caregiving on the parents. Responsibilities can include making meals, caring for siblings, taking responsibilities for pets, transportation, fundraising, listening, companioning, providing respite, watering plants, or actually becoming involved in treatment.

MEDICAL CAREGIVING

There are many different types of care that are necessary for a child with cancer to undergo treatment and maintain emotional and physical health. First, parents participate in medical caregiving that can include medical tasks at home such as changing dressings, administering medicines, cleaning medical equipment, and responding to the debilitating side effects of treatment. Some of the medical care expected of parents is quite high tech and complicated: drawing blood from portable catheters inserted under the skin, assessing the child's medical status, and administering a variety of specific and potentially harmful medicines. Another form of medical caregiving involves transporting the child to clinic visits sometimes daily and providing support during medical procedures including intravenous chemotherapy, radiation, blood draws, spinal taps, and bone marrow aspirations.

When the child is inpatient at the hospital, the parent is usually at the bedside for the entire admission and will accompany the child to all scheduled treatment and medical appointments, consult with the medical team, and constantly monitor the physical and emotional well-being of the child. This type of caregiving can be particularly exhausting for parents who may neglect their own needs for rest, nutrition, personal hygiene, and support due to the demands of inpatient stays. Parents may also feel conflicted by the other "normal" caregiving duties that they usually perform at home with their other children, as a spouse/partner, as a community member, and as an employee. Inpatient stays are an opportunity for the caregiving network to participate in either the hospital or home needs of the family. Social workers can facilitate this arrangement for families who may be too exhausted and or uncomfortable to ask others to create a circle of care for them while their child is in the hospital.

PARENTAL ROLES AND CAREGIVING

Because of societal expectations and typical familial roles, childhood cancer may serve to entrench gender-prescribed roles for fathers and mothers (Young et al., 2002). In most cases, mothers are providing the bulk of the caregiving and letting go of other aspects of their lives to focus on the child in treatment. Mothers of children with cancer report that the caregiving role is extensive and involves a complex set of tasks in order to ensure their will maintain health and well-being (ibid.). In a recent study, mothers indicated that they reorganize their lives in order to maintain proximity as a way to "keep watch" and provide "comfort" during their child's hospital stays (ibid.). This proximity allows mothers little time for self-care and for care of others in the family, especially other children. Proximity is an area of caregiving that is perceived as comforting to the mothers as they fulfill their socially-sanctioned role as protectors of their children (ibid.).

However, some aspects of caregiving for children with cancer are more complicated and stressful for mothers. Issues of treatment compliance places mothers in the difficult emotional bind of knowing that in order for their child to be successful in treatment, the mother must ensure their child's cooperation with medical procedures and treatments which are unpleasant or painful (ibid.). Maintaining a child with cancer's physical well-being takes on new significance as mothers must work diligently to prevent infections while their child is immuno-compromised from chemotherapy and try to ensure adequate nutrition and rest under less than ideal circumstances (ibid.).

According to recent studies, the healthcare system reinforces the traditional roles for fathers and mothers (Faulkner, 1995). This gendering of parental roles can leave fathers in a uniquely different bind as caregivers. They may have less day-to-day information and involvement in their child's care and feel disenfranchised from the healthcare team and/or from their child and spouse. Fathers may feel burdened to maintain or increase the financial caregiving responsibilities for the family. Fathers may feel that they must put on the "public face" and cannot express their emotional responses to their child's illness. Health professionals may be unclear as to how to interact with the father and communicate less information to him, making the father feel more alienated from the experience of his child. Further, strict socially-defined gender roles can be changed in our society when fathers take on the primary caregiving role and are the parent at the bedside. Hospital and healthcare professionals need to remain open to the variety of family structures in modern society that can include non-traditional roles for spouses, single-headed households, blended families, gay and lesbian families, and intergenerational caregiving structures including grandparent-led families.

EMOTIONAL CAREGIVING

From the moment of diagnosis, the child with cancer needs emotional support, developmentally appropriate information, reassurances of safety, and expressions of love and companionship (Jones, 2006; Cincotta, 2004). Providing emotional caregiving is a continuous, complex, and changing task of those who care for the child with cancer. Children are confronted with many new and frightening experiences during their treatment including new surroundings, isolation from peers, extensive hospital stays, developmentally incongruent fears of death, worry about their parents and siblings, painful procedures, difficult and sometimes debilitating treatment, and a general lack of fun and enjoyable childhood activities (Jones, 2006; Cincotta, 2004; Wolfe et al., 2000).

Children's emotional responses can include intense expressions of fear, confusion, loneliness, anger, hopelessness, joy, hope, love, pride, sadness, and a myriad of other emotions. Mothers of children with cancer describe the emotional work of caregiving as intense and complex (Young et al., 2002). Emotional caregiving tasks seem to fall into two categories: managing emotions or communicating with children about what is happening (ibid.). At a time when they are emotionally devastated, mothers must manage their own emotions while trying to support their child. Mothers of children with cancer accomplish this by trying to bolster the child's spirits through positive attitude, establishing "normal" routines, protecting the child's identity, using distraction, and prevention of psychological distress (ibid.). Mothers are also placed in the very conflicting role of having to give their child "bad" news about diagnosis, treatment, hospital stays, and prognosis (ibid.).

Siblings of children with cancer need support for their unique experiences and simultaneously need opportunities to be a caregiver when desired. It is well documented that siblings of children with cancer often have their emotional needs overlooked during the usually extended treatment time (Ballard, 2004; Davies, 1999). Siblings' needs include but are not limited to: reassurance about the health of their sibling, their parents and themselves, opportunities to play and be "normal," information and control, opportunities to express their own feelings including guilt, anger, and resentment, inclusion in the process of care, and social and emotional support for their experiences (Ballard, 2004; Cincotta, 2004; Davies, 1999; Faulkner et al., 1995; Jones, 2006; Martinson et al., 1990). Because siblings typically feel disenfranchised from the care of their brother or sister, they should be given opportunities to participate in caregiving. Siblings can assist in emotional support, activities of daily living, and in some physical caregiving when appropriate. Including siblings as part of the care team of the child with cancer can potentially reduce their feelings of isolation, helplessness, and confusion and respond to siblings' needs for inclusion, information and control.

Medical caregivers such as physicians, nurses, social workers, and child life specialists can assist parents in these caregiving roles through a variety of interventions. Social workers and child life specialists are particularly well-trained to offer the child opportunities to experience the "normal" activities of childhood through play, organizing visits from friends, facilitating connections with other children who are also undergoing cancer treatment, and working with the medical team to allow the child to be able to participate in important activities such as school, field trips, proms, and outings with other children (Jones, 2006).

Children are notorious for protecting their parents from their emotional distress when they are facing a life-threatening condition (Cincotta, 2004;

Jones & Weisenfluh, 2003). Skilled practitioners who can help the child work through the emotions they experience through talk and play therapies will serve as important caregiving allies in the medical setting. Pediatric oncology social workers report that they see the most important part of their role as listening to the child's expression of feelings (Jones, 2005). Doctors and nurses can care for children's emotional needs by providing gentle and developmentally-appropriate medical information throughout care. Mothers report that having hospital staff who are skilled at communicating with children alleviates some of the emotional caregiving burden they may experience (Young et al., 2002). Healthcare professionals also have an important role in helping both the child and the family understand the experiences of children with illness. However, it is important to remember that parents also need to be able to provide support for their child, and the parental role should be augmented, not replaced, by medical caregivers.

In addition to parents and medical caregivers, other family and community members serve important roles in the care of children's emotional needs. Grandparents, in particular, may provide emotional, physical, spiritual, and medical caregiving for the child with cancer. Sometimes the grandparent is the person who brings the child to treatment and sees them through their care. Often, children report that they can talk easily to their grandparents about what their true concerns are because of the unique grandparent-grandchild bond.

Grandparents can be a very important part of the medical-familial team that will provide care and make informed medical decisions. Grandparents are usually torn between their concerns about their grandchild and their concerns about their own child who is experiencing the pain of being a parent of a child with cancer. Grandparents can be critical caregivers by providing support to emotionally-isolated siblings seeking an adult to invest in their life experience. Because of the multiple caregiving roles of grandparents, they can easily feel overwhelmed, helpless, and frightened. Grandparents should receive specific attention and intervention from the psychosocial healthcare providers as they are at risk for intense caregiver burden.

END-OF-LIFE CAREGIVING

When a child is facing the end of life, the role of caregiver for the parent takes on new meaning. Parents often experience their child's impending death as a parental failure to protect their child from harm (Cincotta, 2004; Young et al., 2002). Despite knowing objectively that the child's illness and death is not their fault, the socially-constructed parental role can cause parents to feel culpability in their inability to stop the child from dying. Consequently, parents of children dying from cancer must be allowed opportunities to continue "caring" and "caregiving" for their child. Allowing parents a significant role in physical and medical care can provide them with opportunities to continue this aspect of parenting (Cincotta, 2004). Parents of dying children have many tasks that are part of their caregiving role. These tasks include emotional and spiritual support, advocacy for adequate pain and symptom management, control of amount of stimulation and activity, physical caregiving, and expressions of love and affection and comfort (Jones, 2005; 2006; Cincotta, 2004; Contro, 2002).

THE RESILIENCE OF CAREGIVERS OF CHILDREN WITH CANCER

It is almost impossible to imagine the full magnitude of the impact of a child's cancer diagnosis on the family. Yet, despite the financial, emotional, spiritual, and physical challenges of caring for a child with cancer, many families manage to re-establish a new sense of normalcy and routine. In this "new normal," the family miraculously responds to the ever-changing and often conflicting demands of the medical treatment and family member's health and well-being. This resilience is not often studied and deserves special recognition in understanding caregivers of children with life-threatening conditions. Most studies of caregivers of children with illness have focused on the burden of care for the family. While caring for a child with cancer does present cumulative and ongoing pressure to respond to extensive needs, recent studies have begun to show that parents are successful caregivers and may benefit from the opportunity to provide care (Moore & Beckwitt, 2004; Young et al., 2002; Norberg, 2004).

Concepts of self-care and dependent care are aspects of caregiving frequently discussed in nursing literature as tasks that used to be optional but have now become essential parts of patient care and successful outcome of treatment (Dodd & Miaskowski, 2000). Using Orem's theory of self-care (2001), Moore and Beckwitt (2004) studied self care and dependent care practices of children with cancer and their parents and found that they were "competent agents" of care in the arenas of universal and developmental self care requisites. In care related to healthcare deviation requisites, parents and children performed fewer tasks but still performed well (Moore & Beckwitt, 2004). In universal self-care requisites (Orem, 2001), parents provided dependent care activities related to feeding, activity, rest, normalcy, solitude, social interaction, and hazards (Moore & Beckwitt, 2004). Parents encouraged children to eat, facilitated and monitored activity and rest levels, provided opportunities for social interaction and friendship, protected children as best they could from the hazards of treatment, and made great efforts to foster a sense of normalcy for the child (Moore & Beckwitt, 2004).

In the area of developmental self-care requisites (Orem, 2001), parents provided support, encouragement, continuous presence, vigilance about medical care, opportunities for the child to have some control and power, and provision of services to build academic and social skills. In the area of health deviation self-care requisites (Orem, 2001), parents worked to obtain appropriate healthcare from the initial attempts to secure the correct diagnosis throughout treatment, dealt with negative effects of therapy, provided opportunities for the child to build a new positive self concept, and provided follow-up care to prepare for survivorship (Moore & Beckwitt, 2004).

Families faced with a child with a life-threatening condition do mobilize internal and external strengths to cope with the profound challenges placed before them. Families sometimes adapt by using coping mechanisms and internal resources that they have enlisted in other times of crisis. However, they may also discover familial and community sources of resilience that were previously unknown to them. Understanding familial belief systems, organizational patterns, and communication processes is essential to fostering family resilience in the face of the crisis of a child's life-threatening illness (Walsh, 1998).

FOSTERING FAMILY STRENGTHS AND RESILIENCE

A family resilience perspective is critically helpful in clinical practice with children with cancer because it honors and builds upon the inherent strength of the family in crisis (Greene, 2002). As in a family systems model (see Chapter 1), a family resilience perspective recognizes that when a child is diagnosed with cancer; the entire family is diagnosed, transformed, and ultimately challenged to adapt to the new world (Jones & Weisenfluh, 2003). When viewing childhood cancer as a family disease, the entire family system must be mobilized to foster future functioning regardless of medical outcome.

Families are expected to provide caregiving that is understood as part of normal family development and expectations. As discussed in the functional-age model of intergenerational therapy (FAM), caregiving of an older family member may be a socially expected role. However, caregiving of a child with a life-threatening condition is a non-normative event in the life of the family. Because it is unexpected and traumatic, the family may not be able to readily access their usual adaptive capacity and can be assisted by social workers who can work with the family to identify ways to strengthen resilience and coping.

Walsh (1998, 2003) has delineated a family resilience framework another family therapy model that can be helpful in assisting families facing this crisis. According to Walsh (1998, 2003), the key processes of family resilience occur in three domains of the family life: (1) family belief systems, (2) organizational patterns, and (3) communication and problem-solving. Each of these areas has significant relevance to how a family will respond to the crisis of childhood cancer and how social workers can facilitate family strength and cohesion.

Families come to the crisis of childhood illness with the set of beliefs that have been useful (or not) to them. These beliefs impact how they will approach the diagnosis, treatment, and subsequent outcome of treatment. Familial beliefs are not always shared, such that the child may have a different outlook from the parent, or parents may not agree. Nonetheless, Walsh (1998, 2003) indicates that the belief systems that can enhance family functioning are *making meaning of adversity, positive outlook, and transcendence and spirituality.* For the family of the child with cancer, these belief systems are closely interrelated. First, there many distinct moments at which a family may "make meaning" of childhood cancer. One of the most critical of these, with potential for socially-constructed meaning, is at diagnosis when the family may view cancer as a tremendous but surmountable challenge that will bring them closer together or as a hopeless situation that they cannot handle. At the very first moment of diagnosis, most families experience a range of emotions that may incorporate both hopelessness and determination.

However, the family's belief system about the meaning of adversity in life will likely orient their response to this medical information (ibid.). Additionally, their sense of spirituality and hope will also impact the meaning-making process. One father, when repeatedly confronted with the news that his child had a 1% chance of survival, challenged the medical staff, "How do we know that my child is not the 1%?" This "optimistic bias," as Walsh (1998) would call it, was largely informed by this father's spiritual faith and sense of hope in the future. Medical providers can assist family belief systems by presenting factual information in a culturally congruent way, offering realistic hope, and providing families with the encouragement that they can get through this together. In addition, families' concerns about the cause of their child's cancer can also be alleviated by acknowledgement that, unlike some adult cancers, childhood cancer is not caused by lifestyle choices. Social workers can enhance family belief systems by reflecting on the strengths of the family, giving the family opportunities for social action, and by sharing success stories of families who have successfully coped and even grown through the experience of their child's cancer.

Another key process of family resilience comes in the *organizational patterns* of the family such as *flexibility, connectedness,* and *social and economic resources* (Walsh, 1998, 2003). For families of a child with cancer, the ability to adapt and be responsive to change is an essential part of getting through the rigorous treatments and constant demands on the family. Caregiving responsibilities will change as the treatment changes according the protocol. One month, a family might be faced with daily clinic visits followed by extreme physical and emotional side effects. The next month's treatment could be all outpatient and be less frequent and less intense. The family's ability to respond to these differing needs will be a predictor of their emotional health.

Social workers can facilitate strong family functioning in this area by predicting and preparing families for the trajectory of care and assisting them in creating a plan to handle each part of the treatment regimen. Flexibility in family roles and responsibilities is an important component of the family's resilience. Family roles will often need to be re-negotiated, and the new role of "parent of a child with cancer" or "sibling of a child with cancer" will have to be accommodated into the full functioning of the family system. Most families show remarkable resilience in their ability to be flexible to the treatment demands while remaining connected to each other.

Another aspect of family resilience is identifying and utilizing *social and economic resources* (Walsh, 1998, 2003). For family caregivers of children with cancer, this is an area that is particularly challenged by the onset of the disease. Existing financial resources are hindered by a number of factors. If both parents are employed, caring for the child may require one of them to leave their job thus significantly reducing the family income. Single parents are unable to leave their jobs due to the need for both income and health insurance for treatment. This can put single parents in a significant emotional struggle as they wish to provide full-time caregiving to their child but cannot afford to do so.

Families also experience expenses that they previously did not have, including but not limited to: transportation to/from the hospital, parking fees that can be $10/day in some places, the expense of meals at the hospital, and fees for services to provide extra childcare, household care, or pet care while the parent is in the hospital. If the child needs to travel for treatment, the family may have to relocate to another city for a period of time. Social workers can facilitate financial stability by connecting with the many financial assistance programs at the federal, state, community and hospital level to help families of children with cancer. In addition to economic resources, families need social resources to enhance their own resilience when a child is sick.

Walsh (1998, 2003) identifies a number of strategies for strengthening social resources: *mobilizing extended kin and social support, recruiting mentors*, and *building vital community networks*. Each of these strategies can be employed by families facing the crisis of childhood cancer. Extended kin and social support such as aunts, uncles, grandparents, neighbors, friends, faith community members, and members of the school can all be given parts of the caregiving duties of the family. Tasks that can help include setting up an information line for updates, caring for siblings, providing meals and/or transportation, providing visits in the hospital to give the primary caregiver respite or company, cleaning the home, caring for pets, and so on. Mentors are often found in the form of other parents. Social workers can introduce parents of children with cancer to other parents who have been through the disease to assist in creating this kind of community network for families.

One of the most important aspects of family resilience for families facing childhood cancer is *communication processes* and *problem-solving* (Walsh 1998, 2003). Healthcare practitioners should facilitate families' understanding and informed decision-making by providing clear messages that do not confuse the family (Contro, 2002). In fact, Walsh (1998, 2003) identifies *clarity* in the form of *clear, consistent messages* and *truth-speaking* as essential parts of family resilience. In order for families to have clarity and honesty with each other and the child, they need that quality of information from the healthcare providers.

Walsh (1998, 2003) also discusses the importance of *open emotional expression* for families to function at their highest level. This can be particularly challenging for the family caregivers of a child with cancer. Each member of the family may be experiencing many intense and conflicting emotions simultaneously and while under the watchful gaze of the healthcare team. Parents and children may try to protect each other from the intensity of their own emotions. This can set up a painful situation in which no one is fully able to express their emotions. However, pediatric oncology social workers identify "listening to fears and feelings" as a critical task in their role with children and families (Jones, 2005). And families report that they want their healthcare providers to listen to them and help them with the emotions of childhood illness (Contro, 2002). Ideally, the social worker would facilitate the family's ability to share not only with the practitioners but with each other. These sessions can allow for the full range of emotions to be shared in a way that clears the air and creates mutual empathy and trust. Families also need opportunities for humor, laughter, love, and other pleasurable interactions with each other (Walsh, 1998, 2003; Jones, 2006).

One final aspect of communication as a key to family resilience is *collaborative problem-solving* (Walsh, 1998, 2003). Medical decision-making for families of children with cancer is potentially very loaded with fear and uncertainty. Additionally, families report that they need more involvement, information, and control in the treatment decisions regarding their child with cancer (Contro, 2002; Cincotta, 2004; Jones, 2005). Children, too, may want to participate in the decisions related to their care, and social workers may find themselves helping to negotiate between the family and the medical team, or the family and the child (Jones, 2006). Together, children, families, and healthcare teams can enhance family functioning by sharing in power and decision-making.

CONCLUSION: CARING FOR THE CAREGIVER

Finally, while it is important to honor the strengths of families facing childhood cancer, programs and interventions that address the burden of caring should continue to be developed and enhanced. The diagnosis of childhood cancer comes with enormous emotional, financial, physical, social, and spiritual challenges and consequences. Families cannot handle the burden in isolation. Families need respite, financial assistance, emotional support, skills-based teaching, and at-home nursing care. Perhaps the most important need of the caregiver of the child with cancer is compassion and someone to witness their experience.

REFERENCES

Ballard, K.L. (2004). Meeting the needs of siblings of children with cancer. *Pediatric Nursing.* 30 (5) 394-401.

Bowman, K., Lindahl, A. & Bjork, O. (2003). Disease-related distress in parents of children with cancer at various stages after the time of diagnosis. *Acta Oncologica,* 42, pp.137-146.

Cincotta, N. (2004). The end of life at the beginning of life: Working with dying children and their families. In J. Berzoff & P. R. Silverman (Eds.), *Living with Dying: A handbook for end-of-life healthcare practitioners* (pp. 318-347). New York: Columbia University Press.

Contro, N., Larson J., Scofield, S., Sourkes, B., & Cohen, H. (2002). Family perspectives on the quality of pediatric palliative care. *Archives of Pediatrics and Adolescent Medicine, 156*(1), 14-19.

Contro, N., Larson, J., Scofield, S., Sourkes, B., & Cohen, H. (2004). Hospital staff and family perspectives regarding quality of pediatric palliative care. *Pediatrics, 114* (5), 1248-1252.

Davies, B. (1999). *Shadows in the sun: Experiences of sibling bereavement in childhood.* Philadelphia, PA: Brunner/Mazel.

Dodd, M.J., & Miaskowski, C, (2000). The PRO-SELF program: A self-care intervention program for patients receiving cancer treatment. *Seminars in Oncology Nursing, 16*(4), 300-308.

Faulkner, A., Peace, G., & O'Keefe, C. (1995). *When a child has cancer.* London: Chapman and Hall.

Greene, R.R. (Ed.). (2002). *Resilience: An Integrated Approach to Practice, Policy, and Research.* Washington, DC: NASW Press.

Hewitt, M., Weiner, S.L. & Simone, J.V. (2004). *Childhood Cancer Survivorship: Improving Care and Quality of Life.* Washington, DC: Institute of Medicine, National Academy of Science.

Hoekstra-Weebers, J.E.H.M, Jaspers, J.P.C., Kamps, W.A. & Klip, C. E. (1999). Risk factors for psychological maladjustment of parents of children with cancer. *Journal of the American Academy of Child and Adolescent Psychiatry, 38,* 1526-1535.

Hoekstra-Weebers, J.E.H.M, Jaspers, J.P.C., Kamps, W.A. & Klip, C. E. (2001). Psychological adaptation and social support of parents of pediatric cancer patients: A prospective longitudinal study. *Journal of Pediatric Psychology, 26,* 225-235.

Insook, C. (July, 2004). Initiative for Pediatric Palliative Care Faculty Development Workshop Proceedings. Boston, MA.

Jones, B., & Weisenfluh, S. (2003). Pediatric palliative and end-of-life care: Developmental and spiritual issues of dying children. *Smith College Studies in Social Work: Special Issue on End-of-Life Care, 73*(3).

Jones, B. (2005). Pediatric Palliative and End-of-Life Care: The Role of Social Work in Pediatric Oncology. *Journal of Social Work in End-of-Life & Palliative Care, 1*(4) 35-62.

Jones, B. (2006). Companionship, control and compassion: The psychosocial needs of children and families at the end of life–A social work perspective. *Journal of Pallia-*

tive Medicine Special Series on Social Work in End of Life, G. Christ & S. Blacker (Eds.), *9*(3) 774-788.

Kazak, A.E., Stuber, M.L., Barakat, L.P., Meeske, K., Guthrie, D., & Meadows, A. T. (1998). Predicting posttraumatic stress symptoms in mothers and fathers of survivors of childhood cancer. *Journal of American Academy of Child and Adolescent Psychiatry, 37,* 823-831.

Manne, S., Duhamel, K., & Redd, W.H. (2000). Association of psychological vulnerability factors to post-traumatic stress symptomatology in mothers of pediatric cancer survivors. *Psycho-Oncology, 9,* 372-384.

Martinson, I.M., Gillis, C., Coughlin, Colaizzo, D., Freeman, M., & Bossert, E. (1990). Impact of childhood cancer on healthy school-age siblings. *Cancer Nursing, 13*(3), 183-190.

McCubbin, M.A. & McCubbin, H.I., (1996). Resiliency in families: A conceptual model of family adjustment and adaptation in response to stress and crises. In H. I. McCubbin, A.I. Thompson, & M.A. McCubbin (Eds.), *Family Assessment: Resiliency, Coping and Adaptation, Inventories for Research and Practice* (pp. 1-64). Madison: University of Wisconsin Press.

Moore, J.B., & Beckwitt, A.E. (2004). Children with cancer and their parents: Self-care and dependent-care practices. *Issues in Comprehensive Pediatric Nursing. 27,* 1-17.

National Cancer Institute. (2002). *Cancer facts: National Cancer Institute research on childhood cancers* [on-line]. Available: http://cis.nci.nih.gov/fact/6_40.htm.

National Cancer Institute President's Cancer Panel 2003-2004 Annual Report (2004). *Living beyond cancer: Finding a new balance.* U.S. Department of Health and Human Services National Institutes of Health.

Norberg, A.L., Lindblad, F., & Bowman, K.K. (2004). Coping strategies in parents of children with cancer. *Social Science and Medicine, 60,* 965-975.

Orem, D.E. (2001). *Nursing: Concepts of practice* (6th ed.). St. Louis, MO: Mosby.

Rando, T. (1993). Treatment of Complicated Mourning. Champaign, IL: Research Press.

Ries, L.A.G., Smith, M.A., Gurney, J.G., Linet, M., Tamra, T., Young, J.L., Bunin, G.R. (Eds.). *Cancer incidence and survival among children and adolescents: United States SEER Program 1975-1995,* National Cancer Institute, SEER Program. National Institutes of Health Pub. No. 99-4649. Bethesda, MD, 1999.

Sahler, O.J., Roghmann, K.J., Carpenter, P.J., Mulhern, R.K., Dolgin, M.J., Sargent, J.R., Barbarian, O.A., Copeland, D.R., & Zeltzer L.K. (1994). Sibling adaptation to childhood cancer collaborative study: Prevalence of sibling distress and definition of adaptation levels. *Journal of Developmental and Behavioural Pediatrics, 15(5),* 353-366.

Svavarsdottir, E.K. (2005). Caring for a child with cancer: A longitudinal perspective. *Journal of Advanced Nursing, 50(2),* 153-161.

Tervalon, M. & Murray-Garcia, J. (1998). Cultural humility versus cultural competence: A critical distinction in defining physician training outcomes in multicultural education. *Journal of Healthcare for the Poor and Underserved, 9(2),* 117-124.

Van Dongen-Melman, J.E.W.M., Van Zuuren, F.J. & Verhulst, F.C. (1998). Experiences of parents of childhood cancer survivors: A qualitative analysis. *Patient Education and Counseling, 34,* 185-200.

Walsh, F. (1998). Strengthening Family Resilience. New York: Guilford Press.

Walsh, F. (2003). Family Resilience: A framework for clinical practice. *Family Process, 42(1)*, 1-18.

Wolfe, J., Grier, H., Klar, N., Salem-Schatz, S., Ellenbogen, J.M., Levin, S.B., Emanuel, E.J., & Weeks, J.C. (2000) Symptoms and suffering at the end of life in children with cancer. *New England Journal of Medicine, 342(5)*, 326-333.

Young, B., Dixon-Woods, M., Findlay, M., Heney, D. (2002). Parenting in a crisis: Conceptualising mothers of children with cancer. *Social Science and Medicine, 55*, 1835-1847.

Young, B., Dixon-Woods, M., & Heney, D. (2002). Identity and role in parenting a child with cancer. *Pediatric Rehabilitation, 5(4)*, 209-214.

doi:10.1300/J137v14n01_11

Chapter 12

Families Caring for Persons with HIV/AIDS

Laura M. Hopson

SUMMARY. The extent to which family members are willing and able to assist with daily activities and provide emotional support can greatly affect the quality of life for persons with chronic illness. In the case of HIV/AIDS, the burdens of symptom management and medication are amplified by social stigma. This chapter provides a summary of the physical, psychological, social, and spiritual issues associated with HIV/AIDS along with approaches to assessment and treatment. doi:10.1300/J137v14n01_12 *[Article copies available for a fee from The Haworth Document Delivery Service: 1-800-HAWORTH. E-mail address: <docdelivery@haworthpress.com> Website: <http://www.HaworthPress.com> © 2006 by The Haworth Press, Inc. All rights reserved.]*

KEYWORDS. HIV/AIDS, family care, stigma

Persons living with chronic illness face many challenges in their everyday lives such as pain, fatigue, and complicated medication regimens. Their families must often learn to cope with these challenges as well. The extent to which family members are willing and able to assist with daily activities and provide emotional support can greatly affect the quality of life for persons with chronic illness. In the case of HIV/AIDS, the burdens

[Haworth co-indexing entry note]: "Families Caring for Persons with HIV/AIDS." Hopson, Laura M. Co-published simultaneously in *Journal of Human Behavior in the Social Environment* (The Haworth Press, Inc.) Vol. 14, No. 1/2, 2006, pp. 241-258; and: *Contemporary Issues of Care* (ed: Roberta R. Greene) The Haworth Press, Inc., 2006, pp. 241-258. Single or multiple copies of this article are available for a fee from The Haworth Document Delivery Service [1-800-HAWORTH, 9:00 a.m. - 5:00 p.m. (EST). E-mail address: docdelivery@haworthpress.com].

of symptom management and medication are amplified by social stigma. This stigma creates emotional stress and feelings of isolation that may, in turn, suppress physical health. Because of the complex array of social and emotional issues that accompany a diagnosis of HIV/AIDS, the Functional-Age Model of Family Treatment is especially useful in integrating various aspects of assessment and care. This chapter provides a summary of the physical, psychological, social, and spiritual issues associated with HIV/AIDS along with approaches to assessment and treatment that are consistent with the Functional-Age Model.

PREVALENCE OF HIV/AIDS

More than 750,000 Americans are living with HIV or AIDS (Centers for Disease Control and Prevention [CDC], 2003). The majority of HIV positive males over the age of 13 identify themselves as men who have sex with men. Most females over the age of 13 living with HIV/AIDS were infected through heterosexual contact (CDC, 2003). The primary modes of transmission of HIV are through intravenous drug use and sexual intercourse. During recent years, the number of AIDS cases among intravenous drug users has decreased while the number of those exposed through heterosexual contact has increased. AIDS affects women and minorities at an increasingly disproportionate rate. Although the number of AIDS cases among men has grown 1% between 1999 and 2003, the number of cases among women increased 13% during the same amount of time. AIDS cases among Whites have decreased while increasing among blacks, Hispanics, Asians, and Native Americans (CDC, 2003). An increasing number of parents infected with HIV calls for approaches to treatment that consider the needs of the entire family. These parents are coping with the stressors of parenting as they struggle to live with difficult symptoms of the disease and complicated treatment regimens. Families need help coping with negative social attitudes and discrimination that often accompany an HIV diagnosis (Lee & Rotheram-Borus, 2003; Mok & Cooper, 1997).

THE FUNCTIONAL AGE MODEL: ASSESSMENT

The functional age model encourages the practitioner to plan assessment and intervention by conceptualizing the family as a system in which members have reciprocal roles. The individual is viewed within the context of biopsychosocial functioning. Using the model, the practitioner works to understand an individual's functional age by assessing biological, psychological, social, and spiritual aspects of functioning. The practitioner also assesses the functioning and development of the family system and surrounding social support network. As HIV affects the health of the individual, it also changes family functioning by altering family roles and adding a great deal of stress to family members' daily lives.

An assessment of individuals with HIV/AIDS and their families should include information about physical and psychological functioning, social support, and spirituality. Because HIV/AIDS transmission is associated with risky sexual activity and drug use, those with HIV/AIDS feel stigmatized and ashamed of the diagnosis. As a result, HIV positive individuals are often reluctant to disclose their diagnosis to friends and even family members. In conducting an assessment, it is critical that the practitioner understand who knows about the HIV/AIDS.

Biological Age and HIV/AIDS

According to the Functional Age Model, biological age is understood as a combination of factors that change physical functioning over time. This is important for those living with HIV, because the disease affects the immune system and increases susceptibility to opportunistic infections. The biological age of those with HIV varies because they may experience periods of health followed by periods of acute illness (Greene, Kropf, & McNair, 1994).

Advances in medication during the past decade such as the introduction of antiretroviral therapy (ART) have increased the life span and improved the quality of life for many living with HIV/AIDS. Physical functioning may vary widely based on response to medication regimens, nutrition, physical activity, and other factors associated with a healthy lifestyle. It is therefore important to include an assessment of physical functioning to understand the impact that HIV/AIDS may have on families. Although medications have greatly improved health and life expectancy, they also have troubling side effects. ARTs may cause nausea, headaches, skin rashes, and diarrhea (AIDS Education & Training Centers National Resource Center, 2005). For those living with HIV/AIDS, it is often difficult to distinguish between symptoms of the illness and side effects from the medications. A physical assessment should include questions about medication because the side effects can affect quality of life and can cause individuals to stop taking medications at all. Compliance with medications is critical because many researchers estimate that the medications lose effectiveness when they are not taken correctly at least 95% of the time (Paterson et al., 2000).

Fatigue is commonly associated with HIV along with fever, oral lesions, skin rashes, and diarrhea (UNAIDS, 2005). Fatigue may cause individuals to reduce their activity level, which can lead to even greater weakness and fatigue compounded by additional problems such as depression (Nokes & Kendrew, 2001). In order to understand an individual's physical functioning, it is important for a practitioner to assess areas relevant to a healthy lifestyle. HIV positive individuals who maintain a healthy lifestyle including good nutrition and regular physical activity are likely to sleep better, have improved stamina and less fatigue, and fewer depressive symptoms (Neidig, Smith, & Brashers, 2003).

An assessment of the family's response to changes in physical functioning can help the practitioner determine how well the family is coping and how much support they are giving to the person with HIV. Families may be overwhelmed by health problems that inhibit the ability to perform regular activities and thereby cause a shift in family roles. A mother with HIV, for example, may need to rely on other family members for child care responsibilities when her health wavers. The quality of family support can greatly affect quality of life and health.

Psychological Age and HIV/AIDS

Psychological age, according to the Functional Age Model, is concerned with an individual's adaptation to changes. In the case of HIV/AIDS, psychological age is in part determined by an individual's ability to cope with stressors and whether symptoms of depression and anxiety are present. A diagnosis of HIV may cause individuals and their families to cope with the death of a family member earlier than they would have expected. Such stressors can make it difficult for families to adapt in the face of an HIV diagnosis (Greene, Kropf, & MacNair, 1994).

As with other chronic illness, the psychological effects of HIV/AIDS are closely connected with the physical effects. Those living with HIV/AIDS often suffer from fatigue and sleeplessness, which can amplify physical symptoms of HIV/AIDS (Barroso, Carlson, & Meynell, 2003; Sullivan & Dworkin, 2003). Depression is associated with poor adherence to medication for youth and adults infected with HIV (Barfod et al., 2005; Hosek, Harper, & Domanico, 2005; Lee & Rotheram-Borus, 2003). Among women, depression is associated with more severe symptoms and increases in AIDS related deaths (Cook et al., 2004). Living with the illness causes a great deal of stress for both the individual and family. Research indicates that parents with HIV who experience reductions in anxiety and depression over time after their diagnosis survive longer than those who do not experience such decreases (Lee & Rotheram-Borus, 2003).

Effects of HIV/AIDS on Social Relationships

An individual's social age is defined as the ability to carry out social roles and participate as part of a social network. Determining the strength and size of social networks is critical when a family is coping with HIV/AIDS. Family values, ethnicity, age, income, and education help to shape an individual's social age. The stigma associated with HIV often serves as a barrier to creating healthy social networks and can affect almost every aspect of daily life, including employment, friendships, and family relationships (Greene, Kropf, & MacNair, 1994).

A diagnosis of HIV/AIDS has many social and cultural implications. Among women newly diagnosed with HIV, many have young children and low income (CDC, 2003; Ball, Tannenbaum, Armistead, & Maguen, 2002). It is important to assess the quality of a support network because those who have resources, such as higher income, social support, and a health provider, are more likely to lead a healthy lifestyle than those with few resources. A healthier lifestyle can improve quality of life and functioning for persons with HIV and alleviate some of the stress on their family, as well.

Social support is a critical resource for those diagnosed with HIV. The benefits of social support for those living with HIV include improved emotional well-being and physical health, including slowing the progression of the disease (Leslie, Stein, & Rotheram-Borus, 2002). HIV positive women with fewer people in their social support network report poorer physical functioning and quality of life than those with larger support networks. In addition, those who have few people they can rely on when they need help with money or a place to stay report poorer mental health and quality of life (Gielen, McDonnell, Wu, O'Campo, & Faden, 2001). Social support also has implications for physical functioning. Women with poor social support reported experiencing more pain (Cowdery & Pesa, 2002).

Although the family serves as the primary support network in many cases, friends may play a more important role for others. Many gay men living with HIV regard friends and partners as their primary support system. This support system is often more important than the biological family (Bor, du Pleissis, & Russell, 2004). For this reason, the practitioner needs to understand the individual's definition of family and support network. It may be more helpful to include some friends in family treatment than some family members. Research indicates the importance of social support for gay men with HIV/AIDS. Social support is associated with decreased anxiety, depression, better coping, and fewer symptoms (Leslie, Stein, & Rotheram-Borus, 2002).

In some cases, the caregiver for an HIV positive partner in a gay or bisexual relationship may also be positive. Research indicates that in this case, caregivers who are also HIV positive experience more stress and symptoms of depression than HIV negative caregivers. For this reason, teaching stress management skills may be critical for caregivers in a gay or bisexual relationship, especially if the caregiver is also HIV positive (Land, Hudson, & Stiefel, 2003).

Stigma is related to social support and greatly affects daily life for those living with HIV and their families. Because HIV carries great social stigma, those living with the illness may be reluctant to disclose the diagnosis, thereby limiting the number of people they can turn to for social support. Individuals living with HIV/AIDS report more feelings of stigma than those living with other chronic illnesses. Culture may affect how individuals respond to a diagnosis of HIV/AIDS. In some cultures, the diagnosis may be more stigmatized than others. Religious and spiritual views also affect perceptions about the illness (Miller & Murray, 1999). Behaviors that place an individual at high risk for HIV are unprotected sexual intercourse, having multiple sexual partners, drug use, and combining drug use with sexual activity (Joshi, Hser, Grella, & Houlton, 2001). Because these behaviors are associated with HIV-risk, those who are diagnosed with HIV/AIDS may feel ashamed and stigmatized. They may feel guilt about the way they contracted the illness. Those experiencing more severe symptoms report more perceived stigma, possibly because it is more difficult to conduct daily activities, resulting in greater feelings of isolation and rejection (Fife & Wright, 2000).

Research suggests that stigma has a negative effect on adjustment and quality of life (Brashers et al., 1998). Negative social attitudes about the modes of HIV transmission may foster feelings of shame and isolation for families. Another fear associated with stigma is that of losing a job or a friend if the diagnosis is disclosed. Unfortunately, such fears are sometimes warranted because of social attitudes about those who carry the diagnosis and misperceptions about HIV transmission that leads to fear about working in close proximity with an HIV positive person.

Feeling stigmatized or discriminated against can have serious psychological and physical implications. Stigma causes a great deal of stress for those living with HIV/AIDS and their families (Greene, Kropf, & MacNair, 1994). Feelings of discrimination have been associated with poorer perceptions of health and experiencing more pain (Cowdery & Pesa, 2002). The feelings of rejection and social isolation that accompany stigmatization often result in feelings of low self-worth (Fife & Wright, 2000). It has also been associated with symptoms of depression (Berger, Ferrans, & Lashley, 2001). Women living with HIV report feeling that fear of stigmatization is greater than fear of death (Gray, 1999).

Women living with HIV or at high risk for HIV may experience more stress and use fewer positive coping mechanisms than men. Coping style is important because active, positive coping styles are associated with more satisfaction with health care and less drug abuse. When individuals are unhappy with their health care, they may be less likely to attend appointments and adhere to their treatment regimen (Leslie, Stein, & Rotheram-Borus, 2002).

Spiritual Assessment and HIV/AIDS

Including topics of spirituality in an assessment of persons living with HIV is critical because research indicates that they are more likely to participate in religious and spiritual practices than similar individuals who are not HIV positive (Somlai et al., 1996). Somlai and Heckman (2000) found that many living with HIV place importance on prayer, belief in life after death, belief in miracles, belief that they are cared for by a higher power and belief that HIV/AIDS is not a punishment. In the same study, those who said they placed greater value on formal religion as an asset and reported more frequent prayer and a higher level of spirituality used adaptive coping strategies more often and received more support from family members.

Spirituality may be strongly tied to psychological, social, and even physical functioning for families coping with a diagnosis of HIV/AIDS. It can contribute to feelings of health and well-being, along with providing a sense of meaning to one's life among those living with chronic illness including HIV/AIDS (Fryback & Reinert, 1999). These benefits can also improve physical well-being (Carson & Green, 1992). Spirituality is also associated with improved quality of life, social support, and coping, as well as reduced perceived stress, depression and psychological distress (Simoni & Ortiz, 2003; Tuck, McCain, & Elswick, 2001). Those living with HIV/AIDS often seek alternative therapies that include a spiritual component (Nokes, Kendrew, & Longo, 1995). For many women with HIV, prayer and faith play an important role in daily life (Marcenko & Samost, 1999). Having a spiritual perspective has been shown to help women with HIV/AIDS cope with stress (Gray & Cason, 2002). Often HIV positive individuals may feel that their spiritual beliefs provide emotional support that they cannot find elsewhere. If they are afraid to disclose the diagnosis to friends and family, their spiritual beliefs may serve as their primary support system.

Disclosure of HIV Status

Those living with HIV are often reluctant to disclose their HIV status due to fears of rejection and abandonment. It is important to know whether the HIV status has been disclosed and to whom. Disclosure of HIV status is often important in providing a stronger support system (Bor, du Pleissis, & Russell, 2004). It is also important that HIV status be disclosed to potential sexual partners in order to prevent transmission. Those who would like to disclose their status to partners or family members may need assistance and support from their practitioner (Serovich, 2000). A sense of self-efficacy is an important psychological characteristic in making the decision to disclose HIV status. Because self-efficacy is often difficult to assess, it may be helpful to employ a scale to determine whether individuals feel they are capable of disclosing their HIV status. Kalichman and associates (2001) have developed reliable and valid scales to measure self efficacy for disclosure that can be used for this purpose.

Family Systems Issues

Involving the family in the assessment process is consistent with the Functional Age Model. According to developmental theory, each family member's development is influenced by others in the family (Greene, [1986] 2000). Family members may differ in their perceptions of the functioning of a family member with HIV/AIDS. Learning about a diagnosis of HIV/AIDS may create a crisis not only for the diagnosed individual but for the entire family. In assessing the physical, psychological, social, and spiritual aspects of living with HIV/AIDS, it is important to also assess the effect on the family system. Depending on the individual's level of functioning, there may be considerable changes in family roles. This change in roles can be difficult for families and affect feelings of self-worth. For example, if an HIV positive single mother of two children experiences symptoms of fatigue and depression, a grandparent may need to take on some of the parenting responsibilities. It is important to understand family members' expectations about family roles in order to help the family cope with the changes that occur with chronic illness (Greene, [1986] 2000).

In applying the Functional-Age model to assessment for families affected by HIV/AIDS, the practitioner considers the family to be a resource. Family members may often help to arrange for support services or may be providing a great deal of support in terms of preparing meals, caring for children, and other daily activities. It is important to assess what the family is already doing to support the individual with HIV/ AIDS because it can guide the practitioner's choice of interventions.

Physical symptoms of HIV such as fatigue, nausea, and fevers reduce an individual's capacity to perform daily activities, such as going to the grocery store, driving a child to school, and cooking meals. Psychological symptoms such as depression and anxiety can equally affect an individual's ability to carry out their normal daily routine. The reciprocal relationship between physical, psychological, social, and spiritual aspects of functioning means that physical health can determine whether an individual is able to maintain a support network, family relationships, and employment. At the same time, the resources that are available to a person with HIV which may include family, friends, spiritual beliefs, and employment can, in turn, influence their physical and psychological functioning. Individuals with HIV may be more vulnerable than those with other chronic illnesses because these resources are sometimes limited by stigma and social isolation. For this reason, a family's ability to understand their feelings about the diagnosis, cope with changes that accompany the illness, and provide support are critical in maintaining the health of the entire family system as well as the individual with HIV.

Parents with HIV/AIDS

As the number of women with HIV has increased, so has the number of parents, which has lead to studies examining factors that are associated with longevity among HIV infected parents (Lee & Rotheram-Borus, 2003; Mok & Cooper, 1997). Parents with HIV must cope with the symptoms of the illness, complicated therapy regimens, the emotional stress from having the diagnosis along with the responsibilities that accompany raising children (Rotheram-Borus et al., 2003). Parents with HIV, and mothers in particular, seem to face more stressors than individuals with no children. They often have limited financial and social support compared with parents who do not have HIV. Mothers with HIV may face numerous challenges, such as coping with guilt about behaviors that lead to infection and whether to tell their children about their illness (Marcenko & Samost, 1999). Mothers may also experience great emotional stress over the effect of their HIV status on their children. They may fear rejection by their children when they learn of the disease or worry that their children will face discrimination because of it. They may also feel that they need to make arrangements for others to care for their children in the event of their death (Marcenko & Samost, 1999).

Effect on Children

The stigma associated with HIV/AIDS can have a negative impact on children of HIV-positive parents. Although any type of chronic illness can have a negative effect on the parent-child relationship, HIV/AIDS is associated with unique problems because of the stigma associated with the illness. Parents who contracted HIV/AIDS due to substance abuse may continue to struggle with drug use, which can strain parent-child relationships. A child whose parent is ill due to HIV may be reluctant to disclose this source of stress and anxiety because of negative attitudes associated with the diagnosis. It is often difficult for these children to seek emotional support through schools and community organizations that often provide mental health services to children (Gunther & Crandles, 1998). Children who know about the diagnosis may fear losing their mother or may feel that they need to take care of her (Marcenko & Samost, 1999). Adolescents may feel that they need to care for their siblings or may react to feelings of loss by deciding to have a child of their own (Rotheram-Borus et al., 2003).

TREATMENT APPROACHES
FOR FAMILIES AFFECTED BY HIV/AIDS

The functional age perspective applies multiple modes of treatment to respond to the family's needs. Treatment may include case management, family, couples, and individual counseling, and bereavement counseling.

Stigma and Family

Because of the stigma associated with HIV/AIDS, practitioners may need to conduct outreach activities to engage families. Practitioners may also need to devote a great deal of attention to establishing trust and respecting the need for confidentiality. In some cases, an individual with HIV may not have disclosed the diagnosis to family members and may not want them involved in treatment. In these cases, it is important for the practitioner to respect these wishes. When the family does know about the diagnosis, the practitioner may need to help the family work through their feelings about the way the individual contracted the disease. In some cases, for example, a family may learn that an individual is gay and HIV positive at the same time. They may learn about a history of drug use or risky sexual activity. The family's cultural and religious beliefs may affect their response to this information. All of these issues affect the way the family system defines the problem that brings them to seek help, and the practitioner will need to help them clearly define presenting problems (Greene, Kropf, & MacNair, 1994).

Family Psychoeducational Approaches

Family psychoeducational approaches have been used successfully with families affected by HIV/AIDS. The approach typically includes educational components, coping techniques, and communication skills. Psychoeducational programs have been used with couples in which only one partner is HIV positive (Pomeroy, Green, & Van Laningham, 2002), HIV positive individuals (Pomeroy, Rubin, van Laningham, & Walker), and families with an HIV positive member (Pomeroy & Rubin, 1995). Participation in a psychoeducational group intervention has been associated with improvements in perceived stress, perceptions of stigma, depression and marital satisfaction (Pomeroy & Rubin, 2005; Pomeroy et al., 2002).

Cognitive Approaches

Rotheram-Borus et al. (2003) developed a cognitive behavioral group intervention designed to reduce problem behaviors, substance abuse, emotional distress among parents and children as well as teen pregnancy for families headed by an HIV positive parent. An evaluation of the intervention indicates that children participating in the program were less likely to become a teen parent, experienced decreases in conduct problems and emotional distress and reported increased self-esteem. Parents who were using substances reported less drug dependency and fewer relapses than parents who did not participate in the group. They also experienced less emotional distress and problem behaviors and used more positive coping strategies.

Cognitive behavior therapy has been used successfully to improve coping among individuals who have experienced the death of a loved one to AIDS as well. Individuals participating in a 12-week group cognitive behavioral intervention experienced reductions in psychological distress. Women participating in the group also experienced significant declines in grief and depression (Sikkema, Hansen, Kochman, Tate, & Difrancisco 2004).

Stress Management

Stress management interventions have proven to be helpful for women with HIV in promoting physical and emotional health (Riley & Fava, 2003). Women who are in later phases of HIV infection report higher levels of stress and lower self-efficacy for managing stress than women who are in the earlier stages of this illness (Riley & Fava, 2003). An ability to manage stress is critical for those living with a later stage of HIV because of the negative physical effects caused by stress that could compound the symptoms associated with HIV, such as pain and fatigue. Written emotional disclosure of positive and negative emotions and the ability to process those emotions has been associated with positive physical outcomes and longer survival for persons living with HIV. This intervention involves asking persons with HIV to write about their feelings associated with the stress they have experienced since learning of their HIV diagnosis. Participants who wrote on this topic for 20 minutes and engaged in emotional expression and processing of those emotions experienced greater perceived social support and less stress (O'Cleirigh et al., 2003).

Case Management

Because families affected by HIV/AIDS face a number of stressors that go beyond the symptoms of HIV, case management is often a critical component for any treatment plan. Families may be living in poverty and struggling to juggle child care responsibilities when the individual with HIV is ill. Those living with HIV may need assistance with finding employment, obtaining training, and managing finances (Arns, Martin, & Chernoff, 2004). Because of concerns about others learning of their HIV status, individual may be reluctant to seek employment without assistance. Providing outreach and case management services can also promote retention in primary case services for HIV positive youth and young adults (Harris, Kim, Samples, Keenan, Fox, Melchiono, & Woods, 2003). Multicomponent treatment in which a range of services are provided, often through a team of professionals, is necessary to help individuals and families manage the complex range of issues that are associated with HIV. Providing a combination of case management, mental health, substance abuse, and primary care services results in more positive outcomes for HIV positive adults than if these services were not received (Sherer et al., 2002).

Finally, there are few interventions for individuals with HIV/AIDS and their families that are supported by research. Much of the research on interventions for those living with HIV has focused on improving adherence to medication, increasing HIV testing, and preventing HIV transmission. There is a need for research that expands our knowledge about treatment approaches that can improve the quality of life for families affected by HIV.

EDUCATION AND PREVENTION

The stigma associated with HIV/AIDS has created barriers for intervening with those living with the illness and preventing infection of others. Making a meaningful impact on treatment and prevention requires intervention that goes beyond work with individuals and families. An equally important step involves facilitating an open dialogue in communities and among policy-makers about needed improvements in treatment and reducing stigma associated with HIV/AIDS. Community and social factors related to HIV/AIDS include the political climate, cultural attitudes, such as racism, homophobia, and community beliefs about HIV/AIDS (Chillag et al., 2002). Chillag et al. (2002) found that effective education and prevention efforts are affected by structural factors, such as policy restrictions on needle exchange programs and condom distribution in schools and sociocultural factors, such as stigma and biases against members of a particular race, gender, or sexual orientation, distrust for social service providers, and conservative political environments.

Barriers to Treatment

Reducing barriers to implementing effective prevention programs in community and school settings is critical for increasing knowledge about

HIV and reducing risk. Although many HIV prevention interventions have demonstrated in rigorous research trials that they effectively increase knowledge and reduce risk behavior, few organizations in the community have adopted these interventions. The success of HIV prevention efforts in a community setting depends on its relevance to an organization's mission, ease of implementation, and the opinions of the organization's consumers. In a school setting, successful implementation is influenced by the quality of collaboration between school staff, such as teachers, administrators, and social workers and the support of school leadership. Lohrmann et al. (2001) found that in order for policy-directed HIV prevention programs to be effective in New Jersey schools, school personnel need to be motivated to use the programs, superintendents need to be supportive of policy mandates, and principals need to view the programs as helpful.

Policy Restrictions

In order to improve HIV prevention strategies for schools and communities, it is important to remove policy restrictions on reducing risk, and provide greater funding support for disseminating information and interventions that address HIV/AIDS. Although state policies require most public schools to educate students about HIV and STD, the policies do little to ensure that education is consistent with research on effective prevention (Kirby, 2002). Schools may provide HIV education that only emphasizes abstinence or abstinence until marriage, for example, even though research does not support the effectiveness of such programs. Although many parents support school-based education about contraception, states often restrict schools from providing this information (Kirby, 2002). Such policy restrictions prevent risk reduction even when community attitudes are supportive (Kirby, 2002).

Political Climate

Interventions may not be sustained due to a conservative political climate characterized by cracking down on illicit activities. Providing outreach and services to runaways or those involved with illicit activities, such as prostitution and drug dealing is controversial in many communities (Miller, 2003). Yet, these are the populations most at risk for HIV. Neglecting these issues will prevent interventions from benefiting vulnerable adolescents because they may not be adopted by the organizations that serve them (Miller, 2003).

The stigma associated with HIV has made it difficult for families to cope with the stressors of caring for a family member with the disease while simultaneously creating barriers for prevention efforts that aim to reduce the number of new infections. Changes in federal and state policies and community responses to issues associated with HIV/AIDS are necessary in order to help those already struggling with the disease and prevent its spread. Public awareness campaigns, more effective community outreach, and increased funding for dissemination of accurate information and evidence based practices are examples of strategies that can begin to solve this problem.

CONCLUSION

The functional-age model of family treatment is especially useful for practitioners who are assisting families caring for a member with HIV/AIDS because the illness affects families on multiple ecological levels. The interrelationships between physical, psychological, social, and spiritual functioning mean that deficits in one area are likely to have a negative effect on others. An individual who is experiencing severe symptoms of HIV is likely to become more socially isolated and depressed which can, in turn, exacerbate the physical symptoms. It is therefore critical that the practitioner is able to empower the family to acknowledge and develop their strengths in order to improve functioning in all of these areas.

REFERENCES

AIDS Education & Training Centers National Resource Center (2005). *Side Effects of Antiretroviral Therapy*. Retrieved July 15, 2005 from http://www.aids-ed.org/aidsetc?page=et-30-06&catid=arvteffects&pid=1.

Arns, P. G., Martin, D. J., & Chernoff, R. A. (2004). Psychosocial needs of HIV-positive individuals seeking workforce re-entry. *AIDS Care, 16(3)*, 377-386.

Ball, J., Tannenbaum, L., Armistead, L., & Maguen, S. (2002). Coping with HIV infection in African-American women. *Women & Health, 35(1)*, 17-36.

Barfod, T. S., Gerstoft, J., Rodkjaer, L., Pedersen, C., Nielsen, H., Maller, A., Kristensen, L. Hagelskajaer, Sarensen, H. T., & Obel, N. (2005). Patients' Answers to Simple Questions About Treatment Satisfaction and Adherence and Depression Are Associated with Failure of HAART: A Cross-Sectional Survey. *AIDS Patient Care & STDs, 19 (5),* 317-325.

Barroso J., Carlson J. R., & Meynell, J. (2003). Physiological and psychological markers associated with HIV-related fatigue. *Clinical Nursing Research 12(1),* 49-68.

Berger, B. E., Ferrans, C. E., & Lashley, F. R. (2001). Measuring stigma in people with HIV: Psychometric assessment of the HIV Stigma Scale. *Research in Nursing & Health, 24(6),* 518-529.

Bor, R., du Plessis, P., & Russell, M. (2004). The impact of disclosure of HIV on the index patient's self-defined family. *Journal of Family Therapy, 26 (2),* 167-192.

Carson, V. B., & Green, H. (1992). Spiritual well being: A predictor of hardiness in patients with acquired immunodeficiency syndrome. *Journal of Professional Nursing, 8,* 209-220.

Centers for Disease Control and Prevention. (2003). *HIV/AIDS Surveillance Report: Cases of HIV Infection and AIDS in the United States, 2003.* Atlanta, GA: U.S. Department of Health and Human Services, Centers for Disease Control and Prevention. (pp. 1-9). Retrieved December 18, 2004 from http://www.cdc.gov/hiv/stats/hasrlink.htm.

Chillag, K., Bartholow, K., Cordeiro, J., Swanson, J. P., Stebbins, S., Woodside, C., & Sy, F. (2002). Factors affecting the delivery of HIV/AIDS prevention programs by community-based organizations. *AIDS Education and Prevention, 14 (supplement A),* 27-37.

Cook, J. A., Grey, D., Burke, J., Cohen, M. H., Gurtman, A. C., Richardson, J. L., Wilson, T. E., Young, M. A., & Hessol, N. A. (2004). Depressive symptoms and AIDS-related mortality among a multisite cohort of HIV-positive women. *American Journal of Public Health, 94 (7),* 1133-1140.

Cowdery, J. E., & Pesa, J. A. (2002). Assessing quality of life in women living with HIV infection. *AIDS Care, 14 (2),* 235-245.

Fife, B. L., & Wright, E. R. (2000). The dimensionality of stigma: A comparison of its impact on the self of persons with HIV/AIDS and cancer. *Journal of Health and Social Behavior, 41 (1),* 50-67.

Fryback, P. B., & Reinert, B. R. (1999). Spirituality and people with potentially fatal diagnoses. *Nursing Forum,34,* 13-22.

Geilen, A. C., McDonnell, A. W., Wu, A. W., O'Campo, P., & Faden, R. (2001). Quality of life among women living with HIV: The importance of violence, social support, and self care behaviors. *Social Science and Medicine, 52,* 315-322.

Gray, J. J. (1999). The difficulties of women living with HIV infection. *Journal of Psychosocial Nursing and Mental Health Services, 37(5),* 39-45.

Gray, J. & Cason, C. L. (2002). Mastery over stress among women with HIV/AIDS. *Journal of the Association of Nurses in AIDS Care, 13(4),* 43-57.

Greene, R. (1986). The functional-age model of intergenerational therapy: A social casework model. *Clinical Gerontology,* 335-346.

Greene, R. (1986; 2006) *Social work with the aged and their families.* NY: Aldine de Gruyter.

Greene, R., Kropf, N. P., & MacNair, N. (1994). A family therapy model for working with persons with AIDS. *Journal of Family Psychotherapy, 5 (1),* 1-20.

Gunther, M., & Crandles, S. (1998). A place called hope: Group psychotherapy for adolescents of parents with HIV/AIDS. *Child Welfare, 77 (2),* 251-271.

Harris, S. K., Samples, C. L., Keenan, P. M., Fox, D. J., Melchiono, M. W., & Woods, E. R. (2003). Outreach, mental health, and case management services: Can they help to retain HIV-positive and at-risk youth and young adults in care? *Maternal & Child Health Journal, 7 (4),* 205-219.

Hosek, S. G., Harper, G. W., & Domanico, R. (2005). Predictors of medication adherence among HIV-infected youth. *Psychology, Health & Medicine, 10 (2),* 166-179.

Joshi, V., Hser, Y., Grella, C. E., & Houlton, R. (2001). Sex-related HIV risk reduction among adolescents in DATOS-A. *Journal of Adolescent Research, 16(6),* 642-660.

Kalichman, S. C., Rompa, D., DiFonzo, K., Simpson, D., Kyomugisha, F., Austin, J., & Luke, W. (2001). Initial development of scales to assess self-efficacy for disclosing HIV status and negotiating safer sex in HIV-positive persons. *AIDS and Behavior, 5 (3),* 291-296.

Kirby, D. (2002). The impact of schools and school programs upon adolescent sexual behavior. *The Journal of Sex Research, 39(1),* 27-33.

Land, H., Hudson, S. M., & Stiefel, B. (2003). Stress and depression among HIV-positive and HIV-negative gay and bisexual AIDS caregivers. *AIDS and Behavior, 7(1),* 41-53.

Lee, M., & Rotheram-Borus, M. J. (2001). Challenges associated with increased survival among parents living with HIV. *American Journal of Public Health, 91 (8),* 1303-1309.

Leslie, M. B., Stein, J. A., & Rotheram-Borus, M. J. (2002). The impact of coping strategies, personal relationships, and emotional distress on health related outcomes of parents living with HIV or AIDS. *Journal of Social and Personal Relationships, 19 (1),* 45-66.

Lohrmann, D.K., Blake, S., Collins, T., Windsor, R., & Parrillo, A.V. (2001). Evaluation of school-based HIV prevention education programs in New Jersey. *Journal of School Health, 71(6),* 207-211.

Marcenko, M. O., & Samost, L. (1999). Living with HIV/AIDS: The voices of HIV-positive mothers. *Social Work, 44 (1),* 36-45.

Miller, R.L. (2003). Adapting an evidence-based intervention: Tales of the hustler project. *AIDS Education and Prevention, 15, Supplement A,* 127-138.

Miller, R. & Murray, D. (1999). The impact of HIV illness on parents and children with particular reference to African families. *Journal of Family Therapy, 21 (3),* 284-303.

Mok, J., & Cooper, S. (1997). The needs of children whose mothers have HIV infection. *Archives of Disease in Childhood, 77(6),* 483-487.

Neidig, J. L., Smith, B. A., & Brashers, D. E. (2003). Aerobic exercise training for depressive symptom management in adults living with HIV infection. *Journal of the Association of Nurses in AIDS Care, 14(2),* 30-40

Nokes, K. M., & Kendrew, J. (2001). Correlates of sleep quality in persons with HIV disease. *Journal of the Association of Nurses in AIDS Care, 12(1),* 17-22.

Nokes, K. M., Kendrew, J., & Longo, M. (1995). Alterative/Complementary therapies used by persons with HIV disease. *Journal of the Association of Nurses in AIDS Care, 6,* 19-24.

O'Cleirigh, C., Ironson, G., Antoni, M., Fletcher, M. A., McGuffey, L., Balbin, E., Schneiderman, N., & Solomon, G. (2003). Emotional expression and depth processing of trauma and their relation to long-term survival in patients with HIV/ AIDS. *Journal of Psychosomatic Research,* 54 (3), 225-235.

Paterson, D. L., Swindells, S., Mohr, J., Brester, M., Vergis, E. N., Squier, C., Wagener, M. M., & Singh, N. (2000). Adherence to protease inhibitor therapy and outcomes in patients with HIV infection. *Annals of Internal Medicine, 133,* 21-30.

Pomeroy, E. C., Green, D. L., & VanLaningham, L. (2002). Couples who care: The effectiveness of a psychoeducational group intervention for HIV serodiscordant couples. *Research on Social Work Practice, 12 (2),* 238-252.

Pomeroy, E. C., & Rubin, A. (1995). Effectiveness of a psychoeducational and task-centered group intervention for family members of people with AIDS. *Social Work Research, 19 (3),* 142-152.

Pomeroy, E. C., Rubin, A., & VanLaningham, L. (1997). "Straight Talk": The effectiveness of a psychoeducational group intervention for heterosexuals with HIV/ AIDS. *Research on Social Work Practice, 7 (2),* 149-164.

Riley, T. A., & Fava, J. L. (2003). Stress and transtheoretical model indicators of stress management behaviors in HIV-positive women. *Journal of Psychosomatic Research, 54,* 245-252.

Rotheram-Borus, M., Lee, M., Leonard, N., Lin, Y., Franzke, L., Turner, E., Lightfoot, M., & Gwadz, M. (2003). Four-year behavioral outcomes of an intervention for parents living with HIV and their adolescent children. *AIDS, 17,* 1217-1225.

Serovich, J. M. (2000). Helping HIV-positive persons to negotiate the disclosure process to partners, family members, and friends. *Journal of Marital & Family Therapy, 26 (3),* 365-361.

Sherer, R., Stieglitz, K., Narra, J., Jasek, J., Green, L., Moore, B., Shott, S., & Cohen, M. (2002). HIV multidisciplinary teams work: Support services improve access to and retention in HIV primary care. *AIDS Care, 14, Supplement 1,* 31-44.

Sikkema, K. J., Hansen, N. B., Kochman, A., Tate, D. C., & Difrancisco, W. (2004). Outcomes from a randomized controlled trial of a group intervention for HIV positive men and women coping with AIDS-related loss and bereavement. *Death Studies, 28 (3),* 187-199.

Simoni, J. M., & Ortiz, M. Z. (2003). Mediational models of spirituality and depressive symptomatology among HIV-positive Puerto Rican women. *Cultural Diversity and Ethnic Minority Psychology, 9 (1),* 3-15.

Somlai, A. M., & Heckman, T. G. (2000). Correlates of spirituality and well-being in a community sample of people living with HIV disease. *Mental Health, Religion, and Culture, 3 (1),* 57-69.

Somlai, A. M., Kelly, J. A., Kalichman, S. C., Mulry, G., Sikkema, K. J., McAuliffe, T., Multhauf, K., & Davantes, B. (1996). An empirical investigation of the relationship between spirituality, coping, and emotional distress in people living with HIV infection and AIDS. *Journal of Pastoral Care, 50 (2),* 181-191.

Sullivan, P. S. & Dworkin, M. S.(2003). Prevalence and correlates of fatigue among persons with HIV. *Journal of Pain & Symptom Management, 25 (4),* 329-333.

Tuck, I., McCain, N. L., & Elswick, R. K. (2001). Spirituality and psychosocial factors in persons living with HIV. *Journal of Advanced Nursing, 33 (6),* 776-783.

UNAIDS (2005). About HIV/AIDS: Symptoms. Retrieved July 15, 2005 from http://www.youandaids.org/About%20HIVAIDS/Symptoms/index.asp.

doi:10.1300/J137v14n01_12

Chapter 13

New Challenge to Inner-City Caregiving: What Organizations Must Do to Address Urban-Satellite Mix Communities

Michael A. Wright

SUMMARY. This article discusses how new or emerging city forms present fresh challenges and opportunities for caregiving agencies and institutions. It describes how tapping the resources and assets of inner cities can revitalize the capacity of the community. The way in which religious institutions, traditional social service agencies, and informal caregivers can work together to provide care is explored. doi:10.1300/J137v14n01_13 *[Article copies available for a fee from The Haworth Document Delivery Service: 1-800-HAWORTH. E-mail address: <docdelivery@ haworthpress.com> Website: <http://www.HaworthPress.com> © 2006 by The Haworth Press, Inc. All rights reserved.]*

KEYWORDS. Inner cities, religious institutions, web based initiatives

This article discusses how new or emerging city forms present fresh challenges and opportunities for caregiving agencies and institutions. It

[Haworth co-indexing entry note]: "New Challenge to Inner-City Caregiving: What Organizations Must Do to Address Urban-Satellite Mix Communities." Wright, Michael A. Co-published simultaneously in *Journal of Human Behavior in the Social Environment* (The Haworth Press, Inc.) Vol. 14, No. 1/2, 2006, pp. 259-274; and: *Contemporary Issues of Care* (ed: Roberta R. Greene) The Haworth Press, Inc., 2006, pp. 259-274. Single or multiple copies of this article are available for a fee from The Haworth Document Delivery Service [1-800-HAWORTH, 9:00 a.m. - 5:00 p.m. (EST). E-mail address: docdelivery@haworthpress.com].

Available online at http://jhbse.haworthpress.com
doi:10.1300/J137v14n01_13

describes how tapping the resources and assets of inner cities can revitalize the capacity of the community. The way in which religious institutions, traditional social service agencies, and informal caregivers can work together to provide care is explored. The basis of this modern collaboration is mutual reciprocity, conceptualized beyond the one-to-one personal relationship. Reciprocity in this context is perceived as the core of community building initiatives.

The inner cities themselves face significant environmental challenges in the form of "urban-satellite mix" communities. This chapter details the challenges facing organizations endeavoring to provide support to caregivers in such communities. It discusses opportunities for the use of technology, capacity building, and lessons of successful outcomes that may aid organizations in this evolving milieu. These opportunities can be used to identify reciprocity in caregiving relationships, communicate its usefulness to caregivers and care recipients, and validate the choice of both for formal and informal caregiving relationships. In addition, the chapter draws on the experience of a consultant to three types of inner-city organizations operating on the front lines of helping caregivers, assisting care recipients, and maintaining a sense of balance and reciprocity in the caregiving equation.

INTRODUCTION

The Census Bureau defined *urban areas* for the 1990 census as comprising all territory, population, and housing units in urbanized areas and in places of 2,500 or more persons outside urbanized areas. It defined *urbanized areas* as comprising one or more places, a "central place" and its adjacent densely settled surrounding territory, an "urban fringe," that together have a minimum of 50,000 persons. The urban fringe generally consists of a contiguous territory having a density of at least 1,000 persons per square mile. Territory, population, and housing units not classified as urban constitute *rural areas*.

This classification may not be useful for planning, districting, and funding decisions in today's society because it does not reflect the reality of certain regions. For example, there are a number of small urban areas in southwest Michigan with populations below 13,000. These are only 30 minutes from an urbanized area with a population of about 100,000. Residents of these small cities may live, work, worship, and enjoy recreation in wholly different cities within this cluster of cities. This reality is the geographic foundation of the typical challenges facing cities such as transportation, education, housing, child care, and health care.

A possible term for this geographic entity is *urban-satellite community*. They are typically economically integrated with a nearby urbanized area whose population exceeds 100,000. They are often paired with a city that is economically their polar opposite. This means that the most impoverished of the cities will have an affluent "twin" city nearby. These economic opposites are often separated by a river or train tracks.

The small urban-satellite communities face many of the same issues as the more affluent urbanized center does, but with fewer human and financial resources available to solve them. The satellite communities have the potential for a great amount of hidden or unaddressed poverty. This may be due to their "in between" size and to the fact that they may be overlooked in regional evaluations. Their poor African American and Hispanic residents may constitute a large proportion of a satellite city's population, but a relatively small proportion of the population of the regional population. Residents of impoverished communities may work and spend their disposable income outside of the community. Evaluators may state that "economic indicators have improved for the region," while overlooking the evaluation of each 10,000 person geographic entity as a separate locale. There is growing recognition that there is a need for different strategies of community collaboration (Jeffries, 1999) to provide a different external environment for organizations that serve the inner-city, and perhaps a new front line for inner-city caregiving support.

URBAN-SATELLITE COMMUNITIES: THE NEW CAREGIVING ENVIRONMENT

Urban-satellite communities import many of their community service workers. This means that many of the individuals involved in service to the community do not live in that community. Agency volunteers do not typically live within their service area. Donors and contributors to agencies may not be familiar with the everyday life experience of the community. These commuters may investment little of their personal resources in a community. This problem is exacerbated in urban-satellite communities where as little as a 12-minute commute could mean that an individual lives with a wholly different education and health system, police force, fire department, transportation system, and other public agencies.

In spite of the challenges, many religion-based and secular community service agencies continue to operate within urban satellite mix communities. Some of these agencies are using novel capacity-building strategies to explore how people can contribute to the community. Successful examples are termed *tri-county areas* or sometimes *twin cities*. In addition, technology may be a tool to help integrate and create a virtual larger community out of the interrelated smaller and larger urban areas, keeping residents informed about culture, experiences, and service opportunities.

CAREGIVING AND CAREGIVER SUPPORT IN SATELLITE MIX COMMUNITIES

According to the National Alliance for Caregiving, 44.4 million Americans are providing some form of care. Sixty-two percent of these report having to have made adjustments to their work schedules or report having to give up their work entirely to function as caregivers. In urban areas, caregivers are more likely to be African American aged 18 to 34. African American caregivers are also more likely to say that they receive some form of formal training in caregiving and that they administer medications to their care recipients. One of the most pressing needs expressed by African American caregivers, according to the Alliance, is to have specific information on prescription medications.

Are the problems of caregivers in urban-satellite communities different from those in other communities? Edwards (2001), referring to inner-city communities, suggested that the challenges of these communities include family household management, child adolescent school, adolescent antisocial behavior, family mental health, and physical health challenges. Of these, family household management challenges are the most difficult for these families to address.

In addition, in the past, the deficits stemming from poverty and social isolation were mitigated by connection with networks of upwardly mobile people that poorer individuals might encounter in membership groups or agencies such as NAACP, local churches, the Boys and Girls Club, or other community organizations. Today, that connection is not as usual due to the out migration of more affluent individuals and families (Alex-Assensoh & Assensoh, 2001). Therefore, if caregiving support is to be provided through the agencies like community organizations, innovations must be introduced to respond better to the environment of urban-satellite communities.

RECIPROCITY AND THE CHOICE TO PROVIDE CARE

The choice by individuals to become caregivers is influenced by a host of factors including love, concern, duty, guilt, reciprocity, gender, life cycle positions, and marital circumstances (Cahill, 1999). Of these, reciprocity emerges as one factor that may be amenable to intervention. Increased reciprocity would provide benefits to the caregiver by reducing stress and the perceived burden (Dwyer, Lee, & Jankowski, 1994), supporting sustained caregiving (Sauter, 1997), aiding satisfaction in caregiving (Banerjee & Mann, 1999), and increasing the amount of help given by a caregiver (Horowitz & Shindelman, 1983). The benefits of reciprocity extend to care recipients as well. Care recipients who participate in highly reciprocal relationships and experience less depression than others receiving informal care.

Defining Reciprocity

According to Carruth, Holland, and Larsen (2000), reciprocity is the aggregate of effective and behavioral indicators of the exchange between caregiver, care recipient, and the recipient's family. The authors measured reciprocity using the Caregiver Reciprocity Scale II consisting of four subscales: (1) Warmth and Regard, (2) Intrinsic Rewards of Giving, (3) Love and Affection, and (4) Balance Within the Family. Williams's (1995) work adds to the definition when he points out that the need and desire to reciprocate is not bound by gender, race, or socioeconomic status and is observable in both financial and affective types of support.

There is a considerable amount of literature examining the benefits of reciprocity and its support of the caregiving choice. A number of authors provide advice for supporting caregiving choices. For example, Horowitz, Reinhardt and Howell-White (1996) suggest examining caregiving as a process of mutual exchange between caregiver and care recipient. Similarly, Wright and Aquilino (1998) support enhancing the exchange of emotional support between caregiver and recipients as an identification of reciprocity in the relationship. Hamilton and Sandelowski (2003) believe that elderly people should be allowed to maintain their status as givers as a way of maintaining reciprocity. Carruth, Tate, Moffett, and Hill (1997) suggest that care relationships be extended to the benefit received from a caregiver's increased awareness of his or her reciprocity with all family members. Finally, Bould (1990) proposes that caregiving relationships build social networks that emphasize symmetry and reciprocity.

Limits of Reciprocity

Reciprocity does have its limits. Functional factors represent the most insistent limit to the experience of reciprocity (Antonucci, Fuhrer, & Jackson, 1990). *Functional factors* refer to a care recipient's ability to function effectively in typical human interaction and his or her environment (see Chapter 1). Dementia is an example of a condition that can be most detrimental to functioning, often limiting the ability of the care receiver to reciprocate. Depressive symptoms are another example of factors limiting reciprocity in the caregiving equation (Thomas, Milbrun, Brown, & Gary, 1998).

CULTURE AND COMMUNITY GROUPS OF URBAN-SATELLITE COMMUNITIES

It is commonly understood that culture—the norms, values, and behaviors typical of a group of people—affects a family's mental health (NAMHC, 1996). Reciprocity, too, is a cultural artifact that stems from individual and group values about rules, behavior, and the public good. The cultural environment created by organizations and community affects the potential for individuals and groups to develop reciprocity (Fehr & Gachter, 2000). With this understood, it seems appropriate that organizations recognize the benefits of creating an environment that supports reciprocity and thus aids caregiving.

Urban-satellite communities often have subculture-influenced neighborhood poverty, never-married parent households, perceived social isolation, and people's decreased ability to connect with upwardly mobile role models (Alex-Assensoh & Assensoh, 2001). The culture of the community is also affected by out migration causing underdeveloped networks (Porter, 1995), commuter staffed local organizations, and what is sometimes called "drive by politics." Taken together, this can result in a sense of isolation, which makes even the best of resources hard for residents of such a community to recognize and utilize (Alex-Assensoh & Assensoh, 2001). Therefore, in this type of environment, organizations may need to connect more personally, adopting models of intervention that mirror being a family member or part of the extended family.

The more family-like approach raises an important question: Is maintaining professional distance an ethical consideration or is it a way of negating interdependence? It could be that recognizing and addressing people's need for interdependence is central to alleviate the sense of isolation that members of these communities feel. Reciprocity could ensure that a give and take and mutuality between members of the community and agencies in the community exists: That is, sometimes the community member gives, and the community agency accepts; other times, the community agency gives, and the community member accepts.

Community Groups

Johnson and Mullins (1990) categorize clubs, professional organizations, and churches as "community groups." The concept of community groups encapsulates the idea of groups of people interacting together based on a common set of norms and behaviors. Each of these fits their definition of a community of social networks supporting meaningful relationships through communication of common culture. Churches may be the most likely of these community groups to inspire common attitudes, values, and practices.

There are many similarities in the basic elements of community groups: people, organizing principles, values, and convening schedules are all common characteristics. At the same time, Kilburg (1978) confirms that there are significant differences between churches, schools, social service, and social (membership) organizations. The major difference among groups is their message and the ability to communicate their unique perspective and approach. This may explain why churches that appear to have a clear mission seem more adept at inspiring a cohesive group of attitudes, values, and practices. Though the mission is effectively transmitted, the theoretical perspective of every church system may not support the idea of providing service or volunteering outside of that church (Wilson & Janoski, 1995).

Membership Organizations

Membership organizations are the most general form of community groups. Any community group could be considered a membership organization. The key difference between a membership group and a community group is that membership groups often form for a specific task. For example, they may form to promote social and civic activities, the arts and sciences, and political, religious, and environmental causes. They are typically centralized but may have membership in many geographic locations. The diversity of membership and dispersion of the geographic locations present a significant opportunity, but, they also represent a number of challenges for supporting caregiving urban-satellite communities.

The author's experience with membership organizations is derived from work with a multi-national organization based in New England. The organization has a total membership around 1,700 and over 35 chapters. It was formed to bring an informed perspective to the social work profession regarding Christian themes and spirituality in social work practice. The challenges included dispersed membership, a volunteer and part-time staff, and ambitious goals.

The solution to these problems may have relevance to inner city communities and their relationship to caregiving. The organization needed to connect to its members, in this case, individuals who could literally be all around the globe. The solution had to be intuitive and provide information to users in a readily available form. More than just placing information on a website, the website had to be supportive of an online community.

Since the staff was comprised of volunteers or part-time workers, it was harder to maintain continuity of content production and communication with members. However, a positive feature of the organization was the informal (first name basis) relationship between the executive director, the board, and the membership. A web interface was created that allowed for many of the day-to-day data management and reporting activities of the organization to be accomplished quickly. Functions such as processing new members, listing additional members, changing chapter listings, and posting organization news could be added to the site by a staff member with little web programming knowledge. This allowed part-time staff and the executive director to maintain the web interface focusing less on the technology and more on nurturing the community.

It seems that every organization has big dreams and a substantial vision for its future success. However, it is a tall order to bring a diverse group together in support of a central mission. Success requires correct, centralized, and timely information. Thus, the primary lesson learned from such a membership organization is the need to develop a virtual community into which each member can plug in order to contribute and share in knowledge. By centralizing information, the organization is able to provide each member with a mechanism for reciprocating by sharing information and experience. That is, technology can be used to secure that knowledge base so that only the organization's members have access. Technology can also provide members with the ability to contribute to the knowledge base, which is an important part of growing a membership organization.

Parochial Organizations

Because reciprocity is a common theme in most religious traditions, much has been written about caregiving functions of churches (Adolph, 1995; Boschman, 1987; Haber, 1984; Kopp, 2001; Miller, 1997), including providing care to Alzheimer's patients (Stuckey,1998) and other church-based social programs (Brashears & Roberts,1996). One major conclusion of the aforementioned research is that churches have resources, are natural caregivers, and can serve as support systems for caregivers.

Churches have been discussed as surrogate families for older people (Steinitz, 1981). It is further suggested that small to medium size African American churches can play a vital role in linking secular agencies to at-risk, low income, older adults (Madison & McGadney, 2000). African American churches can also play a vital role in general health-promotion efforts (Thomas, Quinn, & Billingsley, 1994), referral to mental health agencies (Williams et al., 1999; Taylor, Ellison & Chatters, 2000), and community medicine (Levin, 1984). In addition, churches have been suggested as a means of support for persons with developmental disabilities (McNair & Swartz, 1997) and people with other disabilities (Bufford & Buckler, 1987). The African American church service has even been proposed as an effective mental health resource for its participants (Griffith, Young, & Smith, 1984).

Wilson and Janoski (1995), however, caution that the potential of church members to volunteer in secular activities is dependent upon the theological interpretation that faith community holds toward such volunteering. In other words, some churches support volunteering in secular activities as consistent with the purposes of the church and in line with the teachings of the faith. Other churches see volunteering in secular agencies as secondary to volunteering within the church itself. Some hold that only a church-sponsored program should be supported by that faith community. Church size and educational level of the minister are the strongest predictors of church sponsored health promotion (Thomas, Quinn, & Billingsley, 1994).

The author's experience with a church organization involved an African American church located in a city with a population just above 100,000, but the 473 member roster included members from the neighboring satellite cities (with populations of 13,000 or less). The faith tradition is evangelical. Though relatively diverse, much of the membership is African American, lower middle class, relatively well-educated (above the associate level). The pastor holds a Doctor of Theology degree.

The author worked as a church administrator, in charge of non-spiritual matters of the church such as asset, financial, and risk negotiations and management. The key issues faced included the diminishing relevance of church in the community, loss of youth membership, and a lack of new operational models.

There are a number of suggestions to improve the caregiving functions of parochial organizations operating in urban-satellite communities. The first is to work with the community to build upon its natural assets, assisting its members how to contribute to the common good. The second is to challenge the community with a mission of service. Such a mission of service or a reciprocal mission would reconceptualize the church to serve as a repository of service. The members would reciprocate by supporting the enterprise of the church through pledges of time and money to meet the church's service goals, including caregiving.

The third suggestion is to leverage the usefulness of the parochial organization in providing social services, including caregiving, by increasing its collaboration with secular organizations (Boddie, 2002). The city of Deary, New Hampshire, demonstrates an example of this type of collaboration program entitled Community Caregivers of Greater Deary. The organization was created after thorough solicitation and collaborative activity of local faith-based and secular organizations. The program offers friendly visiting, grocery shopping, light chores, and medical support through a network of volunteers. Romualdi and Sandoval (1997) suggest that this model is one of the best for provision of community services.

Community Services

Most people liken community services to already well-established and endowed programs that offer assistance with caregiving such as home and personal care, helping with the activities of daily living (ADLs) such as bathing and using the toilet or meal services, and delivering meals to people's home. However, organizational efficiency and reciprocity may be tenuous at best in newly founded community-based services organizations. Such programs are typified by its principles or direction as well as a consistent staff being engaged in running the business of the organization rather than in training. Lack of documentation is the norm. This leads to a decreased capacity of the organization to sustain its gains. Without a conception of the guiding ideals of the organization, volunteers may implement seemingly innocuous practices that contradict the goals of the organization.

In an environment where resources are scarce, it is important to use every tool to support the efficiency and efficacy of a program. Maintaining documents, conducting evaluations, and training staff to implement best practices are important to demonstrating efficacy. For example, the author's experience with community services is based on work with an after-school program in an urban-satellite community. The basic staff consisted of a husband and wife who are also directors of the program. The program met three times per week with a consistent group of six to nine youth between the ages of 8 and 21, augmented occasionally by five to seven more. The program exists to expose the adolescents to new experiences and to empower them to succeed.

Solutions to promote caregiving reciprocity in the after-school program included developing a system of training-the-trainers as a method of sustaining the staff, the board, and even donors. This mechanism of sharing, support, and informing of the staff, board and the principals is important to maintaining a cohesive organization. Having a version of the training on video tape or CD-ROM supported face-to-face trainings. This was especially important for an organization that has a small staff and relies on volunteers who turnover frequently. The process of evaluation was also computerized, allowing for a step-by-step process of deciding what data is available and valuable. To be of the most benefit, the system should be searchable and indexed.

APPLICATION OF THE LESSONS LEARNED FOR CAREGIVING SUPPORT

The lessons learned from membership, parochial, and community organizations can be summed up as recommendations for innovative organizations to support reciprocity in caregiving. The recommendations are:

- Create a centralized, multi-site accessible depository for caregiving best practices that accepts contributions from caregivers, care recipients, families, and service agencies.
- Provide a forum for face-to-face affirmation and dialogue describing social cues that communicate reciprocity as well as care recipient's contributions to other care recipients.

- Centralize the service planning and availability of trained volunteers to demonstrate the help available for respite, training, and professional services.
- Create a curriculum for "just-in-time" training of caregivers that covers a range of needed topics delivered in individually self-contained modules.
- Connect with professionals to provide specific training such as use of medications.
- Create and utilize awards, annual events, and publications to market, motivate, and provide incentives to organizations that demonstrate effective data management, training, and process.

IMPLEMENTING THE RECOMMENDATIONS

Centralized Best Practices

A web-based or kiosk-type system can effectively centralize best practice information. Web-based interfaces would require Internet access. Kiosk systems are stand-alone systems that may or may not connect to the Internet. They can be located at malls or in community service agencies. Keep in mind that twenty-five percent of caregivers in America get their information from the Internet (NAC, 2005).

Reciprocity Forum

The criticism of kiosks and other methods is that they are not face-to-face and may be better addressed through small group interaction. Within urban-rural mix communities, community groups can convene weekly or monthly help and support groups. Of course, a major function of these groups would be to identify further avenues for reciprocity in caregiving relationships.

Service Central

Volunteer centers are a vital part of communities. A potentially important advance is possible as these centers integrate their information with community groups. Membership organizations, parochial, and community services are fertile grounds for volunteers. An important key to nurturing the crop is providing specific service plans, pre-organized caregiving opportunities where volunteers can plug-in to their communities.

Caregiving Curriculum

Once a centralized system is in place, training can take place. Instead of a linear system that requires completion of every lesson in order, it is more functional to provide shorter lessons that the caregiver can experience as needed. This would make it possible for caregivers with various levels of training to get information at their own pace. A number of training options, from discussions, to games, simulations, and presentations have been implemented with success for churches and social service organizations (Lloyd, McConnell, & Zahorik, 1994).

Professional Connection

An important part of community life is the ability to get information from trusted professionals. Community groups, having already built a level of trust with their communities, may provide professionals with an opportunity to address an expectant audience. Many community service organizations now offer professional services free of charge within communities. Due to the isolation that individual community members feel, it may be up to community groups to connect and provide venue for professionals in urban satellite mix communities.

Market and Motivate

A well-organized annual event can provide a forum for discussion, training, and motivation for sharing best practices. Peer-reviewed information from these events become additional training for the centralized system. The opportunity to provide families with peer support can be substantial.

REFERENCES

AARP. http://www.aarp.org/families/caregiving/caring_help/a2003-10-27-caregiving-communityservices.html. Retrieved 7/5/2005.

Adolph, B. M. (1995). *Caregiving seminar in an African-American church.* Dissertation. Mercy College.

Alex-Assensoh, Y. and Assensoh, A. B. (2001). Inner-city contexts, church attendance, and African-American political participation. *The Journal of Politics, 63*(3). 886-901.

Antonucci, T. C., Fuhrer, R., and Jackson, J. S. (1990). Social support and reciprocity: A cross-ethnic and cross-national perspective. *Journal of Social & Personal Relationships Special Issue: Predicting, activating and facilitating social support, 7*(4). 519-530.

Boddie, S.C. (2002). Fruitful partnerships in a rural African American community: Important lessons for faith-based initiatives. *The Journal of Applied Behavioral Science, 38*(3). 317-333.

Boschman, E. V. (1987). Essentials for caregiving in the church. Dissertation. California Graduate School of Theology.

Bould, S. (1990). The oldest old: Caregiving or social support? *Prevention in Human Services, 9*(1) 235-251

Brashears, F. & Roberts, M. (1996). The Black church as a resource for change. In Logan, S. (Ed.), *The Black family: Strengths, self-help, and positive change* (pp. 181-192).

Bufford, R. K and Buckler, R. E. (1987). *Journal of Psychology & Christianity Special Issue: Lay Christian Counseling, 6*(2), 21-29.

Cahill, S.M. (1999). Caring in families: What motivates wives, daughters, and daughters-in-law to provide dementia care? *Journal of Family Studies, 5*(2), 235-247.

Carruth, A. (1996). Motivating factors, exchange patterns, and reciprocity among caregivers of parents with and without dementia. *Research in Nursing & Health, 19*(5), 409-419.

Carruth, A. K, Holland, C. and Larsen, L. (2000). Development and psychometric evaluation of the Caregiver Reciprocity Scale II. *Journal of Nursing Measurement, 8*(2), 179-191.

Carruth, A. K., Tate, U.S., Moffett, B.S. and Hill, K. (1997). Reciprocity, emotional well-being and family functioning as determinants of family satisfaction in caregivers of elderly parents. *Nursing Research, 46*(2) 93-100.

Clark, M., and Huttlinger, K. (1998). Elder care among Mexican American families. *Clinical Nursing Research, 7*(1), 64-81.

Dwyer, J. W., Lee, G. R., and Jankowski, T. B. (1994). Reciprocity, elder satisfaction, and caregiver stress and burden: The exchange of aid in the family caregiving relationship. *Journal of Marriage & the Family, 56*(1), 35-43.

Edwards, S. (2001). Community-based assessment of social service, physical health, and mental health needs. Dissertation. Bowling Green State University.

Fehr, E. and Gachter, S. (2000). Fairness and retaliation: The economics of reciprocity. *Journal of Economic Perspectives, 14(3)*, 159-181.

Griffith, E. E., Young, J. L. and Smith, D.L. (1984). An analysis of the therapeutic elements in a Black church service. *Hospital & Community Psychiatry, 35(5)*, 464-469.

Haber, D. (1984). Church-based programs for Black care-givers of non-institutionalized elders. *Journal of Gerontological Social Work, 7*(4), 43-55.

Hamilton, J. B. and Sandelowski, M. (2003). Living the golden rule: Reciprocal exchanges among African Americans with cancer. *Qualitative Health Research,* 13(5), 656-674.

Hooker, K., Mannoogian-O'Dell, M., Monahan, D. J., Frazier, L. D. and Shifren, K. (2000). Does type of disease matter? Gender differences among Alzheimer's and Parkinson's disease spouse caregivers. *Gerontologist, 40*(5), 568-573.

Horowitz, A. and Shindelman, L. W. (1983). Reciprocity and affection: Past influences on current caregiving. *Journal of Gerontological Social Work, 5*(3), 5-20.

Horwitz, A. V., Reinhard, S. C. and Howell-White, S. (1996). Caregiving as reciprocal exchange in families with seriously mentally ill members. *Journal of Health & Social Behavior, 37*(2), 149-162.

Ikels, C. (1991). Delayed reciprocity and the support networks of the childless elderly. In B. B. Hess & E. W. Markson (Eds.), *Growing old in America* (4th ed.) (pp. 441-456). New Brunswick, NJ.

Jeffries, C. L. (1999). Development and field-test of an evaluation model for assessing community collaboration. Dissertation. Spalding University.

Jewell, T. C. and Stein, C.H. (2002). Parental influence on sibling caregiving for people with severe mental illness. *Community Mental Health Journal, 38*(1), 17-33.

Johnson, M. A. and Mullins, P. (1990). Moral communities: Religious and secular. *Journal of Community Psychology, 18*(2), 153-166.

Keefe, J. M. and Fancey, P. J. (1998). Work and eldercare: Reciprocity between older mothers and their employed daughters. *Canadian Journal on Aging, 21*(2), 229-241.

Kilburg, R. R. (1978). Scanning the human service environment: A pilot study. *Journal of Community Psychology, 6*(4), 334-343.

Kopp, H. (2001). Soul care: Caregiving in the church. Winnipeg, MB. Kindred Productions.

Levin, J. S. (1984). The role of the Black church in community medicine. *Journal of the National Medical Association, 76*(5), 477-483.

Lewinter, M. (2003). Reciprocities in caregiving relationships in Danish elder care. *Journal of Aging Studies, 17*(3), 357-377.

Lloyd, J. J., McConnell, P. R., & Zahorik, P.M. (1994). Collaborative health education training for African American health ministers and providers of community services. *Educational Gerontology Special Issue: Educational models for reaching underserved older persons, 20*(3), 265-276.

Madison, A., & McGadney, B. F. (2000). Collaboration of churches and service providers: Meeting the needs of older African Americans. *Journal of Religious Gerontology, 11*(1), 23-37.

McNair, J. & Swartz, S.L. (1997). Local church support to individuals with developmental disabilities. *Education & Training in Mental Retardation & Developmental Disabilities, 32*(4), 304-312.

Miller, J. A. (1997). Equipping lay persons in caregiving skills. Dissertation. Stanford University.

Murray, J., Schneider, J., Banerjee, S., & Mann, A. (1999). EUROCARE: A cross-national study of co-resident spouse careers for people with Alzheimer's disease: II–A qualitative analysis of the experience of caregiving. *International Journal of Geriatric Psychiatry, 14*(8), 662-667

National Advisory Mental Health Council. Basic Behavioral Science Task Force Basic behavioral science research for mental health: Family processes and social networks. *American Psychologist, 51*(6), 622-630

National Alliance for Caregiving. http://caregiving.org/data/04execsumm.pdf. Retrieved 07/05/2005.

Neufeld, A. and Harrison, M. J. (1998). Men as caregivers: Reciprocal relationships or obligation? *Journal of Advanced Nursing, 28*(5), 959-968.

Nichols, R. C. (1997). Strengthening the caregiving ministry in a local church. Dissertation. School of Theology, Oral Roberts University.

Parsons, K. (1997). The male experience of caregiving for a family member with Alzheimer's disease. *Qualitative Health Research, 17*(3), 391-407.

Porter, M. E. (1995). The competitive advantage of the inner city. *Harvard Business Review*. 55-71.

Richards, M. (1999). Caregiving: Church and family together. Louisville, KY. Geneva Press.

Romualdi, V., & Sandoval, J. (1997). Community-based service integration: Family resource center initiatives. In Illback, R.J, Cobb, C.T., Joseph, Jr., H.M. (Eds.) Integrated services for children and families: Opportunities for psychological practice. Washington, DC. *American Psychological Association*. 53-73.

Sauter, M.A . (1997). Determinants of quality of the caregiving relationship. *Dissertation Abstracts International: Section B: The Sciences & Engineering, 57*(10-B), 61-81

State of New Jersey Division of Aging and Community Services. Jersey Assistant for Community Caregivers (JACC). http://www.state.nj.us/health/consumer/jacc.shtml. Retrieved 7/5/2005.

Steinitz, L. Y. (1981). The local church as support for the elderly. *Journal of Gerontological Social Work, 4*(2), 43-53.

Stuckey, J. C. (1998). The church's response to Alzheimer's disease. *Journal of Applied Gerontology, 17*(1), 25-37.

Taylor, R. J., Ellison, C. G. and Chatters, L. M. (2000). Mental health services in faith communities: The role of clergy in black churches. *Social Work, 45*(1), 73-87.

Thomas, S. B., Quinn, S. C., and Billingsley, A. (1994). The characteristics of northern black churches with community health outreach programs. *American Journal of Public Health, 84*, 575-579.

Thomas, V. G., Milbrun, N. G., Brown, D. R., and Gary, L. E. (1988). Social support and depressive symptoms among Blacks. *Journal of Black Psychology, 10*, 35-45.

United Way of the Greater Seacoast. http://www.volunteersolutions.org/uwgs/org/223974.html. Retrieved 7/5/2005.

Walker, A. J., Pratt, C. C., and Oppy, N. C. (1992). Perceived reciprocity in family caregiving. *Family Relations: Interdisciplinary Journal of Applied Family Studies, 41*(1), 82-85.

Williams, D. R., Griffith, E. E. H., Young, J. L., Collins, C., and Dodson, J. (1999). Structure and provision of services in Black churches in New Haven, Connecticut. *Cultural Diversity & Ethnic Minority Psychology, 5*(2). *American Psychological Association*. 118-133.

Wilson, J. & Janoski, T. (1995). The contribution of religion to volunteer work. *Sociology of Religion, 56*. 132-152.

Wolff, J. L. & Agree, E. M. (2004). Depression among recipients of informal care: The effects of reciprocity, respect and adequacy of support. *Journal of Gerontology, 59B*(3), 173-S180.

Wood, B. M. (1989). Christian caregiving: An intentional plan for implementing a ministry of care in the local church. Dissertation. School of Theology, Oral Roberts University.

Wright, D. L., & Aquilino, W. S. (1998). Influence of emotional support exchange in marriage on caregiving wives' burden and marital satisfaction. *Family Relations: Interdisciplinary Journal of Applied Family Studies, 47*(2), 195-204.

doi:10.1300/J137v14n01_13

Chapter 14

Older Lesbian and Gay Caregivers: Caring for Families of Choice and Caring for Families of Origin

Harriet L. Cohen
Yvette Murray

SUMMARY. This chapter will explore the experiences of older lesbian and gay men caregivers by examining the socio-historical times in which they have lived, the impact of a lifetime of adverse societal messages about homosexuality, family rejection, and internalized homophobia, as well as their development of resiliency and psychological well-being. Once the contextual issues have been identified, the research on older lesbian and gay caregivers for families of origin and families of choice will be explored. doi:10.1300/J137v14n01_14 *[Article copies available for a fee from The Haworth Document Delivery Service: 1-800-HAWORTH. E-mail address: <docdelivery@ haworthpress.com> Website: <http://www.HaworthPress.com> © 2006 by The Haworth Press, Inc. All rights reserved.]*

KEYWORDS. Lesbian, gay, caregiving, resilience, homophobia

INTRODUCTION

Research on family caregiving has primarily focused on older adults within traditional nuclear family constellations, excluding the experi-

[Haworth co-indexing entry note]: "Older Lesbian and Gay Caregivers: Caring for Families of Choice and Caring for Families of Origin." Cohen, Harriet L., and Yvette Murray. Co-published simultaneously in *Journal of Human Behavior in the Social Environment* (The Haworth Press, Inc.) Vol. 14, No. 1/2, 2006, pp. 275-298; and: *Contemporary Issues of Care* (ed: Roberta R. Greene) The Haworth Press, Inc., 2006, pp. 275-298. Single or multiple copies of this article are available for a fee from The Haworth Document Delivery Service [1-800-HAWORTH, 9:00 a.m. - 5:00 p.m. (EST). E-mail address: docdelivery@haworthpress.com].

Available online at http://jhbse.haworthpress.com
© 2006 by The Haworth Press, Inc. All rights reserved.
doi:10.1300/J137v14n01_14

ences of lesbian and gay men. In addition, most of the research has focused on caregiving to impaired older adults, examining caregiving stress and burden experienced by spouses and children. The majority of research on caregiving responsibilities for lesbians and gay men has focused on a young population caring for people with HIV/AIDS. To date, there has been little research on caregiving issues related to older lesbians and gay men and even less on older lesbians and gay men of color and people with disabilities. This chapter will explore the experiences of older lesbian and gay men caregivers by examining the socio-historical times in which they have lived, the impact of a lifetime of adverse societal messages about homosexuality, family rejection, and internalized homophobia, as well as their development of resiliency and psychological well-being. Once the contextual issues have been identified, the research on older lesbian and gay caregivers for families of origin and families of choice will be explored. The biopsychosocial and spiritual needs of this caregiving population and the dual family systems to which lesbian and gay people belong will be discussed. Policy and clinical suggestions that will help practitioners develop alternative ways of constructing support will be offered.

In the United States, increasing attention has been given to understanding the needs of caregivers and to developing services to support families in their role as informal caregiver to older adults, grandparents raising grandchildren, and older adults providing care for adult children with mental and physical disabilities. A caregiver is one who provides some type of help to an incapacitated person who needs some kind of physical, financial, or emotional assistance, such as bathing, grocery shopping, paying bills, eating, driving, and companionship. Informal caregivers are family members or friends who provide unpaid care (Family Caregiver Alliance, 2001; Pandya, 2005).

A 2004 study entitled *Caregiving in the U.S.* conducted by the National Alliance for Caregiving (NAC) and the American Association for Retired Persons (AARP) found that approximately 21% of the population, or close to 44.4 million Americans, are providing informal caregiving to friends and family over eighteen years old (Pandya, 2005). The Family Caregiver Alliance (FCA) (2001) reported that 52 million Americans provide informal care to someone over twenty who is ill or disabled. An earlier study by the National Alliance for Caregiving and AARP reported that caregiving for people over fifty years of age involved twenty five percent, or one out of every four households in the U.S. (Wagner, 1997). They also found that 15%-24% of caregivers provide care to friends or neighbors rather than family members (FCA, 2001). These staggering figures reveal that 21%-25% of the population is providing care to between 44.4 million and 52 million Americans.

When these figures are broken down by gender, females provide approximately 64% to 75% of the care to older family members and friends (FCA, 2001; Mack & Thompson, 2005). The "typical" caregiver is a female about forty six years old who provides more than 20 hours per week for her mother (Pandya, 2005). Even when men are also involved in caregiving, women caregivers expend 50% more of their time to caregiving than male caregivers (FCA, 2001). In addition to the number of women who are providing care, as mentioned above, women who are widowed make up more than sixty-five percent of the care recipients (Pandya, 2005). With women being the majority of caregivers and care receivers, aging is a woman's issue, both for heterosexual and lesbian providers.

Research on family caregiving has primarily focused on older adults within traditional nuclear family constellations, excluding the experiences of lesbians and gay men. In addition, most of the research has focused on caregiving of impaired older adults examining caregiving stress and burden experienced by spouses and children. To date, there has been little research on caregiving issues related to older lesbians and gay men and even less on older lesbians and gay men of color and with disabilities. Concepts that have been used in the caregiving literature, such as filial responsibility and sandwich generation, may not apply to the caregiving experiences of older lesbians and gay men. They may or may not have children or family members available for assistance in meeting their caregiving needs. In fact, lesbians and gay men may be caring for partners and friends, as well as for older family members and children (Cantor, Brennan & Shippy, 2004; Fredriksen, 1999; Tully, 1989).

Policy makers have turned to the traditional family to provide care for older adults, as technology and medical advances have helped to improve the quality and quantity of life for older adults. However, three social and economic trends are impacting the family and thereby influencing general family caregiving patterns: (1) the increase of women in the workforce, (2) the decrease in the number of children, and (3) greater mobility of family members so that extended families are no longer living close to each other. A fourth trend impacting caregiving is the increasing number of older lesbians and gay men, who may not have children, biological family members, or legal protections to rely upon for assistance in meeting their need for care. According to the Lesbian Gay Bi-sexual and Transgender Persons (LGBT) Aging Project of Massachusetts, "Every week 10,000 more gay, lesbian, bisexual and transgender Americans reach retirement age without equal access to the aging services and economic safety nets their neighbors can take for granted" (LGBT Aging Project, n.d.).

In addition, the caregiving literature has examined caregiving stress and the burden experienced by white, heterosexual, middle-class caregivers, usually adult daughters and presumably heterosexual spouses. Juxtaposed to this body of research is that of caregiving in the lesbian and gay community that has addressed the care of people with HIV/ AIDS by gay men under fifty years of age and the other studies in the LGBT community that focus on issues of concern to younger adults, such as gay and lesbian parenting (Quam, 2001).

The limited studies that do exist in the gay community about caregiving include both older lesbians and gay men in the population sample (Cantor, Brennan & Shippy, 2004; Claes & Moore, 2000; Fredriksen, 1999; Grossman, D'Augelli & Hershberger, 2000; Hash, 2001; Hash & Cramer, 2003; Quam, 2001; Quam & Whitford, 1992). According to Quam (2001), "information about aging issues as they relate to older gay men and lesbian women ranges from scarce to non-existent" (p. 1). Neither the traditional family-focused research nor the studies of lesbians and gay men have examined the caregiving experiences for older lesbians and gay men, who are invisible because of their identities as both homosexual and older adults.

WHAT IS KNOWN ABOUT OLDER LESBIAN AND GAY ADULTS

Recognizing and responding to the needs of lesbian, gay, bisexual and transgender elders will promote better services for ALL elders because it promotes sensitivity and respect for diversity in all its aspects as well as creating space where sexuality and aging in general can be explored and discussed. (Quam, n.d.)

Although there are no exact numbers, the older lesbian and gay population in the United States is estimated at 1 to 3 million (National Gay and Lesbian Task Force Policy Institute, [NGLTF], 2003) or 1.75 to 3.5 million (Woolf, 1998). By 2030, in the general population, approximately one in five people will be sixty five and older, and roughly 4 million of those will be lesbian, gay, and bisexual. No national data exist for the number of transgender people of any age living in the United States. Approximately five percent of older women and four percent of older men have never been married, so it is very probable that many of these are lesbian and gay men. Also, since many lesbians and gay men have been in heterosexual marriages at some time during their lifetime, they may not be counted in national studies (Cantor, Brennan, & Shippy, 2004).

Lesbian and Gay People of Color

While there is little research on lesbian and gay men of color, voter exit polls demonstrate that lesbian and gay people are found among diverse racial categories according to a report by the National Gay and Lesbian Task Force Policy Institute (Cantor, Brennan & Shippy, 2004). The report indicates that seventeen percent of the lesbian, gay, and bisexual (LGB) voters are African American voters; and five percent of LGB voters are Hispanic. While the aging network is planning for an increase in the need for services for older adults as baby boomers move from midlife to retirement age, it can be assumed that the number of lesbian and gay men, including lesbian and gay men of color will increase, and thus the need for services delivered by culturally competent health and human service providers will also increase.

INVISIBILITY AND THE CHALLENGES OF RESEARCH

Lesbians and gays have not only been invisible in the general population, but as *older* adults, they have also been invisible in the gay community. The National Gay and Lesbian Task Force Policy Institute conducted an informal content analysis of nine LGBT East Coast newsletters, involving over 700 pages, and only five articles included references to older LGBT individuals and no pictures of older LGBT were available. An analysis of five LGBT magazines (*The Advocate*, *MetroLife*, *Hero*, *Q.S. F.*, and *Out*), some 542 pages, revealed only two articles referencing older people, and again there were no images of older LGBT. On learning of this information, Apuzzo (2001) emphatically declared, "We will not be re-closeted by our own community" (p. 8).

Because of the double invisibility of this population as older lesbians and gays in the gay community, and as homosexuals in the heterosexual community, studying older lesbians and gay men in general and patterns and issues of caregiving in particular is problematic. The first problem is that there are no national data specifically identifying this population. General information about older people does not include statistics about older lesbians and gay men. In the lesbian and gay community, information about older gays and lesbians is missing (Singer & Deschamps, 1994; Quam, 1997) or is limited to white healthy, middle-class gay men, living in large urban cities, who belong to lesbian and gay organizations and who self-identify (Barranti & Cohen, 2000; Grossman, D'Augelli & O'Connell, 2001; Hash, 2001).

Another challenge in understanding the "gay" population is that there is no one rigid definition of the "gay community." Sometimes the community includes lesbian women and gay men (L/G), sometimes bisexuals are included (LGB) and other times, transgender people are also included (LGBT). While the demographic information is based on the lesbian and gay population, the research studies include lesbian, gay, bisexuals, and transgender people. The third area that limits knowledge development is problematic sampling: Most research data comes from a convenience sample that is from white, middle-class, urban populations who belong to gay and lesbian organizations and groups. Researchers have been challenged to locate older lesbians and gay men of color, as well as those who are rural or lower class (Cantor, Brennan & Shippy, 2004; Quam, 1992, Hash & Cramer, 2003). Fourth, many people do not identify or label themselves by the socially constructed terms "gay," "lesbian," or "bisexual." In fact, the term lesbian was taken from the Greek island Lesbos and reflects its white, Eurocentric origin. Many women of color do not resonate with the term. In addition, some older lesbian and gay men have "been closeted for many years, clutching to their secret due to their sense of vulnerability, and fears of discrimination and social condemnation" (Gewirtzman, 1999).

BIOPSYCHOSOCIAL AND SPIRITUAL ISSUES

Psychological Factors: Homophobia, Heterosexism and Resiliency

This generation of older lesbian and gay men were "labeled 'sick' by doctors, 'immoral' by clergy, 'unfit' by the military, and a 'menace' by police and legislators" (Dawson, 1982). Many older gay people recognized their homosexuality before World War II and long before the 1969 Stonewall Revolution or the 1973 decision by the American Psychiatric Association to declassify homosexuality as a psychiatric disorder. People coming out in the 1930s, 1940s and 1950s were forced to accommodate or hide their identity. *Coming out*, or acknowledging one's sexual orientation, was not experienced as a positive event for many in this population, although many developed resiliency based on their integration into the lesbian and gay community and the extent to which they have revealed their identity to accepting family and friends.

This generation of older lesbian and gay people may be less likely to identify as lesbian and gay. Some lost or feared the loss of job, family, and home. As a result, these lesbians and gay men reacted in different ways. As a way of coping with the homophobic environment, some women learned that it was acceptable to society for them to live together as "room-mates" using the excuse of safety or economic reasons; others chose heterosexual marriage and may have claimed their lesbian identity later in life (Jensen, 1999). Men often chose heterosexual marriages and to have sex with men outside the marriage to hide their homosexuality from society and sometimes from themselves (Cohen, Padilla & Aravena, 2005; Quam, 2001). Because of constantly receiving discounting messages from society and the "strong moral, social, and legal injunctions against homosexuality" (Quam, 2001, p. 2), many lesbians and gay men developed *internalized homophobia* or the phenomenon of a homosexual person accepting and living out the inaccurate myths and negative stereotype applied to her or himself, including feelings of self-loathing.

Throughout their lives, this cohort of lesbian and gay men has fought homophobia and heterosexism. *Homophobia* is the irrational fear and hatred of those who love and sexually desire someone of the same sex. *Heterosexism* is the ideological belief system that stigmatizes or maligns any form of identity, behavior, relationship or community that does not reflect heterosexual beliefs, values and behavior. Ironically, lesbians and gay men have had to "experience the stigma of homosexuality [and heterosexism] usually before they experience the stigma of being old" (Woolf, 1998).

Now, as they are aging, they again confront social and cultural stereotypes and myths about themselves as older lesbians and gay men. Stereotypes of older lesbians and gays define them as more depressed and socially isolated from friends and family than their heterosexual counterparts (Dorfman et al., 1995). These destructive images are harmful to older lesbians and gays and may perpetuate ageism in the gay and lesbian community as well as ageism and homophobia in the general community. A study conducted in California with a sample of older adults who were not randomly selected, but were affiliated with social organizations, and were willing to self-identify as homosexual, demonstrated that there was no significant difference between homosexuals and heterosexuals in terms of levels of depression or social supports; however, what did differ was the type of support that homosexual and heterosexual caregivers received (ibid.). Lesbians and gay men were more likely to receive support from partners and friends called *families of choice*; while heterosexual females and males are more likely to receive support from their biological families referred to as *families of origin* (ibid.; Quam, 2001).

Furthermore, researchers have found that older lesbians and gay men have developed affirming and positive images of themselves as they have deconstructed negative stereotypes from the past and developed *crisis competence*, in which they have restructured homosexuality from something negative to something affirming and positive in their lives (Kimmel, 1978). Kimmel (1978) suggests that as people develop competence in handling a crisis and in dealing with their losses associated with the rejection of heterosexuality, they become more *resilient*–or more able to deal with losses associated with the aging process. As a result, older lesbians and gays have been "described as psychologically well adjusted, vibrant and growing older successfully" (Barranti & Cohen, 2000, p. 349). In addition to developing coping skills to deal with oppression, older lesbian and gay men may have developed more flexibility with nontraditional gender roles than heterosexuals who tend to be more locked into traditional gender roles. This has prepared them for some of the challenges of aging when gender roles become more flexible, taking on tasks of providing physical, emotional, and financial support and assistance to friends and neighbors as they age (Friend, 1990).

Researchers have learned that there are many similarities in the aging process between the homosexual and the heterosexual populations. For example, when reflecting on how older men adjust to aging, Berger (1984) stated that, "Whether you are gay or straight doesn't make a difference, it's your attitude that makes the difference" (p. 60). Like all Americans, lesbians and gays face daunting challenges of aging including experiencing health concerns, receiving reduced income, losing friends and family members, finding suitable housing, engaging in meaningful activities, accessing transportation, and feeling invisible. However, in addition to the universal changes and adjustments that older people make as they age, lesbian and gay older adults face particular problems, such as inadequate health care, income inequities, and lack of access to support services, coupled with experiencing a lifetime of stigmatization in a homophobic and heterosexist environment. On the other hand, since lesbian and gay men have lived with oppression and discrimination all of their lives, they may have learned to develop self-acceptance and a positive sense of who they are. In that case, the negative aging stereotypes may not impact them in the same way that it might affect older heterosexuals who have previously not been challenged by active prejudice.

Biological Factors: Health and Medical Issues

Many lesbian and gay men have patterns of avoiding medical care throughout their lives. They may have sought medical care less often and not received preventative health care because of their fear that their sexual orientation would be discovered by the physician and they would be subject to discrimination (Claes & Moore, 2001). They may have been concerned that their life partner would not be involved in making important medical decisions. Also, there was alarm that health care providers would indicate their sexual orientation in their documentation and that information would get into the wrong hands. Often the lesbians and gay men do not realize that their sexual orientation might be a significant factor in determining the course of treatment. Because most public and private health insurance programs do not recognize same sex partners or offer domestic partner benefits to same sex couples, some lesbians and gay men may not have access to heath insurance that heterosexuals can access. Even those companies that offer domestic partner benefits have not yet extended their coverage to include retirement and death benefits (Table 1).

Lesbians have poorer quality of health care than heterosexual women. Lesbian women have been excluded from medical research and are reluctant to seek medical treatment because of previous negative experiences with the healthcare system or concern about confidentiality. Certain health risk factors may be more common among lesbians such as higher risk for breast cancer as a result of never giving birth, as well as obesity, alcohol, drug and alcohol use. According to a study by Azzuzo (2001), based on the Lesbian Health Study conducted by the National Institute of Health and the Center for Disease Control, more research is needed because "we know virtually nothing about lesbian health issues. . . . Of course, we know even less about *older* lesbian health issues" (pp. 3-4).

Social Factors

One of the perpetual myths about older lesbians and gays are that they are more lonely and isolated from others than their heterosexual counterparts. Researchers have found that heterosexuals tend to turn to family of origin members, while older lesbians and gays are more likely to have a network of close friends or families of choice to whom they turn in need (Bell & Weinberg; Woolf, 1998). Unfortunately, however, "society has not always acknowledged the importance of these 'chosen families' " (LGBT aging project, n.d. p. 8). Grossman, D'Augelli and O'Connell's (2001) study of 416 lesbian, gay, bisexual and transgender people was the largest and most geographically diverse sample to date, but it comprised

TABLE 1

Because lesbians and gay men cannot marry, they have no right to:

- Accidental death benefit for the surviving partner;
- Appointment as guardian of a minor;
- Award child custody in a divorce proceedings;
- Beneficial owner status of securities;
- Bill of Rights benefits for victims and witnesses;
- Burial of service member's dependents;
- Consent to post-mortem examination;
- Control, division, acquisition, and disposition of community property
- Criminal injuries compensation;
- Death benefit for surviving spouse for government employee
- Disclosure of vital statistics records;
- Division of property after dissolution of partnership;
- Eligibility for housing opportunity allowance program of the Housing, Finance and Development Corporation;
- Exemption from claims of Department of Human Services for social services payments, financial assistance, or burial payments;
- Exemption from certain tax;
- Funeral leave for government employees;
- Insurance licenses, coverage, eligibility, and benefits organization of mutual benefits society;
- Legal status with partner's children;
- Making, revoking, and objecting to anatomical gifts;
- Making partner medical decisions;
- Nonresident tuition deferential waiver;
- Notice of probate proceedings;
- Payment of wages to a relative of deceased employee;
- Payment of worker's compensation benefits after death;
- Permission to make arrangements for burial or cremation;
- Qualification at a facility for the elderly;
- Real property exemption from attachment or execution;
- Right of survivorship to custodial trust;
- Right to change names;
- Right to enter into pre-marital agreement;
- Right to file action for nonsupport;
- Right to inherit property;
- Right to support after divorce;
- Right to support from spouse;
- Rights and proceedings for involuntary hospitalization and treatment;
- Rights to notice, protection, benefits, and inheritance under the uniform probate code;
- Sole interest in property;
- Spousal privilege and confidential marriage communications;
- Spousal immigration benefits;
- Status of children;
- Support payments in divorce action;
- Tax relief for natural disaster losses;
- Vacation allowance on termination of public employment by death;
- Veterans' preference to spouse in public employment;
- In vitro fertilization coverage;

Adapted Jan. 07, 2007 Courtesy of PFLAG at http://www.pflag.org/index.php?id=175.

only people who self identified. It found that participants averaged six people in their social network. Lesbians reported higher levels of self esteem and lower levels of internalized homophobia than gay men and lower levels of alcohol consumption. Those living with domestic partners (female and male) reported better physical and mental health and lower rates of loneliness than those living alone.

Another myth is that these older adults do not have children and, therefore, no grandchildren. Lesbians and gays may have children from previous heterosexual marriages, through adoption and through conception by artificial means. Often the children and grandchildren of older lesbians and gay men provide support and some caregiving assistance.

Quam and Whitford (1992) studied eighty lesbians and gays over fifty years old living in the Midwest. Their findings contradict the stereotype of lesbians and gay men as isolated and lonely old people: They found that two thirds of their sample participated in social groups, with a higher rate of participation for lesbians than gay men. While this study demonstrated the importance of social groups for older lesbians and gays, another study revealed some interesting data about living situations for older lesbian and gay men. A 1999 by the National Gay and Lesbian Task Force conducted in New York City found 65 per cent of older lesbians and gay men lived alone compared to thirty six percent of older New Yorkers. Less than 20 percent were living with a partner versus 50 percent of the heterosexual older population who were married. The study also found that 90 percent of the older lesbians and gays had no children compared to 20 percent in the general population.

Lesbians and Gays of Color. Little is known of older lesbians and gays of color. According to one of the few studies by Mays et al. (1998), African American older parents are more likely than other ethnic elders to live in homes of adult family members, with whom they have had childrearing responsibilities rather than in nursing homes. One in four African American lesbians lived with a child for whom they had childrearing responsibilities.

It appears that African American lesbian mothers and grandmothers have a support network that is responsive to the needs of aging family members and that they may be able to rely on these networks for future caregiving needs (Cantor, Brennan, & Shippy, 2004; Mays et al., 1998). Since the number of grandparents raising grandchildren continues to increase, this might predict a trend toward more informal caregivers and social networks in the African American community to care for older lesbians.

Living Arrangements. Regarding living environments, older lesbians and gay men expressed a desire for housing with members of their own community or housing options where the administration and staff were at least sensitive to lesbian and gay aging issues (Claes & Moore, 2001; Lucco, 1987; Quam & Whitford, 1992). Currently older lesbians and gay men may face homophobia from residents and staff in long term care facilities where they are the most vulnerable and may receive poor quality treatment if they reveal their identity. Although there are a number of gay retirement communities being planned, the Palms of Manasota, located in Palmetto, Florida, is the first and only active retirement community specifically for older lesbians and gays (Rosenberg, D. 2001). The Resort on Carefree Boulevard in Fort Myers, Florida, is the only lesbian retirement community. According to Jones (2001), growing old in the gay, lesbian, bisexual, transgender community is positive "if we can work to eliminate ageism, obtain support for dealing with loneliness, and stay in good health, the luck of growing old is good luck" (p. 14).

Economic Concerns. In addition to social discrimination, older lesbians and gay men have faced income discrimination. For example, gay men may receive more than twenty five percent less income than heterosexual men. While there is little income differentiation between lesbian and heterosexual women, all women, lesbian and heterosexual, have consistently made less than men (Cantor, Brennan & Shippy, 2004). Several studies have found that a high percentage of older lesbians and gay men live alone. Because living alone correlates with poverty, more people may face poverty when lower income and living situation are considered.

Religion and Spirituality

Little is known of the religious and spiritual beliefs and practices of older lesbian and gay men. While research on older adults in the general population is growing (Armstrong & Crowther, 2002; Jernigan, 2001; Koenig, Siegler & George, 1989; Moberg, 2001; Wink & Dillon, 2002), and some research has focused on spirituality among younger lesbian and gay men (Simoni & Cooperman, 2000; Sullivan-Blum, 2004; Tan, 2005), there are no studies that focus on older lesbians and gay men. Studies of lesbian and gay men indicate that while some have rejected organized religion, others have found welcoming and inclusive churches and synagogues. There are also churches established to serve the LGBT community, such as the Metropolitan Community Churches (MCC). Most research demonstrates that lesbian and gay men are developing innovative approaches to spirituality resulting in high levels of spiritual well-being, which does not require following a traditional set of religious beliefs or practices.

CAREGIVING

Older Lesbians and Gay Men Caregiving

Similarities in Care. Research with heterosexual caregivers has focused attention on the needs of those giving and receiving care. Many of these are the same concerns that lesbian and gays caregivers confront, such as where to turn for help, how to access services, and what services are available. In addition, Hash and Cramer (2003) found that lesbian and gay caregivers have comparable caregiving concerns and experiences including physical, financial, emotional, social pressure, loss of sleep, depression, conflicts with family members, and tension at work.

With both traditional and lesbian and gay caregivers, the reasons for providing care included the caregiver's sense of responsibility and that the care receiver merited the help. Family of origin more than family of choice caregivers provided care from a sense of obligation and responsibility, "a likely reflection of the long-term and reciprocal nature of parent-child relationships, as well as social norms regarding filial responsibility toward aging parents" (Cantor, Brennan & Shippy, 2004, p. 65). Similar to traditional caregiving situations, lesbian and gay caregivers reported positive outcomes caring for others including a feeling of "emotionally or spiritually nurturing" and providing a sense of meaning in their lives (ibid. p. 66). In addition, about one fifth of the family of origin caregivers shared that providing care created a closer connection with their families.

Differences in Care. In contrast to sharing similar experiences of heterosexual caregivers, lesbian and gay caregivers may face a lifetime of oppression and discrimination and be reluctant to turn to agencies in the community to ask for help. Fear of homophobic and heterosexist attitudes that could affect the quality of care are real concerns. Additional challenges may confront older lesbian and gay caregivers who cannot anticipate what might be a reaction to the disclosure of their sexual orientation. Still other challenges may include planning for long-term health, legal and financial matters.

Several other caregiving challenges affect the gay population. First of all, lesbian and particularly gay older adults may have fewer children who can assist them with caregiving than heterosexuals. Second, because of the large number of young men who died of AIDS, the number of gay caregivers has been dramatically reduced. A third concern is that lacking legal rights and protection of marriage, lesbian and gay men are not entitled to many rights that most heterosexual couples take for granted. For example, lesbian and gay men may be denied access to a life partner because of hospital or nursing home policy that limits visiting or information to family (heterosexual family of origin). Other rights denied include: the right to make arrangements for a funeral or cremation, receive exemption of taxes for homes of totally disabled veterans, and make a partner's medical decisions if that person is incapacitated.

Similarities and Differences. Traditional caregivers report that they are caring for people who are old or frail (15%), have health conditions including cancer, diabetes and heart disease (9% each) and Alzheimer's disease (8%) (Pandya, 2005a). Respondents in a Cantor, Shippy and Brennan (2004) study on gay people caring for a family of origin relative identified similar reasons for providing care: The top three reasons that the family of origin member needed care for physical illness, frailty, and Alzheimer's disease.

When reviewing the type of care given, Cantor, Shippy and Brennan (2004) found that close to one hundred percent of the respondents provided emotional support and advice, including visiting and telephoning, advice on decision making, and financial management. Other services provided consisted of advice-giving and decision-making, serving as liaison with other family members, and acting as care manager, which involved tasks such as assisting with health care providers and arranging for and providing medical care.

Concerning the frequency of care, over half the lesbian caregivers stated that they provided some level of care daily. Two thirds said that they were either the sole provider or provided most of the care (Cantor, Shippy & Brennan, 2004). This study was similar to the traditional caregiving literature in which the responsibility of caregiving was presented in terms of caregiver burden and stress, including placing limits on social life and juggling the demand of being employed and caregiving. Other caregiving burdens included not having enough time for oneself, experiencing difficulty with other care providers and with other family members, and having a lack of privacy (Cantor et al., 2004).

Concerning legal protection, as mentioned earlier, preparing advanced directives for medical and legal authority in decision making is different for lesbian and gay men. Regardless of how long a couple has been together, they are still considered legal strangers. This situation adds a dissimilar type of caregiver stress than that identified in the caregiving literature. Cantor, Brennan and Shippy (2004) found that "eleven percent reported that being a caregiver forced them to come out; while 15% reported that they were forced to conceal their sexual orientation" (p. 50). Many lesbian and gay older adults struggle with the homophobia and heterosexism they encounter in trying to access services. Seventy percent of LGBT reported that they are "tentative" about using services developed by the Area Agency on Aging (AAA), which receives Federal and state monies to administer programs and services to older adults (LGBT Aging Project, n.d.c), although twenty one percent of lesbians sixty and older say that if they are ill, they would turn to an aging service provider (Kehoe, 1988). Nearly half of the AAA admitted that older LGBT individuals would not be welcome, with only 4% indicating that they provide any kind of positive outreach to the LGBT community (LGBT Aging Project, n.d.c).

Support Networks. People outside the partner relationship, families and friends as well as professionals, can impact the caregiving and post-caregiving situation both positively and negatively. Support from family and friends can serve to buffer the pressures of caregiving; however, lack of support from families and professionals can exacerbate the demands of caring for a loved one without any legal or financial protection (Hash, 2001). For example, caregivers often report that support from family and friends helps to relieve them of the stress of providing care to someone with dementia or a chronic illness. Studies of lesbians and gay men indicate that they enjoy the support of a network of friends that helps them to deal with day to day challenges of living in a homophobic culture (Grossman, D'Augelli & Hershberger, 2000; Quam & Whitford, 1992). These same networks can be a source of support and comfort in developing a caring community a chronic illness. In addition to the support from family of friends, some families of origin, including parents and siblings may be positive members of the support network for the lesbian or gay family member. Grossman, D'Augelli and Hershberger (2000) in their study of lesbian, gay, bisexual and transgender older adults found that about one third of their sample mentioned siblings in their social networks and about 40% noted other relatives in their social support networks.

Caregiving for Families of Origin and Families of Choice

The inclusion of research findings on family of origin members and family of choice friends and partners provides a more comprehensive picture of the full range of the challenges and expectations of LGBT caregivers than previously reflected in traditional studies of caregiver burden and stress. The National Lesbian and Gay Task Force Policy Institute surveyed 341 lesbian, gay, bisexual and transgender (LGBT) New Yorkers fifty years of age and older about their caregiving experiences, with particular attention given to the similarities and differences between caregivers for family of origin and family of choice members (Canto, Brennan & Shippy, 2004). The literature suggests that:

- There are similar feelings of providing emotional support among families of origin and families of choice.
- Families of origin are less likely to live with care recipient and so play more of a care manager role, while families of choice caregivers are more likely to give more hands-on care.
- Although both lesbians and gay men are engaged in caregiver activities, women take on more of the stereotypical female tasks.
- Sexual orientation is an issue for a number of family of origin caregivers.
- Both situations, caregivers have to negotiate work and caregiving responsibilities, needing respite, support groups and other services (Cantor, Brennan & Shippy, 2004).
- Family of choice caregivers, according to self-reports, were more likely to reveal their sexual orientation, which may be explained by the fact that they were caring for partners with HIV/AIDS.

Care for Families of Origin. Respondents in Cantor, Brennan and Shippy (2004) indicated that older lesbian and gay adults are being asked and expected to care for family of origin members. Of the 341 respondents, seventy-five respondents indicated they were caring for family of origin members. Half the respondents of family of origin caregivers were female. Of these thirty-seven women respondents, 36% had provided care in the past five year and 41% were currently providing care. For the male respondents, 22% had provided care within the past five years and 39% were currently providing care. For both female and male respondents, the characteristics of the care recipients were similar. About 20% were siblings, children and other relatives; the gender of care recipients for both groups was approximately seventy percent female. Ninety-two percent of the care recipients were heterosexual, three percent lesbian or gay and three percent unknown. The female respondents indicated that thirty-five percent of the family of origin members were living with them.

Care for Families of Choice. Moving from what is known about caring for families of origin to families of choice, Cantor, Brennan and Shippy (2004) found that almost one fourth of the 341 respondents indicated that they had cared for a person who was not a family of origin member in the past five years. Of the 25%, more than fifty percent of the care recipients were identified as the partner or significant other of the respondent. Male caregivers were more likely to be involved with male friends, whereas female caregivers were involved with male and female care recipients. Women were more likely than men to provide care to heterosexual care recipients. Men were more likely to report providing care for someone with HIV/AIDS, while women were twice as likely to report providing care because of physical problems.

Similar to the finding about older lesbian and gay caregivers for family of origin members, close to one hundred percent of the lesbian and gay caregivers for families of choice said that they provided some time of emotional assistance such as telephone calls or in person visits (Cantor, Brennan & Shippy, 2004). Women more often provided household management assistance such as shopping, laundry, cooking, cleaning house and assistance with medical care. Men provided these same services, however, not as frequently.

Since "American educational, religious and other social institutions for the most part do not adequately prepare families to support and affirm their LGBT family members" (Cohen, Padilla & Aravena, 2005, p. 240), it is not surprising that twenty three percent of the family of choice caregivers indicated some kind of difficulty with the care recipient's biological family (Raphael & Meyer, 2000). Thirty percent reported feeling that more was expected of them because of their sexual orientation and sixty three percent indicated that they did not feel their sexual orientation had any impact on the expectations of them as caregivers. Finally, when comparing caregivers' experiences in families of origin and families of choice, Cantor, Brennan and Shippy (2004) concluded "similarities in the amount of caregiving involvement, the reasons for providing care, and the nature of the stress and strain have more to do with the nature of the experience itself than the specific familial relationship between the caregiver and care recipient" (p. 54).

Care for Various Populations. In defining lesbian and gay caregiving, Fredriksen (1999) includes caring for children, as well as caring for an adult with an illness or disability. Her national sample of 1,466 included respondents from 17 to 81 years of age, with a mean of 36.1 years of age. Only 2.8% of her sample was 60 years and older; however, 9.4% were 50 years of age and older. She found that sixteen percent of lesbian and gay men were assisting parents with disability or illness, ten percent were caring for other family members, sixty-one percent were caring for friends, and thirteen percent were caring for partners. Gay men were more likely to be assisting other working-age adults, while lesbians, approximately 60%, were more likely to be providing care to people sixty-five years of age and older (Fredriksen, 1999).

Burden and Rewards of Caregiving. Caregivers have noted the rewards and benefits of caregiving. Caregivers found that providing care for others was an intrinsic part of who they are. It gave them a sense of purpose, and helped them feel emotionally and spirituality nurtured. Caregiving also drew them closer to their family of origin. In a study by Cantor, Brennan and Shippy (2004), respondents reported "relatively high levels of psychological well-being in the domains of self-acceptance, autonomy, and environmental mastery compared with the general population" with women scoring higher scores in the area of self-acceptance and autonomy (p. 78). In addition about 88% indicated that they were at least somewhat satisfied with their lives. However, 30% of respondents in the same study reported being depressed, which is six times higher than the general population. The study also found that caregivers living in New York do not receive the financial, social or emotional support as other caregivers. Cantor, Brennan and Shippy (2004) concluded that

> lesbians and gay men caring for a member of their family of origin go it alone, and depend on other family members, partners and friends to provide support and assistance when needed. Only when the pressures of caregiving become more than their informal systems can accommodate do they turn to formal community organizations, primarily for nursing and home care assistance. (p. 40)

PERCEPTIONS OF OLDER LESBIAN CAREGIVERS

Obviously, while some lesbians have enjoyed positive and supportive relationships with family of origin members, others have experienced more painful and troubled relationships. In an unpublished study by Murray (2005), interviews were conducted with lesbian caregivers that reflected the tension that many may feel as they are torn between taking care of their family of origin member and their family member's negative view of the caregiver's sexual orientation. Study participants expressed a need to protect themselves as they confronted the effects of homophobic and heterosexist environments, also stating that negative societal values led them to feel invisible, socially isolated, and alienated (ibid).

A major theme revealed in Murray's study was that interpersonal family relationships may be strained when there is a lack of acceptance of an adult child's sexual orientation or choice of partner. Robyn, a 46-year-old, single therapist explained,

> *As long as my Dad is alive, I cannot openly live as a lesbian. He has threatened to leave his estate to one of my male cousins if I act 'queer.' I thought that getting married would get him off my case about women, but it didn't. At this point in my life, it's just easier to have female friends rather than lovers.*

Another lesbian caregiver, Carolyn, is a forty-six year old mother and city employee. She is taking care of her elderly mother and shared painfully, *"My mother never treated my partnership as equal to the marriages of my brother and sister. Mom always assumed that I was the one free to drop everything and help her because my siblings had spouses who needed them."* Murray (2005) also found that some lesbian caregivers have been estranged from their families for many years. Yet, when a family member's health affects their ability to care for themselves and to remain in their own homes, the lesbian daughter was asked, expected, or volunteered to assist their family by performing a variety of tasks, such as yard and home maintenance, financial matters, grocery shopping and cooking, and doctors appointments, medication compliance, and filing insurance claims.

Anne, a forty-two year old caregiver who works as a health care administrator and who has been partnered for sixteen years, reflected, *"Although I'm the only one who has taken responsibility for Mom and Dad, they have cut me out of their will. Dad said that he wouldn't leave any money to his queer daughter. "* As Robin, Carolyn, and Anne's stories demonstrate, lesbians may be expected to be caregivers to family members who have been, and sometimes still are, abusive and hostile.

Although some lesbian caregivers experience the additional stress of caring for biological family members who do not accept their sexual orientation, other lesbian caregivers have had a more positive experience in caring for members of their own community. For example, a study by Aronson (1998) provided information on the caregiving experience of fifteen lesbians caring for each other. As a result of her positive findings about mutuality, Aronson redefined the concept of caring for and being cared for in lesbian friendships, partnerships and in the lesbian community: She suggested that in many situations there exists a reciprocal relationship of lesbians caring for each other rather than the traditional view of caregiving as unidirectional in which one person cares for another's needs. Aronson (1998) pointed out that

> we have more language and images for the dilemmas of those who provide care than for those who need it. As a result, we have more language and imagery for the oppressive, unreciprocal and joyless potential for caring than for the possibilities for 'contentment,' 'fun,' and 'satisfaction.' (p. 516)

Aronson's research with lesbian caregivers demonstrates that caregiving relationships are characterized by sharing tasks and responsibilities and creating reciprocity and balanced relationships in which both people receive and give support to each other. This moves the focus from a hierarchal relationship between care receiver and caregiver to a more equitable distribution of power and resources.

CONCLUSION:
POLICY AND CLINICAL RECOMMENDATIONS

This chapter presented research on caregiving in the lesbian and gay community to assist those in the aging network to better understand what makes this group of caregivers different from heterosexual caregivers. It has emphasized that lesbian and gay caregivers may experience adverse societal conditions, rejection by family, and internalized homophobia throughout their lives. They are reluctant to ask for assistance from health and social service providers. Yet they often demonstrate psychological well-being and resiliency in dealing with earlier times of oppression and discrimination. The authors conclude with an overview of policy inequities and clinical concerns.

Inequities in Benefits

Lesbians and gays are denied benefits and rights because they cannot marry or enter into a domestic partnership in most states. For example, retirement and pension plans discriminate against same sex couples, costing the survivor more than $1 million over a lifetime. Social Security pays survivor benefits to spouses in opposite sex marriages when one dies, but not to the life partners in same sex relationships. The Policy Institute of the National Gay and Lesbian Task Force (2003) estimates that this results in lost benefits of $124 million a year (Cahill, 2003).

Clinical Concerns

Because of growing up in a socio-historical time that spread homophobia and heterosexism, many lesbian and gay older adults are fearful of health or social service agencies. Therefore, practitioner understanding of whom older lesbians and gay men are and discerning their needs is even more necessary when providing services and programs. Hash and Cramer (2003) recommend that professionals should spend more time getting to know their clients' needs and receiving diversity training. In addition, the authors suggested that lesbian and gay caregivers should be more open with professionals about the nature of their relationship (Table 2).

TABLE 2. Policy and Clinical Recommendations

Policy
- Understand that older lesbians and gays do not have access to many of the legal protections that heterosexuals enjoy.
- Make the traditional aging network more accessible to older lesbian and gays.
- Assure that older lesbian and gay men are aware of income distribution programs in the area.
- Expand Medicaid spousal impoverishment and Social Security to provide equal access to services to partnered lesbian and gay couples.
- Advocate for an expansion of Family and Medical Leave Act to include partnered lesbian and gay couples.

Clinical
- Develop an inclusive and welcoming service support network for older lesbian and gay caregivers.
- Recognize the diversity within the lesbian and gay community and that we know very little about white, middle class, urban older lesbian and gay caregivers, and even less about those of color or economically struggling.
- Ask culturally competent questions, such as are you partnered rather than are you married? Are there children who are an important part of your life, rather than how many children do you have? Change the intake form to include a check place for partnered, in addition to married, divorced, or single.
- Be sensitive to your client's decision not to come out.
- Make sure to draw the life partner into the health care decision.
- Examine your prejudices. Don't pretend that you know what it is like to live as an older lesbian or gay man in a heterosexist and homophobic society. Be willing to ask questions and let the client teach you.

Adapted from: Hash, L.M. & Cramer, E.P. (2003). *Journal of Gay & Lesbian Social Services*, 15(1/2), 47-63.

REFERENCES

Apuzzo, V. M (2001). A call to action. In D.C. Kimmel and D.L. Martin (Eds), *Midlife and aging in gay America*. (pp. 1-12). New York: Harrington Park Press.

Armstrong, T. & Crowther, M. (2002). Spirituality among older African Americans. *Journal of Adult Development, 9*(1), 3-12.

Aronson, J. (1998). Lesbians giving and receiving care: Stretching conceptualizations of caring and community. *Women's Studies International Forum*, 21(5), 505-519.

Barranti, C. & Cohen, H. (2000). Lesbian and gay elders: An invisible minority. In R. Schneider, N. Kropf and A. Kisor (Eds), *Gerontological Social Work*. (pp. 343-368). Belmont, CA: Wadsworth.

Belden Russmello & Stewart. (2004). Caregiving in the U.S, Retrieved July 25, 2005 from http://www.caregiving.org/data/04finalreport.pdf

Bell, A. P. & Weinberg, M. S. (1981). The Bell and Weinberg study: Future priorities for research on homosexuality. *Journal of Homosexuality, 6*(4), 69-97.

Berger, R. M. (1984). Realities of gay and lesbian aging. *Social Work*, 29, 57-62

Cahill, S. (2003). What do we know about GLBT elders? Retrieved April 4, 2003, from http://www.ngltf.org/issues/agingweknow.htm.

Cantor, M. H., Brennan, M., and Shippy, R. A. (2004). Caregiving among older lesbian, gay, bisexual, and transgender New Yorkers. New York: National Gay and Lesbian Task Force Policy Institute.

Claes, J. A. and Moore, W. (2000). Issues confronting lesbian and gay elders: The challenge for health and human service providers. *Journal of Health and Human Services Administration, 23*(2), 181-202.

Cohen, H. L., Padilla, Y. C., & Aravena, V. C. (2005). Psychosocial support for families of gay, lesbian, bisexual and transgender people. In D. F. Morrow & L. Messinger (Eds.). *Sexual Orientation and Gender Identity in Social Work Practice: Working with Gay, Lesbian, Bisexual and Transgender People* (pp.240-274). New York: Columbian University Press.

D'Augelli, A., Grossman A., Hershberger S., and O'Connell, T. (2001). Aspects of mental health among older lesbian, gay and bisexual adults. *Aging and Mental Health, 5*(2), 149-158.

Dawson, K. (1982). Serving the gay community. SEICUS Report, 11, 5-6.

Dorfman, R., Walters K., Burke P., Hardin, L., Karanik, T., Raphel, J., & Silverstein, E. (1995). Old, sad and alone: The myth of the aging homosexual. *Journal of Gerontological Social Work, 24*(1/2), 28-42.

Family Caregiver Alliance, (2001). Fact sheet: Selected caregiver statistics. Retrieved July 25, 2005 from http://www.caregiver.org/caregiver/jsp/content_node.jsp? nodeid = 439

Fredriksen, K. (1999). Family caregiving responsibilities among lesbians and gay men. *Social Work, 44*(2), 142-155.

Friend, R. A. (1990). Older lesbian and gay people: A theory of successful aging. *Journal of Homosexuality*, 20, 99-118.

Gewirtzman, D. (2000, February 18). Advance planning: Easier than you think. Retrieved July 25, 2005, from http://www.lambdalegal.org/cgi = bin/iowa/documents/records.html?record=591

Gewirtzman, D. (1999, February 1). Better respect for lesbian and gay elders. Retrieved July 25, 2005, from http://www.lambdalegal.org/cgibin/iowa/documents/record2.html?record=377

Grossman, A., Augelli, A., & Hershberger S. (2000). Social support networks of lesbian, gay and bisexual adults 60 years of age and older. *Journal of Gerontology*, 55B(3), 171-179.

Grossman, A., D'Augelli, A. and O'Connell, T. (2001). Being Lesbian, gay, Bisexual and 60 or Older in North America. In D.C. Kimmel and D.L. Martin (Eds), *Midlife and aging in gay America*. (pp. 23-40). New York: Harrington Park Press.

Hash, K. (2001). Preliminary study of caregiving and post-caregiving experiences of older gay men and lesbians.

Hash, L. M. & Cramer, E.P. (2003). Empowering gay and lesbian caregivers and uncovering their unique experiences through the use of qualitative methods. *Journal of Gay & Lesbian Social Services*, 15 (1/2), 47-63.

Jensen, K. L. (1999). *Lesbian epiphanies: Women coming out in later life*. New York: Harrington Park Press.

Jernigan, H. (2001). Spirituality in older adults: A cross-cultural and interfaith perspective. *Pastoral Psychology, 49*(6), 413-437.

Jones, B. E. (2001). Is having the luck of growing old in the gay, lesbian, bisexual, transgender, community good or bad luck? In D.C. Kimmel and D.L. Martin (Eds.), *Midlife and aging in gay America*. (pp. 13-14). New York: Harrington Park Press.

Kehoe, M. (1988). Lesbians over 60 speak for themselves. *Journal of Homosexuality*, 16, 1-111.

Kimmel, D. C. (1978). Adult development and aging: A gay perspective. *Journal of Social Issues, 34*(3), 113-130.

Koenig, H., Siegler, I. & George, L. (1989). Religious and non-religious coping: Impact on adaptation in later life. *Journal of Religion & Aging, 5*(4), 73-94.

LGBT Aging Project. (n.d.a) LGBT aging project: A 3-year plan, and a call for action Retrieved July 25, 2005 from http://www.lgbtaging.org/plan.php

LGBT Aging Project. (n.d.b) Retrieved July 25, 2005, from http://www.lgbtaging.org/

LGBT Aging Project. (n.d.c) Retrieved August 1, 2005 from http://www. lgbtagingproject.org/slide.php

Lucco, A. J. (1987). Planned housing preferences of older homosexuals. *Journal of Homosexuality, 14*,(3/4), 35-36.

Mack, K., & Thompson, L. (2005). A Decade of Informal Caregiving: Are today's caregivers different than informal caregivers a decade ago? Data Profile (Washington, DC: Center on an Aging Society).

Mack, K., & Thompson, L. (2005). How do family caregivers fare: A closer look at their experiences. Data Profile (Washington, DC: Center on an Aging Society).

Mays, V., Chatters L., Cochran S., & Mackness, J. (1998). African American families in diversity: Gay men and lesbians as participants in family networks. *Journal of Comparative Family Studies, 29*(1), 73-87.

McMahan, L. (n.d.) Creating welcoming environments for lesbian, gay, bisexual and transgender elders. Retrieved July 25, 2005, from http://www.lgbtaging.org/guide.php

Moberg, D. (2001). *Guidelines for research and evaluation. Aging and Spirituality: Spirituality Dimensions of Aging Theory, Research, Practice, and Policy* (pp. 211-224). New York: The Haworth Press, Inc.

Mock, S. E. (2001). Retirement intentions of same-sex couples. In D.C. Kimmel & D.L. Martin (Eds.), *Midlife and aging in gay America.* (pp. 81-86). New York: Harrington Park Press.

Murray, Y. (2005). [Interviews with older lesbian caregivers]. Unpublished raw data.

Pandya, S. (2005,April). Caregiving in the United States. Retrieved July 25, 2005 from http://www.aarp.org/research/housing-mobility/caregiving/fs111_caregiving.html

Pandya, S. (2005, June). Racial and ethnic differences among older adults in long-term care service use. Retrieved July 25, 2005 from http://www.aarp.org/research/housing-mobility/caregiving/fs119_ltc.html

PFLAG (2006). Rights, privileges and benefits of marriage. Retrieved June 3, 2003, from http://www.pflag.org/index.php?id=175.

Quam, J. K. (2001). Gay and lesbian aging. SEICUS Report, June/July 1993. Retrieved April 4, 2003, from http://cyfc.umn.edu/seniors/resources/gayaging.html

Quam, J. K. (Ed.). (1997). *Social services for senior gay men and lesbians.* New York: The Haworth Press, Inc.

Quam, J. K., & Whitford, G. (1992). Adaptation and age-related expectations of older gay and lesbian adults. *The Gerontologist, 32*(3), 367-374.

Quam, n.d. Creating welcoming environments for lesbians, gay, bisexual and transgender elders, 3. Retrieved on July 25, 2005, from http://www.lgbtagingproject.org/guide20.php

Raphael, S. M. & Meyer, M. K. (2000). Family support patterns of midlife lesbians: Recollections of a lesbian couple, 1971-1997. In M. R. Marcy. *Midlife lesbian relationships: Friends, lovers, children and parents.* New York: Harrington Park Press.

Rosenberg, D. (2001, January 15). A place of their own. *Newsweek,* 54-55.

Simoni, J. M. & Cooperman, N. A. (2000). Stressors and strengths among women living with HIV/AIDS in New York City. *AIDS Care, 12*(3), 291-297.

Sullivan-Blum, C. R. (2004). Balancing acts: Drag queens, gender and faith. *Journal of Homosexuality, 46*(3-4), 195-209

Tan, P. P. (2005). The importance of spirituality among gay and lesbian individuals. *Journal of Homosexuality, 49*(2), 135-144.

Tully, C. (1989). Caregiving: What do midlife lesbians view as important? *Journal of Gay & Lesbian Psychotherapy, 1*(1), 87-103.

Wagner, D. L. (1997) Comparative analysis of caregiver data for caregivers to the elderly 1987 and 1997. Retrieved July 25, 2005, from http://www.caregiving.org/analysis.pdf

Wenzel, H. V. (2002a). *Fact Sheet: Legal issues for LGBT caregivers.* Retrieved June 6, 2005, from http://www.caregiver.org/caregiver/jsp/content_node.jsp?nodeid=436

Wenzel, H. V. (2002b). *Fact Sheet: LGBT caregiving: Frequently asked questions.* Retrieved June 6, 2005, from http://www.caregiver.org/caregiver/jsp/content_node.jsp?nodeid=409

Wink, P. & Dillon, M. (2002). Spiritual development across the adult life course: Findings from a longitudinal study. *Journal of Adult Development, 9*(1), 79-94.

Woolf, L. (1998). Gay and lesbian aging. Retrieved April 4, 2003, from http://www.webster.edu/~woolfm/oldergay.html

doi:10.1300/J137v14n01_14

Chapter 15

Dementia Caregivers:
Rewards in Multicultural Perspectives

Harriet L. Cohen
Youjung Lee

SUMMARY. Using a strengths-based perspective, the chapter first looks at the positive aspects of dementia caregiving. It then applies the functional age model to the dementia caregiving population. The model allows for a holistic study and assessment of an individual family member's biopsychosocial-spiritual functional capacity in conjunction with the family system's adaptive and coping ability. The role of culture of caregiving practices is also explored. doi:10.1300/J137v14n01_15 *[Article copies available for a fee from The Haworth Document Delivery Service: 1-800-HAWORTH. E-mail address: <docdelivery@haworthpress.com> Website: <http://www.HaworthPress.com> © 2006 by The Haworth Press, Inc. All rights reserved.]*

KEYWORDS. Korean-Americans, functional-age model, adaptive, culture

INTRODUCTION

I have learned a lot about my own strengths . . . having more confidence in my self to make major decisions alone . . . and living in the

[Haworth co-indexing entry note]: "Dementia Caregivers: Rewards in Multicultural Perspectives." Cohen, Harriet L., and Youjung Lee. Co-published simultaneously in *Journal of Human Behavior in the Social Environment* (The Haworth Press, Inc.) Vol. 14, No. 1/2, 2006, pp. 299-324; and: *Contemporary Issues of Care* (ed: Roberta R. Greene) The Haworth Press, Inc., 2006, pp. 299-324. Single or multiple copies of this article are available for a fee from The Haworth Document Delivery Service [1-800-HAWORTH, 9:00 a.m. - 5:00 p.m. (EST). E-mail address: docdelivery@haworthpress.com].

moment. I thought I did that before, but with an Alzheimer's patient in your life, that's very much what you do because you can't really talk about the past a lot. . . . So living in the present is just really important and valuing what we have and enjoying it. (Narayan et al., 2001, p. 24)

With a rising proportion of minority populations among those suffering from dementia, it is increasingly important to understand the cultural conceptualization of dementia and the resilience of their caregivers. Many researchers and clinicians have found the caregiving experience to be associated with long-term exposure to numerous stressful events. However, dementia caregivers also report that they experience growth and a sense of resilience during the caregiving process. Rewards and the beneficial experiences of caregiving to individuals with dementia are described in this chapter. Implications for social work practice with African American, Hispanic, and Asian American dementia caregivers are provided.

Using a strengths-based perspective, the chapter first looks at the positive aspects of dementia caregiving and then applies the functional age model to the dementia caregiving population. The application of the functional age model allows for a holistic study and assessment of an individual family member's biopsychosocial-spiritual functional capacity in conjunction with the family system's adaptive and coping ability (Greene, [1986] 2000). The chapter goes on to discuss family assessment within a multicultural perspective and the general role of culture in dementia caregiving.

DEMOGRAPHICS

Scientists estimate that Alzheimer's disease currently affects up to 4 million people (National Institute of Aging, 2003) and that by 2050, 14 million Americans will be affected by the disease if no treatment becomes available (Hebert et al., 2001). Alzheimer's disease and other forms of dementia are two of the leading diseases that require significant utilization of formal and informal resources (Acton & Kang, 2001; Ory et al., 2000). More than seven million persons in the U.S. currently provide informal care to older adults, with five million informal caregivers providing care for adults fifty years of age and older with dementia (The National Women's Health Information Center, 2004).

The value of the time contributed by dementia caregivers is estimated at 257 billion dollars annually (National Alliance for Caregiving (NAC) & AARP, 2004). The per capita annual cost of providing informal care to elderly people with dementia was estimated to be $18,385 in 1998, and all aspects of costs increased with disease severity (Moore, Zhu, & Clipp, 2001). This is in contrast to privately paid home care or nursing-home care that can cost up to $40,000 a year (Doka & Carter, 2001). Even though Medicare may cover part of the medical cost for the patient, caregiving families still spend an average of $5,800 yearly for nonreimbursable services, and their financial expenditures can increase to more than $10,000 per year until the end of the long caregiving journey (Aoronin, 2004).

NEGATIVE ASPECTS OF CAREGIVING

Practitioners need to distinguish caregiver strain from the positive aspects of caregiving. Although caregiving for a demented family member is typically an expression of love and dedication, it can also be extremely challenging and have adverse effects, such as a sense of burden and feelings of depression, anxiety, and insomnia (Schulz, 2000). Many researchers and clinicians have found the caregiving experience is associated with long-term exposure to numerous stressful events. Caring for a demented relative and coping with the loss of intimate exchanges in the relationship requires many changes in a family's life (Anashen et al., 1995; Connell, Janevic, & Gallant, 2001; Nolan et al., 1996). A national survey of 1,247 caregivers found that most family caregivers experienced physical strain (67 percent), emotional stress (44 percent), or financial hardship (77 percent) as a result of being a caregiver (NAC and AARP, 2004). In short, a long-term disease such as dementia can endanger a caregiving family's general sense of well-being and its financial security.

Ory et al. (1999) analyzed data from 1,509 family caregivers in the 1996 National Caregiver Survey. They argued that the dementia caregiving experience is unlike any other type of caregiving, contributing to a higher level of emotional and physical strain than other type of situation. Controlling for intensity of caregiving involvement and socio-demographic characters such as gender, age, race, education, and income, dementia caregiving status was still a significant predictor of emotional and physical strain (Ory et al., 1999). In another study, McKibbin et al. (1999) found caregivers consume more alcohol than non-caregivers. In addition, Schulz et al. (1995) reported dementia caregivers take more psychotropic drugs than noncaregivers. These research findings indicate the extent to which dementia caregiving can be a high-stress activity.

POSITIVE ASPECTS OF DEMENTIA CAREGIVING

Resilience and Benefit Finding

Despite psychosomatic and negative outcomes that may accompany providing dementia caregiving, caregivers also display resilience. *Resilience*, the ability to overcome adversity, is an innate human characteristic. According to Rutter (1987), human resilience is the "positive pole of individual differences in people's response to stress and adversity, as well as hope and optimism [experienced] in the face of adversity" (pp. 316-317). Greene and Conrad (2002) specified resilience as a biopsychosocial-spiritual phenomenon that occurs across the life course. Resilience also involves competence in daily life. Dementia caregivers exhibit resilience as they continuously shift their role and adapt to a changing family system as their loved one's disease progresses.

Such findings have shifted the caregiving research paradigm to the positive aspects of dementia caregiving (Allen et al., 2003; Boerner, Schulz, & Horowitz, 2004; Roff et al., 2004). Kramer (1997) stated the reasons that positive aspects of caregiving should be investigated: (1) caregivers have reported gains and they want to talk about them; (2) clinicians can work more effectively understanding positive aspects of the experience; (3) older adults may receive increased quality of care; and (4) theorists can build on concepts related to a caregiver's adaptation and psychological health.

Furthering the argument for a strengths perspective, Saleebey (2002) contended that every individual, family, and community has their own capacity for growth. He further remarked that negative experiences and illnesses are part of an individual's culture and personality, and can be a resource for change. The strengths perspective, therefore, can lead practitioners and researchers to focus on client competence rather than on problems, thereby fostering their resilience and well-being (Saleebey, 2002).

Finding Meaning

Research findings generally show that, through caregiving, women can gain a sense of self-worth and mastery, qualities associated with greater family cohesion and marital satisfaction (Martire, Stephens, & Franks, 1997). In addition, caregivers reported that they valued positive aspects of relationships with their impaired family member. Furthermore, they appreciated the feeling of confidence that giving care provided (Farren et al., 1999). For example, Hepburn et al. (2002) conducted a qualitative study of the experiences of 132 spouses giving dementia caregiving. Caregivers talked about the lessons they learned: increased knowledge of self, the importance of "carpe diem" (seizing the day), faith, family unity, idiosyncratic meaning, acquisition of skill, the value of humor, acceptance, and expression of internalized belief. In sum, caregivers found a transformed inner-self through the caregiving process and even received benefit from it.

In Paun's qualitative study (2003), dementia caregivers disclosed that they noticed change, that they took charge, adjusted, or coped. They also made sense of their situation and looked to their future with optimism, projecting strength, determination, and survival. Their interpretations of being a caregiver for their loved one indicated their personal growth. The caregivers were determined not to be victims and to take charge of the caregiving situation.

Similarly, Noonan and Tennstedt (1997) tested the contribution of finding meaning in the caregiving situations of 131 informal caregivers. Findings suggest that caregivers find meaning when they come to terms with their situation. In turn, finding meaning in caregiving had a positive effect on self-esteem, but a feeling of overload or too many responsibilities, could lead to caregiver stress, depression and low self-esteem. It can generally be said that caregivers who more actively sought meaning in their caregiving activity reported greater well-being. This indicates the importance of practitioners exploring the factors related to survivorship and learning what the caregivers perceive as positive coping strategies (Noonan & Tennstedt, 1997).

How do dementia caregivers survive the long journey? Pierce, Lydon, and Yang's study (2001) of 50 caregivers provides insights into how dementia caregivers persist in the sometimes burdensome process. The researchers argued that the better a caregiver's sense of autonomy and self-determination and identification with the dementia caregiving process the greater the caregiver's enthusiasm about caring for their loved one. Such enthusiasm may reduce the caregiver's sense of threat in problematic situations and enhance his or her general well-being.

Coping Styles

Exploring differences in coping styles provides an insight into how dementia caregivers persist. Dementia caregivers present different types of coping styles and develop them through the caregiving process. Lazarus and Folkman (1984) distinguished *problem-focused coping*, which is managing the problem within the stressful environment, from *emotion-focused coping*, which is adjusting the emotional response to the crisis. These coping strategies have complex interrelationships and can be used simultaneously or sequentially (Lazarus & Folkman, 1984).

Garity (1997) used Lazarus and Folkman coping model in his research of seventy-four dementia caregivers to understand their coping styles and their relationship to resilience. The study affirmed that caregivers remained more resilient when they took a proactive coping style. Problem-focused coping strategies used included planning, creating and implementing an action plan, and developing different solutions to each situation. Emotion-focused strategies employed took into account caregivers' need to express anger. Emotion-focused coping strategies were comprised of seeking social support, achieving positive appraisal, confronting oneself, and distancing. Confrontive styles of coping in which the caregiver may express negative feelings towards the care recipient were also found to be beneficial. Garity concluded that the dementia caregivers who made action plans and followed them were more resilient. The results also showed that the caregivers who tried to see the bright side of the situation were more resilient. On the other hand, the caregivers who adopted the emotional coping skills of trying to escape or avoid the situation, wishing the situation would disappear, or increasing their drinking and smoking had a lower resilience score.

An Existential Perspective

Many dementia caregivers have overcome their difficult situations and even grew as a result, being satisfied with being a caregiver for their loved one and receiving benefits from it. However, Farren (1997) has argued that more can be learned about caregiving by combining stress or adaptation models with an existential perspective. Farren took this position because of the belief that existential theory allows for an understanding of a "human's ability to discover and create meaning through transcendence and transformation of the dementia caregiving experience" (p. 255).

Yalom (1995), an existentialist, said that human beings struggle with the ultimate concerns of existence, such as "death, isolation, freedom and meaninglessness" (p. 91). He went on to say that despite these negative conditions, humans are essentially "meaning seeking creatures," fighting to make meaning in a world which does not have inherent meaning (p. 91). He emphasized that when practitioners include existential factors in their practice, such as acknowledging that life is sometimes unfair and recognizing one's ultimate responsibility in a situation regardless of others' help, it is an incredible therapeutic tool in caregiving situations (ibid.). In using an existential perspective, practitioners also learn more about the caregiver's subjective experiences. Thus, the existential perspective can give the practitioner an understanding of why some caregivers grow through the caregiving process, while others do not experience the same benefit.

Burden and Gain

Burden and gain in dementia caregiving are not simply opposites. In a study by Naraya et al. (2001), qualitative interviews with the fifty caregivers supported the coexistence of the seemingly opposite aspects of caregiving. Fifty-eight percent (58%) of respondents disclosed that they experienced "self-fulfilling and affirming" experiences during caregiving, with the same percentage undergoing "losses and difficulties" (p. 27). In addition, positive aspects of caregiving were significantly related to the caregiver's competence.

Similarly, Chappell and Reid (2002) claimed caregivers can experience burden while they maintain high to adequate levels of well-being: namely, positive and negative aspects of dementia caregiving can coexist. The authors went on to suggest that dementia caregivers' quality of life can be enhanced even though they may suppress feelings of caregiving burden. They pointed out that social support is directly related to caregiver well-being while behavioral problems are a main determinant of caregiver burden.

RESEARCH LIMITATIONS

The body of research on gain and positive aspects of dementia caregiving is still growing. However, there are methodological and conceptual issues. Many researchers depend on convenience samples and cross-sectional data (Kramer, 1997). This leaves open questions on the direction of causality among stress, subjective appraisal, and coping. In addition, there are several operational terms for the positive aspect of caregiving including *satisfaction* (Martire, Stephens, & Franks, 1997), *gains* (Kramer, 1997), *meaning making* (Farren, 1999), *benefit finding* (Hepburn et al., 2002; Rapp et al., 1998), *uplifts* (Pinquart & Sorensen, 2003), *reward of meaning* (Cartwright et al., 1994), and *enjoyment*.

Even though there are some limitations in the current research on the positive aspects of dementia caregiving, studies provide important insights for practitioners and researchers. Utilizing a strengths-based perspective, social work practitioners can assess the positive aspects of caregiving and implement interventions to enhance dementia caregiver's well-being. Researchers can investigate the characteristics of dementia caregivers who benefit from the caregiving experience and thereby contribute to the further understanding of family dynamics.

BIOPSYCHOSOCIAL-SPIRITUAL ASSESSMENT

As the research presented suggests, practitioners can best begin their assessment with a view that there may be strengths and challenges in the caregiving experience. A practitioner should have combined this theoretical point of view with a knowledge of biopsychosocial-spiritual factors that influence the dementia caregiver's functional age. These factors are also intertwined in the reciprocal and developing dynamics of the family unit (Greene, [1986] 2000).

Biological Factors

Dementia Defined. Practitioners should first become familiar with the definition and signs of dementia. According to *DSM-IV-TR* (American Psychiatric Association, 2000), dementia refers to

> The development of multiple cognitive deficits that include memory impairment and at least one of the following cognitive disturbances: aphasia (deterioration of language function) apraxia (impaired ability to execute motor activities despite intact motor abilities, sensory function, and comprehension of the required task), agnosia (failure to recognize or identify objects despite intact sensory function), or a disturbance in executive functioning (the ability to think abstractly and to plan, initiate, sequence, monitor, and stop complex behavior). (p. 133)

Dementia progresses slowly: the average length of the disease from observed onset to death is seven years and it ranges from two years to eighteen years (Lichtenberg, Murman, & Mellow, 2003).

Types and Stages of Dementia. There are many types of dementia including "dementia of the Alzheimer's type, vascular dementia, dementia due to HIV disease, dementia due to head trauma, dementia due to Parkinson's disease, dementia due to Huntington's disease, dementia duc to Pick's disease," etc. (American Psychiatric Association, 2000, pp. 163-166). Among the different types of dementias, Alzheimer's disease is the most common, accounting for 50% to 70% of all dementias (Agronin, 2004).

Health and Physical Impact on Caregivers. The major population of dementia caregivers is older adults who have biologically-based concerns of their own. When they experience the burden of caregiving for a long period of time, their health can be threatened. Caregivers providing care for family members over fifty years of age routinely underestimate the length of time they will spend as caregivers. Only forty six percent expected to be caregivers longer than two years. In reality, because of the physical, medical, or frailty issues of the older adult, the average length of time spent on caregiving is about eight years, with approximately one third of respondents providing care for 10 years or more (MetLife Mature Market Institute, November 1999).

Research suggests that dementia care status does not appear to have a consistent physical health impact on dementia caregivers. For example, Schulz and Beach (1999) conducted a population-based prospective study from 1993 to 1998 with a total of 392 caregivers and 472 noncaregivers. They examined four-year mortality rates and found out that caregivers who experienced caregiving strain had a 63% higher mortality rate than noncaregivers, after controlling for sociodemographic factors, prevalent disease, and subclinical cardio-vascular disease (Schulz, & Beach, 1999).

On the other hand, the Canadian study of health and aging working group (2002) studied a nationally representative sample of 948 dementia caregivers. The research was conducted longitudinally with a 4 to 5.9 year interval between the two measurement points. They found that caregiving burden does not directly translate into deteriorating health. Therefore, practitioners need to obtain specific information from caregivers on their health concerns.

Psychological Factors

Cohen, Colantonio, and Vernich (2002) also conducted research on the positive aspects of caregiving. They reported that positive feeling about caregiving is negatively related to depression, burden, and poor health.

Two hundred and eighty nine (289) dementia caregivers were asked about their perceptions of positive aspects of cargiving. Two hundred and eleven (211) caregivers (73%) answered that they could find a positive aspect of caregiving. Positive aspects of giving care included experiencing companionship (22.5%), feeling a sense of fulfillment and reward (21.8%), experiencing enjoyment (12.8%), and achieving a sense of duty and obligation (10.4%).

Tarlow et al. (2004) developed a new measure for evaluating the positive aspects of caregiving with dementia caregivers. Their statistically reliable and valid measure was used to examine the perceptions of 1,229 dementia caregivers. Dementia caregivers who participated in the study mentioned that "caregiving made them feel needed, useful, and good about themselves" (p. 446). They also said that "it enabled them to appreciate life more, to develop a more positive attitude toward life, and strengthened their relationships with others" (p. 449). Such research outcomes emphasize the necessity of the practitioner conducting comprehensive assessments including how the caregiver perceives the negative and positive aspect of dementia caregiving.

Problem Behaviors, Burden and Depression. A dementia patient's severe and early problem behaviors may have harmful and long term effects on his or her caregiver (Gaugler et al., 2005). In Gaugler et al.'s study (2005), caregivers who experience the care recipient's deleterious behaviors in the early stages of dementia showed increased burden and depression over the three year research period. Covinsky et al.'s cross-sectional (2003) study of 5,627 dementia family caregivers reported that almost one-third (32%) of the caregivers presented six or more symptoms of depression on the 15-item Geriatric Depression Scale (GDS). Conducted with a geographically and ethnically diverse population, this study was one of the largest investigating dementia caregivers' depression. The independent factors which predicted caregiver depression were low income, the relationship to the patient (being daughter or wife compared to son of male patient), more hours spent on caregiving, and poor caregiver functional status (Covinsky et al., 2003).

In Schulz et al. (1995) review of forty-one dementia caregiving studies from 1990 to 1995 all reported increased depressive symptoms compared to nondementia caregivers. Across forty-one studies, psychiatric mobility (mostly depression and anxiety) was related to patient problem behaviors and income. In a similar vein, Pinquart and Sorensen's (2003) meta-analysis with 228 studies showed dementia caregivers are most burdened when care recipients exhibit problem behaviors despite the amount of care provided. Caregivers' self-rated health, perceived stress, and life satisfaction were also linked with their psychological health (Schulz et al., 1995).

Depression or Anticipatory Grief. Since dementia is long-time disease, it is sometimes called an *ongoing funeral.* Through the ongoing process, caregivers experience anticipatory grief that can even be beneficial when, as practitioners put it, anticipatory grief supports early expressions of loss of the familiar behaviors of a loved one. The assessment question becomes whether the depression is solely depression or an expression of anticipatory grief.

Walker and Pomeroy (1996) attempted to distinguish dementia caregivers' anticipatory grief from depression. A hundred dementia caregivers' anticipatory grief and depression were measured by the Grief Experience Inventory (GEI) and the Beck Depression Inventory (BDI). The intensity of grief explained almost half of the variance in depression when controlling for length of caregiving time, support group attendance, gender, relationship with care receiver, and knowledge of dementia (ibid.). This study reveals the importance of an accurate assessment of a client's feelings and sense of despair in the long-term caregiving process and the need for timely intervention.

The Role of Appraisal. Much of the literature shows that the caregiver's appraisal of the caregiving experience can play a central role in how the caregiving relationship is experienced (Harwood et al., 2000; Hooker et al., 2002; Rapp & Chao, 2003). Therefore, practitioners will need to assume that the relationship between caregiving and the psychological health of the caregiver is neither simple nor linear and depends on the caregiver's appraisal process. Caregiving appraisal may be thought of as "all cognitive and affective appraisals and reappraisals of the potential stressor and the efficacy of one's coping effort" (Lawton et al., 1989, p. 61).

Lazarus and Folkman (1984) also emphasized that appraisal of the caregiving situation contributes to adaptation during the caregiving experience. They conceptualized a transactional, process-oriented model comprised of three types of cognitive appraisal: (1) primary, (2) secondary, and (3) reappraisal. *Primary appraisal* includes the caregiver's judgment about the unexpected onset of a condition that it is "irreverent, benign-positive, or stressful" (p. 32). *Secondary appraisal* refers to the caregiver's evaluation of how he or she may cope within that perceived context. *Reappraisal* is a changed appraisal when new resources are provided or perceived within one's environment. *Personal factors,* such as commitment and belief, and *situational factors,* including novelty, predictability, event uncertainty, and timing of the stressful event, also determine the appraisal process.

Harwood et al. (2000) showed that appraised burden mediated the relationship between objective stressors, caregiving resources, caregiver ethnicity, and adaptational outcome of depression. In this study of 114 dementia caregivers, the authors argued that subjective appraisals of stress, rather than the role of objective stressors, is important in determining a dementia caregiver's well-being. Hooker et al.'s (2002) study with sixty-four dementia patient-caregiver dyads showed that care receivers' increased problem behaviors and prolonged caregiving were strongly associated with a caregiver's worsening mental and physical health. However, the relationship between the dementia patient's behavioral and psychological symptom and the caregiver's mental and physical health is again mediated through stress appraisal.

Social Support Factors

Because social support has been found to be an important determinant of a dementia caregiver's well-being, the extensiveness of such support is another area for practitioners to assess. In Chapell and Reid's (2002) research, 243 Canadian caregivers showed that perceived social support was positively related to their general well-being. In another study of depression, quality of life, and perceived benefit among caregivers, Rapp et al. (1998) found that social resources were the most significant factor related to a caregiver's well-being. Controlling for socio-demographic characteristics of the caregivers and care receivers' problem behaviors, caregivers reported that they felt less depressed, experienced better quality of life, and perceived more benefit from caregiving when they were able to use their skills to obtain more resources.

Despite the benefit of social support, many caregivers are left alone until their physical and mental health are in danger. Loneliness and social isolation are often associated with dementia caregivers' increasing depression. Secondary analysis of 242 caregivers by Beeson et al. (2000) showed that caregivers' depression is significantly predicted by loneliness, relational deprivation, quality of the current relationship, and distance from supports due to caregiving. Tebb and Jivanjee (2000) maintain the view of the importance of early intervention on dementia caregivers' isolation and lack of social support. Their qualitative study on dementia caregivers' isolation articulated multidimensional causes of isolation including

- *environmental isolators*–encompassing lack of provider's information on dementia and caregiver needs, negative societal views on aging, and lack of community support;
- *individual isolators*–including role changes, loss of companionship and social relationships, limited knowledge of resources, and inadequate income to access social activities.

In the assessment of a caregiver's social functional capacity, it is important to investigate caregivers' perceived social support and social ties/integration separately. Thoit (1995) held that social integration is positively related with physical/mental health but cannot buffer physical or emotional effects of continuing difficulties in one's life. Perceived emotional social support, however, is directly related with good physical and mental health and also buffers the damages a person receives from major life crisis. A further distinction can be made about caregiver support systems. In Stuckey and Smyth's (1997) study of 203 dementia caregivers, functional support was distinguished conceptually from social support. A caregiver's subjective awareness of social ties was a stronger predictor of positive health outcome than their objective amount of social ties.

Spiritual Factor

Many studies have shown the role of spirituality–a universal human phenomenon (Chiu et al., 2004)–in reducing dementia caregivers' burden (Picot et al., 1997; Farran, Paun, & Elliott, 2003; Roff et al., 2004). It is therefore another pertinent area to assess in caregiving situations. For example, Crowther et al. (2002) argued that positive spirituality enhances elders' physical and psychological well-being. They also suggested that Rowe and Kahn's (1998) successful aging model, which is based on the older adult's ability to engage in active life, minimize risk and disability, and maximize physical and mental abilities, should be extended to incorporate positive spirituality.

Farran, Paun, and Elliot (2003) provided a spiritual model for dementia caregivers based on their qualitative research with multicultural caregivers including African American, Latino, Caucasian, and other ethnicities. The 43 respondents in the study articulated the importance of their faith in their life and how they benefited from spirituality during the dementia caregiving experience. Researchers concluded that the combination of a prior experience of faith and more recent gains from spirituality can contribute to positive meaning in the caregiving experience (Farran, Paun, & Elliot, 2003).

Research suggests that minority caregivers experience increased religiosity in the caregiving process and benefit from it more than majorities (Navaie-Waliser et al., 2001; Haly et al., 2004). In a study by Picot et al. (1997), the fact that African-American caregivers perceived greater reward than their white counterparts was thought to be associated with burden being mediated by religiosity. Haley et al. (2004) also found that

African-American caregivers make greater use of religion in coping and appear to have better psychological well-being than white caregivers.

In a similar qualitative study by Koening's (2005), ethnic minority dementia caregivers disclosed that spirituality gave them a "sense and meaning and purpose as a caregiver" (p. 164). Caregivers went on to state that they would feel guilty if they relied on outside help since caring for their loved one is their "soul" responsibility. That is, spirituality helped them resolve their ethical caregiving dilemmas. Caregivers also used spirituality as a way of transcending complicated decision-making issues. One interviewee said "I am just so happy and grateful that she (the care receiver) is still here with me. I just wouldn't consider nothing hard" (p. 167). In a similar study by Paun (2003), spirituality was an important factor that empowered African American caregivers to find ultimate meaning to overcome harsh caregiving situations (Paun, 2003).

Family System Factors

Due to the interdependence of each family member in the system, exploring a family's functioning along with the caregiver's and the care recipient's biopsychosocial-spiritual functioning is an important assessment process. This task may be complicated because in some cases multiple family members are involved in the caregiving process even though there is one primary caregiver.

Several studies point to the family characteristics that enhance or detract from caregiving situations. For example, Heru, Ryan, and Iqbal (2004) reported that dementia caregivers with poor family functioning report higher levels of strain and burden. This in turn disrupted communication. Poor problem-solving skills were also related to high strain, while good problem-solving skills were an important component in family resilience (Greene & Livingston, 2002).

Role Transitions

In the functional age model, the family is considered a system with family roles reflecting the family's developmental patterns. Role changes and transitions are inevitable as the family moves through the developmental process (Greene, [1986] 2000). In multigenerational families, caring for an aging or ill parent is a developmental task. When caregiving tasks are successful, caregivers' self-esteem and resilience are enhanced.

Sherrell, Buckwalter, and Morhardt (2001) studied the midlife developmental task of adult child caring their older parents. They argued that when parents need an adult child's protection, he or she should "shift their own identity toward consolidation of an adult sense of self and individualism" (p. 387). This perspective of caring for a parent during midlife is different from views that suggest midlife is a time of personal freedom and autonomy.

Sandwich-Generations. An example of potential role conflict can be found among sandwich generation female caregivers who simultaneously care for a frail parent and their own children at home. These women are also predisposed to health and psychological problems (Tebes & Irish, 2000). Along with potential health issues for the caregiver, younger children of the caregiver are also vulnerable given their mother's stressful situation. Tebes and Irish (2000) explored family-focused mutual help intervention for such families. These interventions were found to reduce depressive symptoms and decrease the negative impact of caregiving. In addition, the children who participated in the intervention group showed increased global functioning along with an increase in social competence.

Family Decision-Making

The following case illustrates how a family's culture, decision making and coping style influences its response to a parent with dementia:

Mr. Kim was diagnosed as having Alzheimer's disease two years ago. He showed several disturbing behaviors and he was recently hospitalized due to a stroke. Even though Mrs. Kim has been his main caregiver, their married daughter, Mrs. Park who works full time and has two young sons, has been heavily involved in the caregiving. Mr. Kim's two sons, who live in other states, have contributed financially. On the day of Mr. Kim's discharge from the hospital, some concerns emerged. First, his primary doctor did not include Mr. and Mrs. Kim in the discussion process even though their bilingual daughter was trying to translate. This insulted Mr. and Mrs. Kim in front of their children. The experience of being left out of the discussion depressed the Kims and made them believe they hade lost their parental authority. The daughter, Mrs. Park, felt caught between her obligation to her parents and to her two children. Caring for her parent with dementia and taking care of her two boys were strenuous work for the full-time working mom. Mrs. Park wished her brothers would provide more than financial support.

Research suggests that families can be guided in making positive decisions as the parent with dementia becomes increasingly ill. For example, in Liberman and Fisher's (1999) study of 211 dementia caregivers, families that used positive methods of conflict resolution and handled the decision-making process well, provided better care to their ill parents than those who did not. Family members' mutual help and supportive personal relationships in the caregiving context are imperative for the caregiver's resilience and healthy family functioning.

MULTICULTURAL PERSPECTIVES

Culture

In 2003, minorities represented 17.6% of the U.S. elderly population, and the proportion is expected to increase to 26.4% by 2030 (Administration on Aging, 2004). With the growing population of minority caregivers in the U.S., it is necessary to better understand a cultural conceptualization of caregiving (NAC & AARP, 2004). Culture plays an important role through entire period of dementia caregiving, including designating a main caregiver, decision-making during the experience, utilizing outside help, institutionalizing a loved one, and healing through the bereavement process. Moreover, it is necessary to use cultural information to teach minority dementia caregivers problem-solving skills and active coping skills to improve their well-being.

Comparison studies of dementia caregivers from multiple cultures reveals the role of culture in appraisal and coping on the caregivers' psychological well-being (Adam, Aranda, Kemp, & Takagi, 2002). For example, Dilworth-Anderson, Goodwin, and William (2004) explained that the cultural socialization and sense of duty to family members of African-American caregivers play important roles in the perception of dementia caregiving along with their general health. The findings of Dilworth-Anderson, Goodwin, and William (2004) coincide with other researchers who have found that African-American caregivers are less depressed and or burdened in the caregiving role than white caregivers (Haley et al., 2004; Janevic & Connell, 2001); that they perceive more reward from caregiving than white caregivers (Haley et al., 2004; Picot et al., 1997), and that they are more positive than white counterparts in the caregiving situation (Roff et al., 2004). In addition, African-American dementia caregivers have been shown to use less psychotropic medication than white caregivers (Haley et al., 2004).

Similarly, Knight et al. (2000) sociocultural stress and coping model emphasized the significant effect of culture on caregiving. (The model refers to ethnicity as a culture as well as a structural status variable). In their research, African-Americans appraised the caregiving situation as less stressful than their white counterparts. The authors emphasized that minority ethnicity culture as well as differences in gender influence the demand, appraisal, coping, and health outcome of dementia caregiving. According to Roth, Haley, Owen, Clay, and Goode (2002), African American caregivers show better adaptation and less deterioration than white caregivers over the caregiving period. Both of the caregiver groups, however, present decreased physical health caused by chronic caregiving stresses. Clearly, these studies show that even though minority caregivers are resilient through the caregiving journey, they are still vulnerable and face many challenges (Roth et al., 2002).

Economic Hardship

Still another consideration is the economic level of the caregiving family. Regardless of the caregiving status, many minorities struggle with financial hardship. Almost half of unmarried elderly Hispanic females (49%) and forty-one percent (41%) of unmarried elderly African American women are poor. Even though African-American caregivers have heavier caregiving workloads than white caregivers (Naviae-Waliser et al., 2001), they are only half as likely to have paid home care service as are white caregivers (Women's Institute for Secure Retirement, 2002).

Familism

For many reasons, some minority family caregivers try to handle the issue of dementia within their family network. From a biomedical perspective, within western culture, dementia is viewed as an abnormal and pathological condition that is distinct from the process of normal aging. Among many Asian-American families, however, memory loss and slightly demented behaviors are openly viewed as a 'normal' part of the aging process (Hinton et al., 2000; Braun et al., 1995). Adult children find no reason to announce their parent's memory loss. This is why Asian-American caregivers tend to not seek outside help until they have arrived at the point when the patient and the family require professional intervention.

Minority families put *familism*, known as "the perceived strength of family bonds and sense of loyalty to family" (Luna et al., 1996, p. 267), as a top priority and prefer not to disclose sensitive family issues (Bullock, Crawford, & Tennstedt, 2003; Hinton, Guo, & Hillygus, 2000). This involves the widely-held cultural value whereby families will be the first, and often the only, place to turn to for help (Hicks & Lam, 1999). Many studies support the idea that minority caregivers prefer to rely on extended family networks rather than to use formal services in the caregiving process (Bullock, Crawford, & Tennstedt, 2003; Dilworth-Anderson, Williams, & Gibson, 2002).

Similarly, John, Resendiz, and Vargas (1997) found that Mexican-American families view eldercare as "an affirmation and fulfillment of core Mexican American cultural values" (p. 159). They want to take care of their frail parent in their family network despite the personal cost or other negative consequences. The researchers concluded that the ethnocultural family value of care is a salient factor that guides them in continuing to care for aging parents and not to use institutions as services (John, Resendiz, & Vargas, 1997).

Although familism is an important cultural factor in dementia caregiving, the role of familism in caregivers' psychological and physical well-being is still unsettled. For example, in a study by Youn et al. (1999), the amount of stress among recent Korean immigrants, Korean, Korean American, and white caregivers was compared. Familism was found to be highest among Korean immigrants and lowest among white participants. At the same time, the study showed inconsistent relationships among the familism, burden, and distress along ethnic lines, leaving more research to be done. The lack of conclusive research further suggests that the practitioner must learn more about a particular family's caregiving practices and beliefs.

Filial Piety

In large measure, family cultural expectations explain who is selected as the main decision-maker when a parent is ill. Such cultural tradition is rooted in filial piety that teaches that children should respect their parents and take care of their old parents (Lee & Sung, 1998). However, in mainstream culture, it is a spouse who is more likely to be the main caregiver (Janevic & Connell, 2001). In Asian culture, in keeping with the values of

Confucianism, it is common for the eldest son and his wife to provide care and make decisions for a parent (Braun & Browne, 1998). Even when the first son and his wife do not reside with the parent, it is they who are assumed to be the decision-makers (Youn et al., 1999).

Currently, the concept of filial piety in the Asian family and in society at large is changing. Yeh and Bedford (2003) have proposed a modern dual filial piety model: They compare *reciprocal filial piety,* emotional and spiritual attending to the fact that one was raised by their parents, and *authoritarian filial piety*, suppressing one's own wishes and following parent's wishes. Interestingly, the authors concluded that because it is self-reinforcing, reciprocal filial piety is applicable in other than Asian cultures (Yeh & Bedford, 2003).

CONCLUSION

This chapter provided the rationale supporting the coexistence of positive and negative aspects of caregiving, highlighting the importance of exploring both these aspects in the assessment process. Despite the growing body of literature on the coexistence of positive and negative aspects of dementia caregiving, many researchers continue to focus on negative aspects of dementia caregiving, while social work practitioners far too frequently overlook the positive aspect of dementia caregiving (Greene, [1986] 2000). The authors urge that, first and foremost, social workers begin their assessment of client families by asking about their perceptions of dementia caregiving and expectations for care in their culture.

The importance of practitioners understanding social norms and the specific culture of a client family system cannot be overemphasized. Heterogeneity of each subculture even within the same ethnic group should be respected. This is achieved by attending to such factors as a caregiver's country of origin, reason for immigration to the U.S., length of residence in the U.S., socioeconomic status, educational attainment, and acculturation status. In addition, the need for practitioners to be culturally competent and to promote a caregiver's resilience was discussed. Finally, the authors portrayed dementia caregivers as increasingly important to the overall well-being of people with dementia at a time when the cost of health care continues to increase. Such care may not be given a price.

REFERENCES

Acton, J.G., & Kang, J. (2001). Interventions to reduce the burden of caregiving for an adult with dementia: A meta-analysis. *Research in Nursing & Health, 24,* 349-360.

Adams, B., Aranda, M., Kemp, B., & Takagi, K. (2002). Ethnic and gender differences in distress among Anglo American, African American, Japanese American, and Mexican American spousal caregivers of persons with dementia. *Journal of Clinical Geropsychology, 8*(4), 279-301.

Administration on Aging (AoA). (2004). *A Profile of Older American: 2004.* U.S. Department of Health and Human Service. Washington, DC.

Agronin, M. (2004). *Practical guides in psychiatry: Dementia.* Philadelphia, PA: Lippinncott Williams & Wilkins.

Allen, R., Kwak, J., Lokken, K., & Haley, W. (2003). End-of-life issues on the context of Alzheimer's disease. *Alzheimer's Care Quarterly, 4,* 312-330.

American Psychiatric Association. (2000). *Diagnostic and statistical manual of mental disorders IV.* Washington, DC: American Psychiatric Association.

Aranda, M. (2001). Racial and ethnic factors in dementia care-giving research in the U.S. *Aging and Mental Health, 5*(supplement 1), S116-S123.

Beeson, R., Horton-Deutsch, S., & Farran, C. (2000). Loneliness and depression in caregivers of persons with Alzheimer's disease or related disorders. *Issues in Mental Health Nursing, 21*(8), 779-806.

Boerner, K., Schulz, R., & Horowitz, A. (2004). Positive aspects of caregiving and adaptation to bereavement. *Psychology and Aging, 19*(4), 668-675.

Braithwaite, V. (2000). Contextual or general stress outcomes: Making choices through caregiving appraisals. *The Gerontologist, 40*(6), 706-717.

Brown, K., & Browne, C. (1998). Perceptions of dementia, caregiving, and help seeking among Asian and Pacific Islander Americans. *Health and Social Work, 23*(4), 262-275.

Bullock, K., Crawford, S., & Tennstedt, S. (2003). Employment and caregiving: Exploration of African American caregivers. *Social Work, 48*(2), 150-162.

Cartwright, J., Archbold, P., Stewart, B., & Limandri, B. (1994). Enrichment processes in family caregiving to frail elders. *Advanced Nursing Science, 17*(1), 31-43.

Chappell, N., & Reid, R. (2002). Burden and well-being among caregivers: Examining the distinction, *The Gerontologist, 42*(6), 772-780.

Chee, Y., & Levkoff, S. (2001). Culture and dementia: Accounts by family caregivers and health professionals for dementia-affected elders in South Korea. *Journal of Cross-Cultural Gerontology, 16,* 111-125.

Chiu, L., Emblen, J., Hofwegen, L., Sawatzky, R., & Meyerhoff, H. (2004). An integrative review of the concept of spirituality in the health science. *Western Journal of Nursing Research, 26*(4), 405-428.

Chow, J. (2001). Assessment of Asian American/Pacific Islander organization and communities. In R. Fond & S. Furuto (Eds.), *Culturally competent practice: Skills, interventions, and evaluations* (pp. 211-225). Needham Heights, MA: Allyn & Bacon.

Cohen, C., Colantonio, A., & Vernich, L. (2002). Positive aspects of caregiving: Rounding out the caregiver experience. *International Journal of Geriatric Psychiatry, 17*(2), 184-188.

Connell, C., Janevic, M., & Gallant, M. (2001). The costs of caring: Impact of dementia on family caregivers. *Journal of Geriatric Psychiatry & Neurology, 14*(4), 179-187.

Covinsky, K., Newcomer, R., Fox, P., Wood, J., Sands, L., Dane, K., & Yaff, K. (2003). Patient and caregiver characteristics associated with depression in caregivers of patients with dementia. *Journal of General Internal Medicine, 18*, 1006-1014.

Cox, C. (1995). Comparing the experiences of Black and White caregivers of dementia patients. *Social Work, 40*(3), 343-349.

Crowther, M., Parker, M., Achenbaum, W., Larimore, W., & Koenig, H. (2002). Rowe and Kahn's model of successful aging revisited: Positive spirituality–The forgotten factor. *The Gerontologist, 42*(5), 613-620.

Dilworth-Anderson, P., Williams, I., & Gibson, B. (2002). Issues of race, ethnicity, and culture in caregiving research: A 20-year review (1980-2000). *The Gerontologist, 42*(2), 237-272.

Doka, K., & Carter, R. (2001). *Caregiving and loss.* Washington; Hospice Foundation of America.

Farren, C. (1997). Theoretical perspectives concerning positive aspects of caring for elderly persons with dementia: Stress/adaptation and existentialism. *The Gerontologist, 37*(2), 250-256.

Farran, C., Keane-Hegerty, E., Salloway, S., Kupferer, S., & Wilken, C. (1991). Finding meaning: An alternative paradigm for Alzheimer's disease family caregivers. *The Gerontologist, 31*(4), 483-489.

Farren, C., Miller, B., Kaufman, J., Donner, E., & Fogg, L. (1999). Finding meaning through caregiving: Development of an instrument for family caregivers of persons with Alzheimer's disease. *Journal of Clinical Psychology, 55*(9), 1107-1125.

Farren, C., Paun, O., & Elliott, M. (2003). Spirituality in multicultural caregivers of persons with dementia. *Dementia, 2*(3), 353-377.

Frankl, V. (1962). *Man's search for meaning.* Boston: Beacon Press.

Frankl, V. (1967). *Psychotherapy and existentialism: Selected papers on logotherapy.* New York: Simon & Schuster.

Frankl, V. (1978). *The unheard cry for meaning: Psychotherapy and humanism.* New York: Simon & Schuster.

Frankl, V. (1990). Facing the transistorizes of human existence. *Generations, 14*(4), 7-10.

Frankl, V. (2004). *On the theory and therapy of mental disorders: An introduction to logotherapy and existential analysis.* New York: Brunner-Routledge.

Fredriksen-Goldsen, K., & Farwell, N. (2004). Dual Responsibilities Among Black, Hispanic, Asian, and White Employed Caregivers. *Journal of Gerontological Social Work, 43*(4), 25-44.

Garity, J. (1997). Stress, learning style, resilience factors, and ways of coping in Alzheimer family caregivers. *American Journal of Alzheimer's Disease, July/August*, 171-178.

Gaugler, J., Kane, R., Kane, R., & Newcomer, R. (2005). The longitudinal effects of early behavior problem in the dementia caregiving career. *Psychology and Aging, 20*(1), 100-116.

Greene, R. R. ([1986] 2000). *Social work with the aged and their families.* Hawthorne, NY: Aldine de Gruyter.

Greene, R. R. & Livingston, N. (2002). A social construct. In R. R. Greene (Eds.). *Resiliency Theory: An Integrated Framework for Practice, Research, and Policy* (pp. 63-94). Washington, DC: NASW Press.

Greene, R.R. & Conrad, A. (2002). Basic assumptions and terms. In R. R. Greene (Eds.). *Resiliency Theory: An Integrated Framework for Practice, Research, and Policy* (pp.29-62). Washington, DC: NASW Press.

Haley, W., Gitlin, L., Wisniewski, S., Mahoney, F., Coon, D., Winter, L., Corcoran, M., Schinfeld, S., & Ory, M. (2004). Well-being, appraisal, and coping in African-American and Caucasian dementia caregivers: Findings from the REACH study. *Aging and Mental Health, 8*(4), 316-329.

Harwood, D., Ownby, R., Burnett, K., Barker, W., & Duara, R. (2000). Predictors of appraisal and psychological well-being in Alzheimer's disease family caregiver. *Journal of Clinical Geropsychology, 6*(4), 279-297.

Hebert, L.E., Beckett, L.A., Scher, P.A., & Evans, D.A. (2001). Annual incidence of Alzheimer disease in the United States projected to the years 2000 through 2050. *Alzheimer Disease and Associated Disorders, 15*(4), 169-173.

Hepburn, K., Lewis, M., Narayan, S., Tornatore, J., Bremer, K., & Sherman, C. (2002). Discourse-derived perspective: Differentiating among spouses' experience of caregiving. *American Journal of Alzheimer's Disease and Other Dementias, 17*(4), 213-226.

Heru, A., Ryan, C., & Iqbal, A. (2004). Family functioning in the caregivers of patients with dementia. *International Journal of Geriatric Psychiatry, 19,* 533-537.

Hicks, M., & Lam, M. (1999). Decision-making within the social course of dementia: Accounts by Chinese-American caregivers. *Culture, Medicine & Psychiatry, 23*(4), 415-452.

Hinton, L., Guo, Z., & Hillygus, J. (2000). Working with culture: A qualitative analysis of barriers to the recruitment of Chinese-American family caregivers for dementia research. *Journal of Cross-Cultural Gerontology, 15*(2), 119-137.

Hooker, K., Bowman, S. R., Coehlo, D., Lim, S., Kaye, J., Guariglia, R., & Li, F. (2002). Behavioral change in persons with dementia: Relationships with mental and physical health of caregivers. *Journal of Gerontology: Psychological Science 57*(5), 453-460.

Hwang, K. (1999). Filial piety and loyalty: Two types of social identification in Confucianism. *Asian Journal of Social Psychology, 2,* 163-183.

Janevic, M. & Conell, C. (2001). Racial, ethnic, and culture differences in the dementia caregiving experience: Recent findings. *The Gerontologist, 41*(3), 334-347.

John, R., Resendiz, R., & Vargas, L. (1997). Beyond familism? Familism as explicit motive for elder care among Mexican American caregivers. *Journal of Cross-Cultural Gerontology, 12,* 145-162.

Knight, B., Robinson, G., Longmire, C., Chun, M., Nakao, K., & Kim, J. (2002). Cross cultural issues in caregiving for persons with dementia: Do familism values reduce burden and distress? *Ageing International, 27*(3), 70-94.

Knight, B., Silverstein, M., McCallum, T., & Fox, L. (2000). A sociocultural stress and coping model for mental health outcomes among African American caregivers in southern California. *Journal of Gerontology: Psychological Sciences, 55B*(3), 142-150.

Koening, T. (2005). Caregivers' use of spirituality in ethical decision-making. *Journal of Gerontological Social Work, 45*(1/2), 157-174.

Kramer, B. (1997). Gain in the caregiving experience: Where are we? What next? *The Gerontologist, 37*(2), 218-232.

Lawton, M., Kleban, M., Moss, M., Rovine, M., & Glicksman, A. (1989). Measuring caregiving appraisal. *Journal of Gerontology: Psychological Science, 44*, P61-P71.

Lazarus, R., & Folkman, S. (1984). *Stress, appraisal, and coping.* New York: Springer.

Lee, Y., & Sung, K. (1998). Cultural influences on caregiving burden: Cases of Koreans and Americans. *International Journal of Aging & Human Development, 46*(2), 125-141.

Lichenburg, P., Murman, D., & Mellow, A. (2003). Handbook of dementia: Psychological, neurological, and psychiatric perspective. Hoboken, New Jersey: John Wiley & Sons.

Lieberman, M., & Fisher, L. (1999). The effect of family conflict resolution and decision making on the provision of help for an elder with Alzheimer's disease. *The Gerontologist, 39*(2), 159-166.

Luna, I., Ardon, E., Lim, Y., Cromwell, S., Phillips, L., & Russell, C. (1997). The relevance of familism in cross-cultural studies of family caregiving. *Western Journal of Nursing Research, 18*(3), 267-274.

Martire, L., Stephens, M., & Atienza, A. (1997). The interplay of work and caregiving: Relationships between role satisfaction, role involvement, and caregivers' well-being. *Journals of Gerontology: Series B: Psychological Sciences & Social Sciences, 52B*(5), 279-289.

McKibbin, C.L., Walsh, W., Rinki, M., Koin, D., & Gallagher-Thompson, D. (1999). Lifestyle and health behavior among female family dementia caregivers: A comparison of wives and daughters. *Aging & Mental Health, 3*(2), 165-172.

McMillen, J. (1999). Better for it: How people benefit from adversity. *Social Work, 44*(5), 455-468.

MetLife Mature Market Institute, (November, 1999). *The MetLife juggling Act study: Balancing caregiving with work and the costs involved.* New York: Metropolitan Life Insurance Company.

Miller, B., & Guo, S. (2000). Social support for spouse caregivers of persons with dementia. *Journal of Gerontology: Social Science, 55B*(3), S163-S172.

Miller, B., Townsend, A., Carpenter, E., Montgomeray, R., Stull, D., & Young, R. (2001). Social support and caregiver distress: A replication analysis. *Journal of Gerontology: Social Sciences, 58B* (4), S249-S256.

Moon, A., Lubben, J., & Villa, V. (1998). Awareness and utilization of community long-term care services by elderly Korean and non-Hispanic White Americans. *The Gerontologist, 38*(3), 309-316.

Moore, M. J., Zhu, C. W., & Clipp, E.C. (2001). Informal costs of dementia care: Estimates from the national longitudinal caregiver study. *Journal of Gerontology: Social Science, 56B* (4), S219-S228.

Morano, C., & King, D. (2005). Religiosity as mediator of caregiver well-being: Does ethnicity make a difference? *Journal of Gerontological Social Work, 45*(1/2), 69-84.

Narayan, S., Lewis, M., Tornatore, J., Hepburn, K., & Corcoran-Perry, S. (2001). Subjective responses to caregiving for a spouse with dementia. *Journal of Gerontological Nursing, 27*(2), 19-28.

National Institute of Aging (2003). 2001-2002 Alzheimer's Disease Progress Report (NIH Publication No. 03-5333). Washington, DC: U.S. Department of Health and Human Services.

National Alliance for Caregiving & AARP. (2004). Caregiving in the U.S. Washington, DC: AARP.

Navaie-Waliser, M., Feldman, P., Gould, D., Levine, C., Kuerbis, A., & Donelan, K. (2001). The experiences and challenges of informal caregivers: Common themes and differences among Whites, Blacks, and Hispanic. *The Gerontologist, 41*(6), 733-741.

Noonan, A.E. & Tennstedt, S.L. (1997). Meaning in caregiving and its contribution to caregiver well-being. *The Gerontologist 37*(6), 785-794.

Ory, M., Hoffman, R., Yee, J., Tennstedt, S., & Schulz, R. (1999). Prevalence and impact of caregiving: A detailed comparison between dementia and nondementia caregiver, *The Gerontologist, 39*(2), 177-185.

Ory, M.G., Yee, J.L. Tennstedt, S.L., & Schulz, R. (2000). The extent and impact of dementia care: Unique challenges experienced by family caregivers. In R. Schulz (Eds.), *Handbook on Dementia Caregiving: Evidence-based interventions in family caregiving.* New York: Springer Publishing Company.

Paun, O. (2003). Older women caring for spouses with Alzheimer's disease at home: Making sense of the situation. *Health Care for Women International 24,* 292-312.

Pearlin, L., Mullan, J., & Semple, S. (1990). Caregiving and the stress process: An overview of concepts and their measures. *The Gerontologist, 30*(5), 583-594.

Picot, S., Debanne, S., Namazi, K., & Wykle, M. (1997). Religiosity and perceived rewards of black and white caregivers.*The Gerontologist, 37*(1), 89-101.

Pierce, T., Lydon, J., & Yang, S. (2001). Enthusiasm and moral commitment: What sustains family caregivers of those with dementia. *Basic & Applied Social Psychology, 23*(1), 29-41.

Pinquart, M., & Sorensen, S. (2003). Associations of stressor and uplifts of caregiving with caregiver burden and depressive mood: A meta-analysis. *Journal of Gerontology: Psychological Science, 58B*(2), 112-128.

Rapp, S., & Chao, D. (2000). Appraisals of strain and gain: Effects on psychological wellbeing of caregivers of dementia patients. *Aging and Mental Health, 4*(2), 142-147.

Rapp, S., Shumaker, S., Schmidt, S., Naughton, M., & Anderson, R. (1998). Social resourcefulness: Its relationship to social support and wellbeing among caregivers of dementia victims. *Aging and Mental Health, 2*(1), 40-48.

Roff, L., Burgio, L., Gitlin, L., Nichols, L., Chaplin, W., & Hardin, M. (2004). Positive aspects of Alzheimer's caregiving: The role of race. *Journal of Gerontology: Psychological sciences, 59B*(4), 185-190.

Rose-Rego, S.K., Strauss, M.E., & Smyth, K.A. (1998). Differences in the perceived well-being of wives and husbands caring for persons with Alzheimer's disease. *The Gerontologist, 38,* 224-230.

Roth, D.L., Haley, W.E., Owen, J.E., Clay, O.J.,& Kathryn, T. (2001). Latent growth model of the longitudinal effects of dementia caregiving: A comparison of African American and White family caregiver. *Psychology & Aging, 16*(3), 427-436.

Rowe, J.W. & Kahn, R.L. (1998). *Successful aging.* New York: Pantheon Books.

Rutter, M. (1987). Psychological resilience and protective mechanisms. *American Journal of Orthopsychiatry, 57,* 316-331.

Saleebey, D. (2002). Introduction: Power in the People. In D. Saleebey (Eds.), *The strengths perspective in social work practice (3rd ed.)*(pp.176-194). Boston, MA; Allyn and Bacon.

Schulz, R. (2000). *Handbook on dementia caregiving: Evidence-based interventions for family caregivers.* New York: Springer Publishing.

Schulz, R., & Beach, S. (1999). Caregiving as a risk factor for mortality: The caregiver health effects study. *Journal of American Medical Association, 282* (23), 2215-2219.

Schulz, R., O'Brien, A., Bookwala, J. & Fleissenger, K. (1995). Psychiatric and physical morbidity effects of dementia care-giving: Prevalence, correlates, and causes. *The Gerontologist, 35,* 771-791.

Sherrell, K., Buckwalter, K., & Morhardt, D. (2001). Negotiating family relationships: Dementia care as a midlife developmental task. *Families in Society, 82*(4), 383-392.

Smerglia, V., & Deimling, G. (1997). Care-related decision-making satisfaction and caregiver well-being in families caring for older members. *The Gerontologist, 37*(5), 658-665.

Stuckey, J. (2001). Blessed assurance: The role of religion and spirituality in Alzheimer's disease caregiving and other significant life events. *Journal of Aging Studies, 15,* 69-84.

Stuckey, J., & Smyth, K. (1997). The impact of social resources on the Alzheimer's disease caregiving experience. *Research on Aging, 19*(4), 423-441.

Sung, K. (1997). Filial piety in modern times: Timely adaptation and practice patterns. *Australasian Journal on Ageing, 17*(1, Supplement), 88-92.

Tarlow, B., Wisniewski, S., & Belle, S. (2004). Positive Aspects of Caregiving: Contributions of the REACH project to the development of new measures for Alzheimer's caregiving. *Research on Aging, 26*(4), 429-453.

Tebb, S., & Jivanjee, P. (2000). Caregiver isolation: An ecological model. *Journal of Gerontological Social Work, 34*(2), 51-72.

Tebes, J., & Irish, J. (2000). Promoting resilience among children of sandwiched generation caregiving women through caregiver mutual help. *Journal of Prevention & Intervention in the Community, 20*(1/2), 139-158.

Tennen, H. & Affleck, G. (2002). Benefit-finding and benefit-reminding. In C. Snyder, & S. Lopez (Eds.), *Handbook of positive psychology* (pp.584-597). New York: Oxford University Press.

The Canadian Study of Health and Aging Working Group. (2002). Patterns and health effects of caring for people with dementia: The impact of changing cognitive and residential status. *The Gerontologist, 42*(5), 643-652.

The National Women's Health Information Center. (2002). *What is caregiving?* Retrieved January 25, 2005, from http://www.4woman.gov/faq/caregiver.pdf

Thoits, P. (1995). Stress, coping, and social support processes: Where are we? What next? *Journal of Health and Social Behavior, 36*(Suppl.), 53-79.

Wagnild, G., & Young, H. (1993). Development and psychometric evaluations for pediatricians. *Developmental and Behavioral Pediatrics, 1*(2), 165-179.

Walker, R., & Pomeroy, E. (1996). Depression or grief? The experience of caregivers of people with dementia. *Health & Social Work, 21*(4), 247-254.

Watari, K., & Gatz, M. (2004). Pathways to care for Alzheimer's disease among Korean Americans. *Cultural Diversity and Ethnic Minority Psychology, 10*(1), 23-38.

Yalom, I. (1995). *The theory and practice of group psychotherapy* (4th ed.). New York, NY: Basic Books.

Yeh, K., & Bedford, O. (2003). A test of the dual filial piety model. *Asian Journal of Social Psychology, 6,* 215-228.

Yong, F., & McCallion, P. (2003). Hwabyung as caregiving stress among Korean-American caregivers of a relative with dementia. *Journal of Gerontological Social Work, 42*(2), 3-19.

Youn, G., Knight, B., Jeong, H., & Benton, D. (1999). Differences in familism values and caregiving outcomes among Korean, Korean American, and White American dementia caregivers. *Psychology & Aging, 14*(3), 355-364.

Zuniga, M. (2001). Latinos: Cultural competence and ethics. In R. Fond & S. Furuto (Eds.), *Culturally competent practice: Skills, interventions, and evaluations* (pp. 211-225). Needham Heights, MA: Allyn & Bacon.

doi:10.1300/J137v14n01_15

Chapter 16

Community Caregiving Partnerships in Aging: Promoting Alliances to Support Care Providers

Nancy Kropf

SUMMARY. Although greater numbers of families are providing support to older adults, a lack of comprehensive programming in resource allocation continues to exist at the social policy level. This chapter explores how community caregiving partnerships may contribute to a solution. doi:10.1300/J137v14n01_16 *[Article copies available for a fee from The Haworth Document Delivery Service: 1-800-HAWORTH. E-mail address: <docdelivery@haworthpress.com> Website: <http://www.HaworthPress.com> © 2006 by The Haworth Press, Inc. All rights reserved.]*

KEYWORDS. Community partnerships, older adults, caregiving

Contemporary social trends have created additional demands for families and community organizations that work to provide support to older generations. One change is the demographic shifts that are occurring

---

[Haworth co-indexing entry note]: "Community Caregiving Partnerships in Aging: Promoting Alliances to Support Care Providers." Kropf, Nancy. Co-published simultaneously in *Journal of Human Behavior in the Social Environment* (The Haworth Press, Inc.) Vol. 14, No. 1/2, 2006, pp. 325-338; and: *Contemporary Issues of Care* (ed: Roberta R. Greene) The Haworth Press, Inc., 2006, pp. 325-338. Single or multiple copies of this article are available for a fee from The Haworth Document Delivery Service [1-800-HAWORTH, 9:00 a.m.- 5:00 p.m. (EST). E-mail address: docdelivery@haworthpress.com].

within the older population. The 2000 Census reports that 35 million people in the U.S. are over 65 years of age, which is an increase of 3.8 million from 1990 (U.S. Bureau of the Census, 2003). In addition to the greater number of older adults generally, the most dramatic increase is in the number within the over 85 year old population. At this point in the life course, it is probable that an older adult will be experiencing some health-related or functional impairment. As the number in the oldest cohort increases, families and society will have additional responsibility to provide assistance and care for these older adults.

A second trend is the changing profile of those family members who provide support to older adults. In a recent national study (AARP & National Alliance for Caregiving, 2005), the number, description, and impact of care upon the caregivers were highlighted. Some of the key findings from this national study were:

- There are 44.4 million caregivers (over age 18) who provide unpaid care to another adult.
- A profile of the "typical" care provider is a 46 year old female with some college education, is in the labor force, and spends more than twenty hours per week caring for her aged mother.
- Over half (59%) of caregivers work full- or part-time, and 62% report that they have had to make adjustments in their work schedule to accommodate care tasks.
- Excluding spousal care providers, about half of the caregivers report that they spend an average of $200 per month on costs related to care provision.
- Caregivers cope with demands of care in various ways. The most common was by praying (71%), which was used most frequently by African-American (84%) and Hispanic caregivers (79%). Other typical coping mechanisms that were reported included talking with friends or relatives (71%), reading (44%), and exercising (41%).
- Formal sources of support vary by location. Those who are caring for someone in an urban area are more likely to report using formal services (58%) than those caring for someone in suburban (42%) or rural settings (44%).

Taken together, there is a clear picture that caregiving is a task assumed by significant numbers of adults, especially women. As a result of caregiving tasks, other life experiences of the care provider may be affected such as the quality of the relationship with the care recipient or the relationships with other family members. For adult children, role dynamics may become confusing for both the parent and adult child, such as when a son or daughter has to feed or bathe an older parent. Caregiving partners or spouses may lose a source of companionship as the care recipients' levels of functioning decreases with a possible outcome of feeling isolated and lonely within their caregiving role (Li, 2004). While the role of caregiver is becoming more statistically normative, care providers may feel very alone with these multiple and diverse tasks.

A particular challenge of caregivers is the balance of family and workplace responsibilities. As the NAC/AARP study indicates, most caregivers work and many are expending hundreds of dollars per month on related expenses. For these families, it is important that the care provider remains in the labor force. Yet from an organizational perspective, studies have documented the costs associated with caregiving within the workplace such as absences, decreased morale, and decreased productivity (Barnett, Marshall & Singer, 1992; Singer, Yegidis, Robinson, Barbee & Funk 2001; Robinson, Barbee, Martin, Singer & Yegidis, 2003). As greater numbers of women have jobs and careers, the stress of family versus labor force roles seems especially acute for females (Field and Bramwell, 1998; Frederiksen & Scharlach, 1999; Pavalko & Artis, 1997).

Although greater numbers of families are providing support to older adults, a lack of comprehensive programming and resource allocation continues to exist at the social policy level. This third trend–the lack of a comprehensive system of long term and community-based support–leaves some families without access to appropriate supportive services (Morgan, Semchuk, Stewart & D'Arcy, 2002; Palley, 2003; Wiener, Tilly, & Alecxih, 2002). Without availability of formal sources of support, some families may face dire economic, social and physical hardships as a result of assuming care for an older adult.

At face value, changes in current federal policy, such as funding of faith-based initiatives, appear to broaden the circle of service providers within social welfare. In fact, during President Bush's first week in office, he laid the groundwork for the White House Office of Faith-Based and Community Services (Fact Sheet, 2003). With this new policy focus, various organizations are becoming more integrated into service delivery operations. Coupled with this trend, however, governmental agencies are receiving less public support for traditional service roles (Dluhy, 1990). In addition to decreased funding for established programs, the lack of coordination between the various sources of support can create a more chaotic environment for the care provider. Within the context of shrinking fiscal resources, families who require support in care provision are unable to access services to help them with caring for an older family member.

Within this environment, community partnerships can assume a critical role in coordinating disparate services and issues across multiple networks and social agencies. In addition, partnerships can provide an opportunity to collaborate on needed community programs and promote a political agenda (Armbruster, Gale, Brady & Thompson, 1999). This chapter describes issues related to construction of caregiving partnerships, and presents models to identify ways to successfully plan and implement partnerships to address family care provision.

COMMUNITY PARTNERSHIPS

Types of Partnerships

The literature on partnerships has developed over the past forty years as changes within social services have occurred. In fact, there are various types of community relationships that represent formalized partnerships among agencies (Bailey & Koney, 2000; Reilly, 2001). A *cooperation* is a relatively informal process that exists without a defined structure or a systematic planning effort. An example is a group of neighborhood families that bring groceries to older adults who live alone. While there may be some discussion or information exchange between the families, this system is informal and is based upon the characteristics, motivation, and overall "goodwill" of those who are involved.

A second type of alliance is a *coordination* between different groups. This type of alliance is more formalized and involves a modest amount of planning and information exchange. Most often, these types of alliances are constructed around a single issue. For example, a task force was created to deal with elder abuse prevention and prosecution in Oregon (DeMonnin & Schneider, 2005). This multidisciplinary task force was successful in bringing about legislation to better enforce and prosecute perpetrators of abuse, as well as to raise awareness of elder abuse in the community and increase protective options for older adults within the state.

The most formalized type of partnership is a *collaboration*. This type of structure brings together diverse groups in order to achieve a new structure for a shared mutual purpose. Examples of collaborations are coalitions, consortia, or alliances. These types of partnerships seek to create a unified agenda, promote a particular position, or work to increase competence within the community. During the 1960s, community collaborations began to form as a way to create a power base for social services through political advocacy initiatives (Armbruster et al., 1999). Currently, collaborations may serve various functions, including the opportunity for networking, sharing of information and resources, and realigning community activities to achieve maximum benefit (Wolff, 1993).

Successful Partnerships

While building relationships among individuals and organizations has the potential to ameliorate some of the stresses experienced by caregivers, building effective partnerships is complex. Just as the Functional Age Model specifies, interdependence exists between systems such as a care recipient and care provider, a family and the community, and a community and the larger socio-political environment. The application of this tenet to the community level provides a framework for determining the factors that are associated with those partnerships that are successful, as well as challenges in implementing effective partnerships.

Mizrahi and Rosenthal (2001) have constructed a conceptual framework based upon a study of social change coalitions, which is a common type of partnership in social services. Through interviews with coalition leaders, four major factors were related to successful functioning of coalitions. *Conditions* include the level of resources of the coalition, community climate to support the coalition, and feasibility of the coalition to exert some influence within the environment. Successful coalitions seemed to select the "right issue and timing" that fit with the priorities of the external environment.

A second dimension, *commitment*, is the tension between the degree of power and influence exerted by the coalition and the dominant ideology that is represented. Coalitions that were evaluated as being successful were able to strike a balance between action and ideals. The third dimension in the conceptual framework was *contribution*. Successful coalitions are able to share resources and assets among members, thereby contributing in meaningful ways to one another. The final factor, *competence*, primarily addresses the leadership role. Successful, or competent, leaders demonstrated skillful management of internal dynamics (e.g., decision-making, sharing responsibility) along with a goal orientation to promote sustained positive movement of the coalition.

Other research has focused on how talents, skills, and knowledge combine to promote "partnership synergy" within community collaborations

(Weiss, Anderson & Lasker, 2002). *Synergy* was conceptualized as the process wherein members' abilities combine to enhance thinking and actions of the group and therefore enhance the partnership productivity within the community. The results indicated that two factors were primarily responsibility for creating synergy. *Leadership effectiveness* was the most influential factor and involved the leader's ability to facilitate productive interactions among the members, promote open dialogue, and bring together partnership members from diverse backgrounds and experiences. The second dimension was *partnership efficacy* which included the degree of resources available to the group, as well as the level of expertise that the various members contributed.

Alternate frameworks to address success of partnerships have also been constructed. Reilly (2001) offers several factors through a synthesis of existing research on collaborations. In his analysis, five essential components are: (1) an articulated and *meaningful purpose* to the collaborative, (2) *membership* across multiple constituencies, (3) roles, rules and communications that provide a *structure* for the partnership, (4) a *process* for the partnership that allows investment of the members and leaders towards successful outcomes, and (5) *resources* such as funding and staff. As identified, these factors span the leadership, composition, and methodology of the partnership in working toward goals and outcomes.

Challenges in Forming Partnerships

The process of bringing together disparate entities to share a process, goals and outcomes is not always successful. Unfortunately, many partnerships are unable to function effectively or sustain involvement over time. Regardless of the degree of formality of the partnership, an internal structure is necessary to ensure that all members are moving in the same direction. In an attempt to identify threats to effective functioning, an analysis of decision making within community coalitions was constructed using recorded minutes of group meetings (Speer & Zippay, 2005). This study determined that many principles of good leadership and organizational functioning were applied unevenly in the least effective partnerships. Examples of particular problems included a lack of specific tasks and a lack of delegation of authority to move the agenda forward. One particular finding was a lack of assignment of particular tasks to individuals or sub-groups. In partnerships where there is no accountability or responsibility, it is not surprising that outcomes are compromised.

Leaders must also be aware of how accurately a partnership's agenda corresponds to priorities within the community. This issue is one of validity and representation, as partnerships may be effective for a segment of the population or a dimension of a particular problem without addressing the issue more comprehensively. In an analysis of how needs of family caregivers were defined, for example, the process of needs assessment techniques undertaken by Area Agencies on Aging (AAA) were examined (Kietzman, Scharlach, & Dal Santo, 2004). The findings indicated that the AAAs were successful in determining needs of certain profiles of caregivers, including White/non-Hispanic, grandparent care providers, people caring for individuals with cognitive impairments, and low income caregivers. AAAs were less successful identifying harder to reach populations, such as needs of gay/lesbian caregivers, those individuals who did not speak English, and people living in rural communities.

In research on partnerships in child welfare services, a conceptual model of environmental stressors was constructed (Mulroy, 2003). The model included the following components: *uncertain funding streams* such as changing priorities in ways funding sources made decisions about allocating their resources, *existence of conflicting policies* which creates tension and competition between potential members of the partnership, and *changing demographics* within the community that can create different community needs. These factors can have an impact on the ability of the partnership to establish a structure that is responsive to caregiver needs within the community.

COMMUNITY PARTNERSHIPS IN CAREGIVING

Various types of partnerships have been implemented and evaluated within aging services. Three models of community partnerships will be highlighted as examples of ways that various community systems can work together to enhance and improve the quality of care provision. Each of these three examples provides a different type of focus: a statewide initiative to provide a comprehensive network for caregiving, an effort to bridge aging and disability networks, and a lasting advocacy coalition. While this certainly is not an exhaustive list, it provides some examples of efforts to promote care provision at the community level.

CARE-NETs

The CARE-NET project is a statewide effort to establish caregiving coalitions across the State of Georgia. Initiated by the Rosalynn Carter Institute (RCI) for Caregiving at Georgia Southwestern State University and funded by a grant from the Administration on Aging. This initiative formed partnerships within twelve regions of the state. Each CARE-NET is a collaborative network of representatives from a variety of constituencies, including family care providers, aging agencies, educational institutions, businesses, and other interested groups (Dodd, Talley & Elder, 2004). The initiative was also an effort to raise awareness of caregiving issues and needs, within the context of diverse communities around the state. The purpose of these groups was to develop a comprehensive statewide system that would further caregiving capacity within all communities of the state.

Each CARE-NET represents an autonomous coalition that is connected to the others by an infrastructure initially supported by the RCI. As a beginning step in developing the coalition, each CARE-NET elected formal leaders, established by-laws, and held membership meetings. In addition, each coalition crafted a purpose and focus that fit with the needs of the particular region of the state. For example, several coalitions in rural areas included non-traditional members such as funeral home directors. Another coalition formed solely around faith-based service providers. While the individual coalitions maintained statewide connections, there was great variability in the structure and membership overall depending on the needs within the particular region.

In a formative evaluation of the coalition development that was undertaken midway through the grant, findings indicated that the majority of the CARE-NET participants perceived that their coalition was effective in reaching their goals (Kropf, 2003). In addition, the membership of the CARE-NETs was diverse and included aging service providers, family members of older adults, local business, faith-based and religious organizations, and health care providers. The overall reason that the members participated in the statewide coalition initiative was an avowed commitment to improving the experience of caregivers, by being connected to others with an interest in care.

Several different initiatives have been undertaken by the various CARE-NETs to enhance the resources within local communities. Several coalitions have sponsored seminars on caregiving within their areas, such as *Caring for You, Caring for Me* (Haigler, Mims & Nottingham, 1998), which is a leadership preparation curriculum to promote self care skills for care providers. Other programs have included public service announcements to raise awareness of care-related issues, and sponsoring health fairs for caregivers. In the faith-based coalition, the focus was on using untapped resources within the religious organizations and raising awareness of religious leaders to issues of aging within their congregations.

An additional part of the grant was to construct a community-level assessment tool to determine strengths and limitations in helping caregivers and their families. Termed the Community Caregiving Capacity Index (CCC-I), the focus of the instrument is on community-wide resources and services. Through rigorous development and field testing (Holland & Kim, 2004), the CCC-I is a multifactorial assessment protocol that includes the dimensions of available and useful health care resources, social services, in home and community services, and caregiver supports. The purpose is to provide a tool that can be used to determine the "competence" of a community to support individuals in care provision roles. As the CCC-I is more widely used, it has the potential of providing a sound assessment tool at the community level.

Aging and Developmental Disabilities

Another statewide initiative was undertaken in Georgia to bridge aging and developmental disabilities networks. Due to increased life expectancies and community-based forms of service provision, more parents and other family members are in caregiving roles for family members with disabilities into late life (Doka & Lavin, 2003; Heller, Miller & Hsieh, 1999; Malone & Kropf, 1996). This situation, the simultaneous aging process of both the parent and caregiver, is a fairly recent line of inquiry within research and practice. Although the needs of the family may straddle multiple service sectors, linkages often do not exist between aging and disability networks, the lack of which creates service gaps and unmet needs (Kropf, 1997).

In an effort to bridge these service networks, a statewide coalition initiative was undertaken between aging and developmental disability service providers. Through a series of nine coalition meetings in different parts of the state, service providers from both networks were brought together to learn more about ways to work together to bridge services. In day-long sessions, a series of panels, activities, and presentations were aimed at promoting interaction between the aging and DD providers. As a concluding segment, time to establish local planning coalitions was included so that the groups could interact beyond the course of the formal session.

At the conclusion of the initiative, an evaluation was undertaken to determine if these statewide planning meetings increased coordination across service systems (Smith, Thyer, Clements, & Kropf, 1997). Some successes were found such as increased awareness of services that are delivered by the aging and DD service sectors and enhanced professional relationships that crossed service sector boundaries. However, long-lasting structural changes to service delivery were not sustained. The goal to develop more permanent coalitions within the various regions of the state was not achieved. Participants reported that a planning infrastructure, such as a coordinating entity, was needed, and, sadly, momentum to sustain relationships was thwarted without this additional type of support.

Advocacy

In addition to partnerships that focus on services within the community, some initiatives focus on creating relationships for advocacy purposes. One of these alliances is the Southwestern Pennsylvania Partnership for Aging (SWPPA) (Kelly, 2004). This interorganizational entity was formed in 1990 and started with 24 members. Currently, there are 398 members that include family caregivers, non-profit and for-profit aging providers, long term care and healthcare providers, businesses, governmental entities and universities committed to improving the social, emotional, physical and psychological well being of older adults.

A goal of SWPPA is to bring together diverse segments of the community to improve the context for care within this region, which has a high density for older adults. In addition to providing a forum for networking, the coalition holds an annual regional conference on some aspect of care. Due to its size and longevity, the coalition has become a recognizable force within the community, serving as a catalyst to promote positive change in programs, policies, and care systems that can improve the quality of life for older adults.

The Functional-Age Model Applied to Community Partnerships

As developed by Greene (1986; 2000), the Functional Age Model (FAM) provides a framework for assessment and intervention with older adults and their families. Although this model has been primarily used with smaller social systems, such as the individual and family, this model has potential to help practitioners understand larger systems such as community-level dynamics. Using the content on community partnerships contained within this chapter, particular ways of blending the FAM into more macro-practice principles is suggested.

As the literature on community partnerships indicates, there are two major dimensions for assessment. One area is the experience of care providers and older adults within a particular community; that is, what are the major priorities that are facing the families in this area? A second is an assessment of the effectiveness of the partnerships that are established, and ways to determine if these alliances are able to promote competent communities to support caregiving.

As the Functional Age Model states, assessment must contextualize the individual in the perspective of his or her social system. On a more macro-practice level, an analysis of the community includes the strengths, resources, and challenges that exist in supporting care providers in their roles. Using that framework, partnerships can be established around the gaps that exist within community-based and long-term care support systems. In addition, there also may be a need to raise awareness of the needs of families within the context of other organizations and roles. For example, the NAC/AARP report indicates that religious practices are important to many care providers, especially those who are African American. The Black Church, which has historically promoted social justice, is an important partner in providing emotional and spiritual support to caregiving families.

Partnerships can also promote political strength by crafting a unified political agenda. Due to the increase in the numbers of adults who hold caregiving roles, the business community needs to consider how care for older adults impacts workers. For example, childcare facilities have become a common fixture in community and corporate life. In fact, some industries have childcare on site so parents have a convenient and accountable option while they are at work. Sadly, counterpart supports are lacking for older adults. Partnerships can form around both political and economic agendas to increase support and access to resources for caregivers such as respite, in-home services, and adult day care options.

At the level of community practice, social workers can make an important impact in creating relationships among systems that can support older adults and their caregivers. Case managers work to link families with resources within the environment, and this type of practice is critical within the fragmented service systems that exist. However, there is a need to move beyond this practice model to transform service systems. Initiatives such as the partnerships highlighted within this chapter provide examples of innovative ways to change *how* services are provided to care providers. The leadership within a community partnership must be effective at using the internal resources to transform the service structure by forging new alliances, opening up new pathways into services (such as the aging and DD initiative), and raising the consciousness of the community about the experience of care provision. While case management will continue to be an important social work method, there is a dire need to devote energy to transform the service networks themselves.

In summary, the impacts of a changing demographic will be felt at all levels of social systems. At an individual level, a greater number of people will live longer lives than ever before. For families, this change will signal a need to provide support and assistance to older family members within their advanced years. Age-related changes also impact communities and organizations, as care providers hold other social roles and require assistance and support from employers, formal service providers, and voluntary organizations such as religious and civic organizations.

The Functional Age Model has been used as a framework for assessment and practice with older adults and their families. Within this chapter, the Model has been used to distinguish community partnerships that can potentially bridge gaps within the aging service system. Several factors that are related to successful partnerships were highlighted, as well as partnership models in aging. As our society ages, communities and formal resources will be crucial to support families who will be involved in providing even greater degrees of support to their older family members.

REFERENCES

AARP & National Alliance for Caregiving (2005). *Caregiving in the U.S.* Washington DC: AARP.

Armbruster, C., Gale, B., Brady J. & Thompson, N. (1999). Perceived ownership in a community coalition. *Public Health Nursing, 16*(1), 17-22.

Bailey, D. & Koney, K. M. (2000). *Strategic alliances among health and human service organizations: From affiliations to consolidations.* Thousand Oaks, CA: Sage.

Barnett, R. C., Marshall, N. L. & Singer, J. D. (1992). Job experiences over time, multiple roles, and women's mental health: A longitudinal study. *Journal of Personality and Social Psychology, 62*, 634-644.

DeMonnin & Schneider (2005). Elder abuse prevention in Oregon. *Victimization of the Elderly and Disabled, 7*(6), 81-85.

Dluhy, M. J. (1990). *Building coalitions in the human services.* Newbury Park: Sage Publications.

Dodd, J., Talley, R. & Elder, T. (2004). *Caregivers together: Establishing your own CARE-NET.* A program of the Rosalynn Carter Institute for Caregiving.

Doka, K. J. & Lavin, C. (2003). Paradox of ageing with developmental disabilities: Increasing needs, declining resources. *Ageing International, 28*(2), 135-154.

Fact Sheet (2003). White House Office of Faith-Based and Community Initiatives. [http://www.whitehouse.gov/news/releases].

Field, S. & Bramwell, R. (1998). An investigation into the relationship between caring responsibilities and the levels of perceived pressure reported by female employees. *Journal of Occupational and Organizational Psychology, 71*(2), 165-170.

Fredriksen, K. I. & Scharlach, A. E. (1999). Employee family care responsibilities. *Family Relations, 48*(2), 189-206.

Greene, R. R. (1986; 2000). *Social work with the aged and their families.* (2nd ed.). New York: Aldine De Gruyter.

Haigler, D., Mims, K., & Nottingham, J. (1998). *Caring for you: Caring for me: Education and support for caregivers.* Athens, GA: University of Georgia Press.

Heller, T., Miller, A. B. & Hsieh, K. (1999). Impact of a consumer-directed family support program on adults with developmental disabilities and their family caregivers. *Family Relations, 48*(4), 419-427.

Holland, T. & Kim, H.Y. (2004). *The Community Caregiving Capacity Index: Instrument Design, Field Test Results, and Recommendations.* A report to the Rosalynn Carter Institute, Georgia Southwestern State University, Americus, Georgia.

Keitzman, K. G., Scharlach, A. E., & Dal Santo, T. S. (2004). Local needs assessment and planning efforts for family caregivers: Findings and recommendations. *Journal of Gerontological Social Work, 42*(3/4), 39-60.

Kelly, M. A. (2004). Developing an advocacy coalition with varied interests and agendas: A Pennsylvanian experience. *Generations, 28*(1), 83-85.

Kropf, N. P. (2003). *A Formative Evaluation of the CARE-NET Coalitions.* A report to the Rosalynn Carter Institute, Georgia Southwestern State University, Americus, Georgia.

Kropf, N. P. (1997). Older parents of adults with developmental disabilities: Practice issues and service needs. *Journal of Family Psychotherapy, 8*(2), 35-52.

Li, L. (2004). Caregiving network compositions and the use of supportive services by community dwelling dependent elders. *Journal of Gerontological Social Work, 43*(2/3), 147-164.

Malone, D. M. & Kropf, N. P. (1996). Growing older. In P. McLaughlin & P. Wehmann (Eds.). *Mental retardation and developmental disabilities.* (2nd ed.) (pp. 83-107). Austin, TX: Pro-Ed.

Mizrahi, T. & Rosenthal, B. B. (2001). Complexities of coalition building: Leaders' successes, strategies, struggles, and solutions. *Social Work, 46*(1), 63-78.

Morgan, D. G., Semchuk, K. M., Stewart, N. J., & D'Arcy, C. (2002). Rural families caring for a relative with dementia: Barriers to use of formal services. *Social Science and Medicine, 55*(7), 1129-1142.

Mulroy, E. A. (2003). Community as a factor in implementing interorganizational partnerships: Issues, constraints, and adaptations. *Nonprofit Management & Leadership, 14*(1), 47-66.

Palley, H. A. (2003). Long-term care policy for older Americans: Building a continuum of care. *Journal of Health & Social Policy, 16*(3), 7-18.

Pavalko, E. K & Artis, J. E. (1997). Women's caregiving and paid work: Causal relationships in mid-life. *The Journals of Gerontology, 52B*(3), S170-S179.

Reilly, T. (2001). Collaboration in action: An uncertain process. *Administration in Social Work, 25*(1), 53-74.

Robinson, M. M., Barbee, A. P., Martin, M., Singer, T. L. & Yegidis, B. (2003). The organizational costs of caregiving: A call to action. *Administration in Social Work, 27*(1), 83-102.

Singer, T. L., Yegidis, B. L., Robinson, M. M., Barbee, A. P. & Funk, J. (2001). Faculty in the middle: The effects of family caregiving on organizational effectiveness. *Journal of Social Work Education, 37* (2), 295-307.

Smith, G. S., Thyer, B.A., Clements, C. & Kropf, N.P. (1997). An evaluation of coalition building training for aging and developmental disability service providers. *Educational Gerontology, 23*, 105-114.

Speer, P. W. & Zippay, A. (2005). Participatory decision-making among community coalitions: An analysis of task group meetings. *Administration in Social Work, 29*(3), 61-68.

U.S. Bureau of the Census (2003). The U.S. Population is Growing Older. American Fact Finder. [http://factfinder.census.gov].

Weiss, E. S., Anderson, R. M. & Lasker, R. D. (2002). Making the most of collaboration: Exploring the relationship between partnership synergy and partnership functioning. *Health Education & Behavior, 29*, 683-698.

Wiener, J. M., Tilly, J. & Alecxih, L. M. B. (2002). Home and community-based services in seven states. *Health Care Financing Review, 23*(3), 89-114.

Wolff, T. J. (1993). Coalition building: Is this really empowerment? Paper presented at the American Public Health Association, Annual Meeting. San Francisco, CA.

doi:10.1300/J137v14n01_16

Appendix

The Assessment and Intervention Planning Workbook

Roberta R. Greene

The University of Texas at Austin

To be used in conjunction with CD-ROM.

[Haworth co-indexing entry note]: "The Assessment and Intervention Planning Workbook." Greene, Roberta, R. Co-published simultaneously in *Journal of Human Behavior in the Social Environment* (The Haworth Press, Inc.) Vol. 14, No. 1/2, 2006, pp. 339-377; and: *Contemporary Issues of Care* (ed: Roberta R. Greene) The Haworth Press, Inc., 2006, pp. 339-377. Single or multiple copies of this article are available for a fee from The Haworth Document Delivery Service [1-800-HAWORTH, 9:00 a.m.- 5:00 p.m. (EST). E-mail address: docdelivery@haworthpress.com].

Available online at http://jhbse.haworthpress.com/
doi:10.1300/J137v14n01_17

Contents

Part 1: ASSESSMENT

Section I

• Self-Awareness

Section I is intended to build your self-awareness as you begin your work with families who are in caregiving situations. Do you approach clients from a strengths perspective? Are you culturally sensitive? How do you approach your own resiliency? You may want to rate yourself? Three self-assessment instruments are presented below.

Reading to facilitate this section includes:

Greene, R. R., Watkins, M., Evans, M., David, V., & Clark, E. J. (2003). Defining diversity: A practitioner survey. *Arête*, *27*(1), 51-71.

Activity 1

When you finish the short Likert test you may want to explore more about a strengths-based resilience perspective. Do you agree philosophically with a strengths-based approach to practice? Rate yourself using the following questions in Table 1 to see how you approach some of your practice strategies.

TABLE 1
To What Extent Do I Assess Client Strengths?

Using a Likert scale, answer the following questions about your approach to social work practice.

When I meet with a client, I

1. give preeminence to client's understanding of the facts.

Low 1   2   3   4   5 High

2. believe the client.

Low 1   2   3   4   5 High

3. discover what the client wants.

Low 1   2   3   4   5 High

4. move the assessment towards personal and environmental strengths.

Low 1   2   3   4   5 High

5. make the assessment of strengths multidimensional.

Low 1   2   3   4   5 High

6. use the assessment to discover uniqueness.

Low 1   2   3   4   5 High

7. use language the client can understand.

Low 1   2   3   4   5 High

8. make assessment a joint activity between social worker and client.

Low 1   2   3   4   5 High

9. reach a mutual agreement on the assessment.

Low 1   2   3   4   5 High

10. avoid blame and blaming.

Low 1   2   3   4   5 High

11. avoid cause-and-effect thinking.

Low 1   2   3   4   5 High

12. assess do not diagnose.

Low 1   2   3   4   5 High

Adapted from: Cowger, C.D. (1994). Assessing client strengths: Clinical assessment for client empowerment. *Social Work, 39*(3), 262-268.

Activity 2

To learn more about your own understanding of culture, use Ho's (1991) Ethnic-Sensitive Inventory for self-assessment. See Table 2.

TABLE 2
Ethnic-Sensitive Inventory

In working with ethnic minority clients, I

☐ realize that my own ethnic and class background may influence my effectiveness.

☐ make an effort to assure privacy and/or anonymity.

☐ am aware of the systematic sources (racism, poverty, and prejudice) of their problems.

☐ am against speedy contracting unless initiated by them.

☐ assist them to understand whether the problem is of an individual or a collective nature.

☐ am able to engage them in identifying major progress that has taken place.

☐ consider it an obligation to familiarize myself with their culture, history, and other ethnically related responses to the problems.

☐ am able to understand and "tune in" to the meaning of their ethnic dispositions, behaviors, and experiences.

☐ can identify the links between systematic problems and individual concerns.

☐ am against highly focused efforts to suggest behavioral change or sensitivity.

☐ am aware that some techniques are too threatening to them.

☐ am able at the termination phase to help them consider alternative sources of support.

☐ am sensitive to their fears of racism or prejudiced orientations.

☐ am able to move more slowly in the effort to actively "reach for feelings."

☐ consider the implications of what is being suggested in relation to each client's ethnic reality (unique dispositions, behaviors, and experiences).

☐ clearly delineate agency functions and respectfully inform clients of my professional expectations of them.

☐ am aware that lack of progress may be related to ethnicity.

☐ am able to understand that the worker-client relationship may last a long time.

☐ am able to explain clearly the nature of the interview.

☐ am respectful of their definition of the problem to be solved.

☐ am able to specify the problem in practical concrete terms.

☐ am sensitive to treatment goals consonant to their culture.

☐ am able to mobilize social and extend family networks.

☐ am sensitive to the client's premature termination of service.

Adapted from: Ho (1991). Use of Ethnic-Sensitive Inventory (ESI) to enhance practitioner skills with minority clients. *Journal of Multicultural Social Work, 1*(1), 60-61. Compiled by Roberta R. Greene.

Activity 3

As you read and answer the questions in Table 3, you should become more aware of your own beliefs about risk and resilience. How resilient are you? What contributed to your sense of well-being?

TABLE 3
A Resiliency Questionnaire

1. What is your position in the family? Oldest? Youngest? Oldest boy?
2. Do you have any memories or recollections about what your mother or father said about you as a young baby? Or other members of the family or friends?
3. Did anyone ever tell you about how well you ate and slept when you were a baby?
4. Do members of your family and friends seem happy to see you and to spend time with you?
5. Do you feel like you are a helpful person to others? Does your family expect you to be helpful?
6. When life becomes difficult, do you consider yourself a happy and hopeful (optimistic) person?
7. Tell me about some times when you overcame problems or stresses in your life. What do you think about them now?
8. Do you think of yourself as alert most of the time? Do others see you that way?
9. Do you like to express new ideas and try new life experiences?
10. Tell me about some plans and goals you have for yourself over the next three to five years.
11. When you are in a stressful, pressure-filled situation, do you feel confident that you will work these difficulties out or do you feel depressed and hopeless?
12. What was the age of your parents when you were born? Your mother? Your father?
13. How many children are in your family? How many years are there between children in your family?
14. What do you remember about how you were cared for when you were little by mom and dad?
15. When you were growing up, were there rules and expectations in your home? List some?
16. Did any of your brothers or sisters participate in raising you? Tell how?
17. When you felt upset or in trouble, to whom in your family did you turn for help? Was there someone outside the family?
18. From whom did you learn about the values and beliefs of your family?
19. Do you sometimes feel it is your responsibility to help others? Or your community?
20. Do you feel that you have self-understanding?
21. Do you like yourself? How about today? Yesterday? Last year?
22. When you are under stress, what skills do you use to cope?
23. Tell me about a time when you assisted others.
24. Do you see yourself as confident? Even when stressed?
25. How do you feel about this interview/questionnaire?

Adapted from: Rak, C. & Patterson, L. (1996). *Journal of Counseling & Development, 74*, 360-368.

Activity 4

Write a one-page reflection paper on your feelings of readiness to serve caregiving families.

Section II

• Theoretical Frameworks

Section II examines several of the theoretical frameworks available to practitioners who are delivering social work services to families in caregiving situations. While we will emphasize systems theory and risk and resilience theory, you may want to review various schools of thought you may also consider.

Readings to facilitate the completion of this section include:

Greene, R. R. (1999). Systems. In R. R. Greene, *Human behavior and social work practice* (pp. 215-249). New York: Aldine De Gruyter.

Greene, R. R. (2002). *Resiliency theory: An integrated framework for practice, research, and policy.* Washington, DC: NASW Press. Chapters 1-3.

Activity 1

Read Table 4. What clinical approaches do you want to learn more about?

TABLE 4
Premises of Schools of Thought Relevant to Risk and Resilience Theory

Existential

1. People are not victims of circumstances; rather they have the freedom to choose what they want to be.

2. As people make choices, they grow.

3. To be adaptive, people need a reason to live. That is, they develop meaning.

4. People must learn to accept themselves to relate to and love others. Helping others in community efforts validates the self.

5. People's thoughts and behavior are not fixed. People may not be able to change an event, but they can change what they think about it.

6. Practitioner's help clients consider and initiate new choices.

Cognitive

1. People's emotions are based on how they think about themselves.

2. Most people have irrational or erroneous conceptions about themselves and their social situation.

3. People can overcome irrational beliefs and self-defeating patterns of behavior.

4. Practitioners facilitate a cognitive process that identifies and challenges misconceptions.

5. Helping strategies are primarily educational.

6. The purpose of intervention is to help the client develop cognitive tools that foster their sense of mastery and control.

Systems

1. Systemic interventions focus on group membership and affiliations.

2. Family and community systems have the ability to adapt to stress.

3. Adaptability rests on a systems' organizational and communication patterns.

4. Belief systems influence the capacity to maintain continuity and tolerate change.

5. Practitioners foster positive group organization and communication patterns.

6. Family members have the ability to transform and explore alternative solutions.

Ecological

1. Stress is brought about when people believe they have inadequate internal and external resources to meet environmental demands.

2. When people perceive stress, they engage in a coping process.

3. Stress can be reduced by improving the level of person-environment fit; this involves a change in people's behaviors, perceptions, and environmental response.

4. Social systems also play an important role in enhancing person-environment fit.

5. The practitioner can help clients manage stressors by reinforcing client's natural problem-solving skills, optimism, and resilience.

Social Constructivism

1. This approach assumes that there are no universal truths or singular reality. Rather, knowledge is created through interaction at the local level.

2. Constructivists provide a safe environment in which individuals and families explore their own meaning of events.

3. Reflective questions help clients construct and reconstruct their sense of self.

4. Clients are asked to externalize their problem or view themselves as "free" from a difficulty, developing alternative understandings and solutions.

5. Clients may choose not to accept negative attributions, such as racism or victimization.

6. Language and culture is the vehicle for the exchange of ideas and meaning.

7. By creating new meaning, individuals and communities can overcome life challenges.

Narrative

1. People are proactive and self-organizing.

2. People's behavior is shaped by the meaning they give to events.

3. As people create meaning in interaction with others, they develop a life story.

4. A person's life story contains information about how they have met life's critical events. The story gives life coherence and continuity.

5. If a story is problem-saturated, the client can be helped to reauthor it and discover alternative solutions.

6. Practitioners aim to broaden the client's view of reality and find alternatives ways to overcome an impasse.

Solution-focused

1. The focus of therapy is to create future solution.

2. Practitioners explore what the client hopes to achieve by going step by step to find positive solutions.

3. Client-social worker conversation help the client gain control by imagining a positive self-chosen direction.

4. Practitioners help clients explore alternative ways of gradually achieving success.

Adapted from: Greene, R. R. (2007). *Social Work Practice: A Risk and Resilience Perspective* (with CD-ROM). Belmont, CA: Wadsworth.

Section III

Part A. Assessment; Ecological Aspects

Section III is intended to guide you through ecological aspects of assessment.

Ecological approaches emphasize the multiple systems of influence in which people live. Bronfenbrenner's (1979) description of the ecological metaphor has frequently served as a multilevel visualization of the connections among individuals at various systems levels (Greene & Watkins, 1998). The visualization is like "a set of nested structures, each inside the next, like a set of Russian dolls" (Bronfenbrenner, 1979, p. 22). It describes a person's environment in terms of *microsystems*, including the immediate, personal, day-to-day activities and roles, such as in the family; *mesosystems*, which encompass the linkages between two or more settings involving the developing individual, such as family and school; *exosystems*, which include the linkages between two or more systems that do not involve the developing individual, such as parents and the workplace; and *macrosystems*, which encompass overarching societal systems, such as cultural and societal attitudes. See Figure 1.

Readings to facilitate the completion of this section include:

Carter, B. & McGoldrick, M. (1999). *The expanded family life cycle: Individual, family, and social perspectives* (3rd ed.). Boston: Allyn & Bacon. Chapter
Greene, R. R. (2000). *Social work with the aged and their families*. New York: Aldine De Gruyter. (pp. 51-58).
Greene, R. R. (1999). Ecological perspective. In R. R. Greene, *Human behavior theory and social work practice* (pp. 259-300). New York: Aldine De Gruyter.
Greene, R. R. & Watkins, M. (1998). *Serving diverse constituencies: Applying the ecological perspective*. New York: Aldine de Gruyter.
Meyer, C. (1993). *Assessment in social work practice*. New York: Columbia University Press.

Activity 1

When you complete this exercise you will know your chosen family's place within other social systems and the social supports available to them. For example, are they eligible for Medicaid? Medicare? Do they receive support from members of a religious congregation? Their neighbors? People at the office?

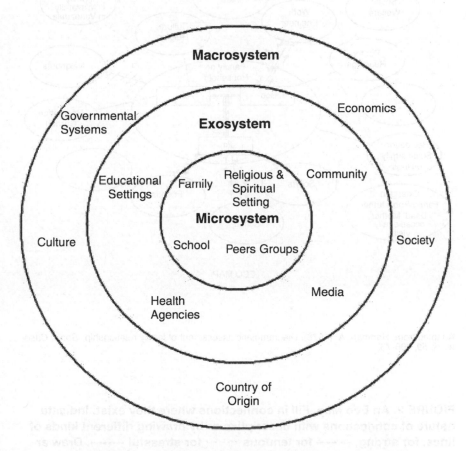

FIGURE 1. An Ecological Model of Human Development.

Adapted from: Bronfenbrenner, U. (1979). The ecology of human development. Cambridge, MA: Harvard University Press.

Assignment: To depict your assessment of the family's place within other social systems, complete the ecomap in Figure 2. See Figure 3 for a sample Eco Map.

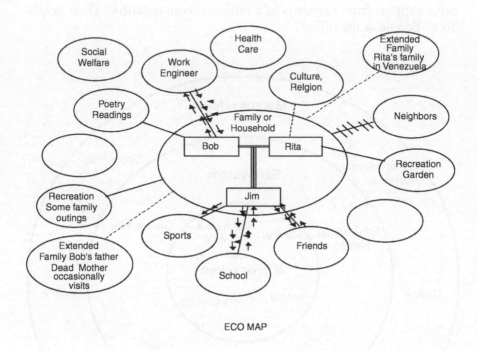

ECO MAP

Adapted from: Hartman, A. (1978). Diagrammatic assessment of family relationship. *Social Casework, 59*, 465-76.

FIGURE 2. An Eco Map. Fill in connections where they exist. Indicate nature of connections with descriptive or by drawing different kinds of lines: for strong, ——— for tenuous ········ for stressful --------. Draw arrows along lines to signify flow of energy, resources, etc. Identify significant people and fill in empty circles as needed.

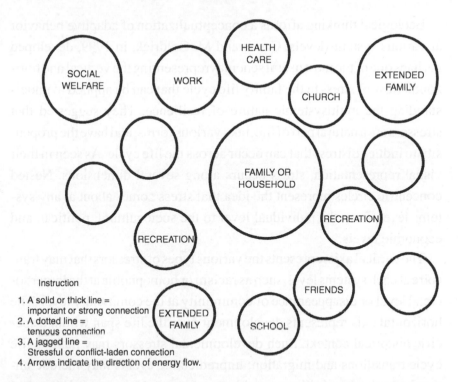

Adapted from: Hartman, A. (1978). Diagrammatic assessment of family relationships. *Social Casework, 59*, 465-476.

FIGURE 3. A Sample Eco Map.

Directions for using an eco map: The eco map simulates the family in its life space, namely the major systems that are apart of a family's life as well as the nature of those relationships—whether they are nurturant or conflict-laden. Connections between the family and the various systems are indicated by drawing different types of lines between the family and those systems: a solid or thick line depicts an important or strong connection; a dotted line, a tenuous connection; and a jagged line, a stressful or conflict-laden connection. Arrows indicate the direction of the flow of energy. Educational, religious, health, recreational, political, economic, neighborhood, and ethnic systems usually are graphically represented (Swenson, 1979). The relative flow of resource to the family is the paramount concern.

Ecological thinking affords a conceptualization of adaptive behavior at various systems levels. Carter and McGoldrick, in 1999, developed perhaps one of the most useful schemas representing the vertical and horizontal flow of stress in the family life cycle that can be applied to understanding the multisystemic nature of resilience. They suggested that stressors are a natural part of life, take various forms, and have the propensity to induce distress that can occur across the life cycle. As seen in their visual representation, stress occurs along several dimensions. Nested concentric circles represent the idea that stress comes about at any systems level, from the individual level to the sociocultural, political, and economic levels.

The vertical axis represents the various types of stressors that may transpire at each systems level, such as racism or homophobia at the larger societal level or disappearance of community at the community level. The horizontal axis represents development over the life span within a specific historical context. Such developmental stressors may include life cycle transitions and migration; unpredictable events may include untimely death, chronic illness, accidents, or unemployment; and historical events may encompass economic depression, war, or political oppression, and natural disasters.

For practitioners to assess resilience requires an understanding of the mutual influences of various systems in which clients participate: family, school, peer, work, neighborhood, community, and the larger society. At the same time, practitioners must evaluate whether families and communities can be considered resilient in their own right—"if they provide collective adaptation strategies for their members to confront risks or adverse circumstances" (Bartelt, 1994, p. 101), such as a community offering summer park programs as a means of enhancing peer relationships and reducing risk. Social systems-level resilience has not received as much attention as individual-level resilience and social institutions have been vaguely defined as neutral, supportive, or oppressive.

Section III

Part B. Family Dynamics

Activity 2

Families who give care are under some degree of stress that is derived from various personal and social conditions. When you finish assessing your family, you should be able to identify how various stressors are influencing caregiving. Did the caregiver have to leave paid employment? Is the care recipient experiencing homophobia?

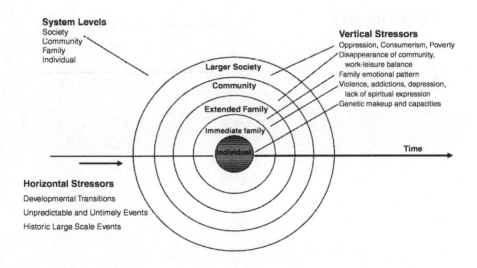

Adapted from: Carter, B., & McGoldrick, M. (Eds.). (1999). *The expanded family life cycle: Individual, family, and social perspectives*. Boston: Allyn & Bacon.

FIGURE 4. Flow of Stress Through the Family.

Assignment: To facilitate the understanding of how multisystemic stressors affect family caregiving, use Carter and McGoldrick's schema (Figure 4) to assess your family. What are two examples of events that fit the horizontal stressors and two that fit vertical stressors categories that you think produce stress?

Horizontal stressors: 1._____

                                        2._____

Vertical stressors: 1._____

                                        2._____

Section IV

• Assessment: Functional Age

Section IV is intended to guide you through a functional age assessment. *Functional age assessment* involves an understanding of the biopsychosocial-spiritual behaviors that affect a person's ability/competence to perform behaviors central to everyday life (see Figure 5). *Biological factors* are related to functional capacity and include health, physical capacity, or vital life limiting organ systems; *Psychological factors* encompass an individual's affect state or mood, cognitive or mental status, and their behavioral dimensions; and *sociocultural aspects* to consider involve the cultural, political, and economic aspects of life events (Greene, 2000). *Spiritual factors* may include a person's relationship with his or her faith/religious community and or an inner system of beliefs. The importance of spiritual functioning is that spirituality contributes to a person's ability to transcend the immediate situation and to discover meaning in seemingly meaningless events.

When assessing an older adult for example, biological facts to remember are that older adults are less likely to have an acute sense of smell, touch, vision, and hearing. Psychological facts to remember when conducting assessment involve prior mental health conditions. Older adults may have a history of tiredness, loss of interest and appetite, weight loss, or inability to sleep. They may be disoriented to time and place or not be able to take stock of their situation. Social functioning following an adverse event is related to how a person has made role transitions across his or her lifetime. The various events across the life course may be *normative*, referring to events that most people experience over their lifetime or *nonnormative*, encompassing situations that are not expected to occur and are experienced by an entire cohort such as the Great Depression, the Nazi Holocaust, or September 11th.

Readings to facilitate the completion of this section include:

Greene, R. R. (2000). *Social work with the aged and their families*. New York: Aldine De Gruyter. Chapters 3, 4, & 5.
Berger, R. & Federico, R. (1982). *Human behavior: A social work perspective*. New York: Longman.

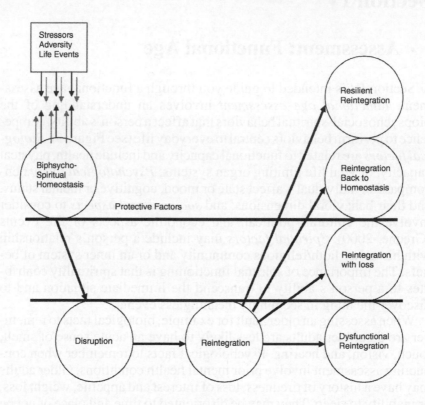

Richardson, G. E. (2002). Metatheory of resilience and resiliency. *Journal of Clinical Psychology*, *58*(3), 307-321. Reprinted with permission of John Wiley & Sons, Inc.

FIGURE 5. The Resiliency Model.

Assignment: To gather information on the care recipient's functional age, select questions from Tables 5, 6, 7, 8.

TABLE 5
Framework for Biological-Age Assessment

I. **Common Physical Symptoms**

Pain

Fatigue

Shortness of breath

Swelling of ankles

Change in skin-pallor

Constipation-diarrhea

Incontinence or bladder problems

Bowel control

Fainting, dizziness

Bleeding

Other (client's self-report)

II. **Physical Limitations**

Hearing loss-hearing aid

Vision loss-glasses, cataracts, glaucoma

Dentures

Gait-cane, walker, wheelchair

Prosthetic devices

Posture

III. **Cognitive Ability, Judgment, and Communication**

Use of telephone

Knowledge of news events

Financial management

Memory

Intellect

Orientation: use of calendar, appointments

IV. **Medical Regimes**

General medical history

Chronic illnesses

Acute illnesses

Prescription drugs and over-the-counter drugs (e.g., laxatives, aspirin)

Special diets: low-sodium, low-sugar, low-fat, low-cholesterol

V. Daily Living Habits

Alcohol and drug use

Water intake

General nutritional requirements, vitamins, and protein

Eating and self-feeding skills and general appetite

Grooming: shaving, hair, teeth, nails, skin, clothes

Bathing/washing

Caffeine use

Smoking

Exercise/activity: regular, exertion level

Sleep patterns: difficulties, naps, average number of hours, sleeping pills, day-night reversals, insomnia

Sexual activities: desires, changes, outlets

VI. Mobility and Safety

General speed of motion

Home environment (manipulation of) lighting, stairs, bathtub, locations of toilet and bedroom

Architectural barriers: accessing ramps, curbs

Ability to handle emergencies: fire, medical

Safety: lighting, security of carpets

VII. Home Management

Housecleaning

Kitchen activities: e.g., open cans and meal preparation

Ability to shop for groceries

Adapted from: Greene, R. R. (2000). *Social Work with the Aged and their Families.* New York: Aldine De Gruyter.

TABLE 6
Person-in-Environment System Coping Index

☐ Outstanding coping skills: The client's ability to solve problems; to act independently; and to use ego strength, insight, and intellectual ability to cope with difficult situations is exceptional.

☐ Above-average coping skills: The client's ability to solve problems; to act independently; and to use ego strength, insight, and intellectual ability to cope with difficult situations is more than would be expected in the average person.

☐ Adequate coping skills: The client is able to solve problems; can act independently; and has adequate ego strength, insight, and intellectual ability.

☐ Somewhat adequate coping skills: The client has fair problem solving ability, but has major difficulties in solving the presenting problems; acting independently; and using ego strength, insight, and intellectual ability.

☐ Inadequate coping skills: The client has some ability to solve problems but it is insufficient to solve the presenting problems; the client shows poor ability to act independently; and the client has minimal ego strength, insight, and intellectual ability.

☐ No coping skills: The client shows little or no ability to solve problems; lacks the capacity to act independently; and has insufficient ego strength, insight, and intellectual ability.

Adapted from: Karls & Wandrei (1994). *Person-in-Environment System.* Washington, DC: NASW Press, (p. 33).

TABLE 7
Framework for Social Relationship Assessment

---

1. Is there any one person you feel close to, whom you trust and confide in, without whom it is hard to image life? Is there any one else you feel very close to?

2. Are there other people to whom you feel not quite that close but who are still important to you?

3. For each person named in (1) and (2) above, obtain the following:

   a. Name

   b. Gender

   c. Age

   d. Relationship

   e. Geographic Proximity

   f. Length of time client knows the individual

   g. How do they keep in touch (in person, telephone, letters, combination)

   h. Satisfaction with amount of contact–want more or less? If not satisfied, what prevents you from keeping in touch more often?

   i. What does individual do for you?

   j. Are you satisfied with the kind of support you get?

   k. Are there other things that you think he or she can do for you?

   l. What prevents him or her from doing that for you?

   m. Are you providing support to that individual? If so, what are you doing?

4. Now thinking about your network, all the people that you feel close to, would you want more people in it?

5. Are there any members of your network whom you would not want the agency to contact? If so, who? Can you tell us why?

6. Are you a member of any groups or organizations? If so, which ones?

7. Are you receiving assistance from any agencies? If so, what agency and what service(s)?

Biegel, D., Shore, B., & Gordon, E. (1984). *Building Support Networks for the Elderly.* Beverly Hills, CA: Sage. Used with permission.

TABLE 8
Framework for Spiritual Assessment

Initial Narrative Framework

1. Describe the religious/spiritual tradition in which you were raised. How important was spirituality to your family? Extended family? How were spiritual beliefs expressed?

2. What sort of personal experiences (practices) stand out to you during your years at home? What made these experiences special? Have they informed your later life? How?

3. Have you changed or matured from those experiences? How? Can you describe your current spiritual or religious orientation? Does your spirituality or religion serve as a personal strength? If so, describe how?

Interpretive Anthropological Framework

1. Affect: What aspects of your spiritual life give you pleasure? What role does your spirituality play in handling life's sorrows? How does spirituality give you hope for the future?

2. Behavior: Are there particular spiritual rituals or practices that help you deal with life's obstacles?

3. Cognition: What are your current spiritual/religious beliefs? On what are they based? What beliefs do you find particularly meaningful? How does this belief help you overcome obstacles?

4. Communion: Describe your relationship to the Ultimate. How does your relationship help you face life challenges? How would the Ultimate describe you?

5. Conscience: How do you determine right or wrong? What are your key values?

6. Intuition: To what extent do you experience intuitive hunches (flashes of creative insight, premonitions, spiritual insight)? Have these insights been strength in your life? If so, how?

Adapted from: Hodge, D. R. (2001). Spirituality assessment: A review of major qualitative methods and a new framework for assessing spirituality. *Social Work, 46*(3), 203-207. p. 208.

Activity 2

When you have finished your functional age assessment, you will want to conclude with your overall rating of the care recipient's well-being. Do you know what successes the care recipient has had over his or her life? How does he or she feel about his or her well-being? Use Ryff and Springer's (2002) instrument in Table 9.

TABLE 9
Definitions of Theory-Guided Dimensions of Well-Being

Self-Acceptance
High scorer: possesses a positive attitude toward the self; acknowledges and accepts multiple aspects of self, including good and bad qualities; feels positive about past life.
Low scorer: feels dissatisfied with self; is disappointed with what has occurred in past life; is troubled about certain personal qualities; wishes to be different than what he or she is.

Positive Relations with Others
High scorer: has warm satisfying, trusting relationships with others; is concerned about the welfare of others; capable of strong empathy, affection, and intimacy; understands give-and-take of human relationships.
Low scorer: has few close, trusting relationships with others; finds it difficult to be warm, open, and concerned about others; is isolated and frustrated in interpersonal relationships; is not willing to make compromises to sustain important ties with others.

Autonomy
High scorers: is self-determining and independent; is able to resist social pressures to think and act in certain ways; regulates behavior from within; evaluates self by personal standards.
Low scorer: is concerned about the expectations and evaluations of others; relies on judgments of others to make important decisions; conforms to social pressures to think and act in certain ways.

Environmental Mastery
High scorer: has a sense of mastery and competence in managing the environment; controls complex array of external activities; makes effective use of surrounding opportunities; is able to choose or create contexts suitable to personal needs and values.
Low scorer: has difficulty managing everyday affairs; feels unable to change or improve surrounding contexts; is unaware of surrounding opportunities; lacks sense of control over external world.

Purpose in Life
High scorer: has goals in life and a sense of directedness; feels there is meaning to present and past life; holds beliefs that give life purpose; has aims and objectives for living.
Low scorer: lacks a sense of meaning in life; has few goals or aims; lacks sense of direction; does not see purpose in past life; has no outlooks or beliefs that give life meaning.

Personal Growth
High scorer: has a feeling of continued development; sees self as growing and expanding; is open to new experiences; has a sense of realizing his or her potential; sees improvement in self and behavior over time; is changing in ways that reflect more self-knowledge and effectiveness.
Low scorer: has a sense of personal stagnation; lacks a sense of improvement or expansion over time; feels bored and uninterested with life; feels unable to develop new attitude or behaviors.

Ryff, C. & Singer, B. (2002). From social structure to biology. In C. R. Snyder & S. J. Lopez (Eds.), *Handbook of positive psychology* (p. 543). New York: Oxford University Press. By permission of Oxford University Press, Inc.

Section V

• Assessment: Family

Section V explores the family's ability to provide care. Specifically its development over time, role allocation, communication, and organizational properties. Students will assess how a family copes with or is responsive to stress.

Readings to facilitate the completion of this section include:

Farran, C., Miller, B., Kaufman, J., Donner, D., & Fogg, L. (1999). Finding meaning through caregiving: Development of an instrument for family caregivers of persons with Alzheimer's disease. *Journal of Clinical Psychology, 55*(9), 1107-1125.

Greene, R. R. (2000). *Social work with the aged and their families*. New York: Aldine De Gruyter. Chapters 6 & 7.

McCubbin, H. I., Thompson, E. A., Thompson, A. I., Elver, K. M., & McCubbin, M. A. (1994). Ethnicity, schema, and coherence: Appraisal processes for families in crisis. In H. McCubbin, E. A. Thompson, A. I. Thompson, & J. E. Fromer (Eds.), *Stress, coping and health in families: Sense of coherence and resiliency* (pp. 41-70). Madison: University of Wisconsin Press.

Walsh, F. (1998). *Strengthening Family Resilience*. New York: Guilford Press.

• Role Allocation

Activity 1

Students may choose elements from three frameworks mentioned below in developing a family assessment.

1. Greene's Functional-Age Model of Intergenerational Therapy addresses the interplay between the care recipient's biopsychosocial functioning and the adaptive capacity of the family. The mutual interdependence among family members, and the dynamic development of family structure and organization throughout the life course is assessed. The social worker processes and integrates diagnostic information to arrive at family-centered interventions. See Chapter 1.
2. Another well-known clinical approach to promoting family resilience was developed by Walsh (1997, 2002). Her metaframework on relational resilience is based on risk and resilience research suggesting that severe challenges influence the whole family. Therefore, the framework is comprised of interventions to fortify the family relationship network. The model concentrates on how a family has developed over time, how it responds to a crisis event, and uses multiple systems interventions.

The model has several elements that the practitioner can use to foster family resilience and addresses three key domains of family functioning:

(1) *family belief systems*, referring to what meaning a family gives to the crisis;
(2) *organizational patterns*, involving the family's structure and supports; and
(3) *communication processes*, including problem-solving ability (Walsh, 1998)

Select elements from Table 10 to use in your assessment.

TABLE 10
Key Processes in Family Resilience

Belief Systems
Making meaning of adversity
- Affiliative value: resilience as relationally based
- Family life cycle orientation: normalizing, contextualizing adversity and distress
- Sense of coherence: crisis as meaning, comprehensible, manageable challenge
- Appraisal of crisis, distress, and recovery: facilitative versus constraining beliefs

Positive outlook
- Active initiative and perseverance
- Courage and en-courage-ment
- Sustaining hope, optimistic view: confidence in overcoming odds
- Focusing on strengths and potential
- Mastering the possible; accepting what can't be changed

Transcendence and spirituality
- Larger values, purpose
- Spirituality; faith, communion, rituals
- Inspiration: envisioning new possibilities, creativity, heroes
- Transformation: learning and growth from adversity

Organizational Patterns
Flexibility
- Capacity to change: rebounding, reorganizing, adapting to fit challenges over time
- Counterbalancing by stability: continuity, dependability through disruption

Connectedness
- Mutual support, collaboration, and commitment
- Respect for individual needs, differences, and boundaries
- Strong leadership: nurturing, protecting, guiding children and vulnerable members
- Varied family forms: cooperative parenting/caregiving teams
- Couple/coparent relationship: equal partners
- Seeking reconnection, reconciliation of troubled relationships

Social and economic resources
- Mobilizing extended kin and social support; community networks
- Building financial security; balancing work and family strains

Communication Processes
Clarity
- Clear, consistent messages (words and actions)
- Clarification of ambiguous situation; truth-seeking/truth-speaking

Open emotional expression
- Sharing range of feelings (joy and pain; hopes and fears)
- Mutual empathy; tolerance for differences
- Responsibility for own feelings, behavior: avoid blaming
- Pleasurable interactions: humor

Collaborative problem solving
- Creative brainstorming; resourcefulness
- Shared decision making: negotiation, fairness, reciprocity
- Conflict resolution
- Focusing on goals: taking concrete steps, building on success, learning from failure
- Proactive stance: reinventing problems, crises; preparing for future challenges

3. McCubbin, Thompson, Thompson, Elver, and McCubbin (1994) identified five fundamental levels involved in the family appraisal processes at times of crisis known as the FARR Model. The Resiliency Model of Family Stress, Adjustment, and Adaptation Levels of family functioning that may be addressed include:

Level 5. *Family schema:* A generalized structure of shared values, beliefs, goals, expectations, and priorities, shaped and adopted by the family unit, thus formulating a generalized informational structure against and through which information and experiences are compared, sifted, and processed. A family schema evolves over time and serves as a dispositional worldview and framework to evaluate crisis situations and legitimate adherence to and change in the family's established patterns of functioning. . . .

Level 4. *Family coherence.* A construct that explains the motivational and cognitive bases for transforming the family's potential resources into actual resources, thereby facilitating coping and promoting the health of family members and the well-being of the family unit. . . .

Level 3. *Family paradigms.* A model of shared beliefs and expectations shaped and adopted by the family unit to guide the family's development of *specific* patterns of functioning around *specific* domains or dimensions of family life (for example, work and family, communication, spiritual/religious orientation, child rearing). . . .

Level 2. *Situational appraisal.* The family's shared assessment of the stressor, the hardship created by the stressor, the demand upon the family system to change some established patterns of functioning. The appraisal occurs in relation to the family's capability for managing the crisis situation. . . .

Level 1. *Stressor appraisal.* The family's definition of the stressor and its severity is the initial level of family assessment. . . . (pp. 43-46)

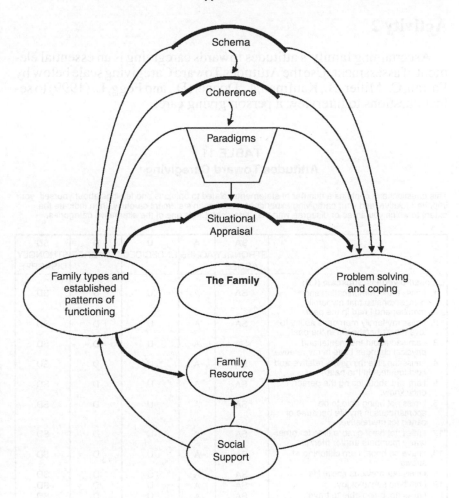

FIGURE 6. Focus on Appraisal Processes in the Resiliency Model of Family Adjustment and Adaptation

From "Ethnicity, Schema, and Coherence: Appraisal Processes for Families in Crisis," by H.I. McCubbin, E.A. Thompson, A.I. Thompson, K.M. Elver, and M.A. McCubbin, (1994). In *Stress, Coping and Health in Families: Sense of Coherency and Resiliency* (p. 44). Thousand Oaks, CA: Sage Publications. Reprinted by permission of Sage Publications, Inc.

Activity 2

Ascertaining family's attitudes towards caregiving is an essential element of assessment. Use the Attitudes Toward Caregiving scale below by Farran, C., Miller, B., Kaufman, J., Donner, D., and Fogg, L. (1999) to select questions to interview a person giving care.

TABLE 11
Attitudes Toward Caregiving

This questionnaire contains a number of statements related to opinions and feelings about yourself, your impaired relative, and your caregiving experience. Read each statement carefully, then indicate the extent to which you agree or disagree with the statement. Circle one of the alternative categories.

	SA STRONGLY AGREE	A AGREE	U UNDECIDED	D DISAGREE	SD STRONGLY DISAGREE
1. Loss/Powerless Subscale (LP)					
1. I miss the communication and companionship that my family member and I had in the past.	SA	A	U	D	SD
2. I miss my family member's ability to love me as he/she did in the past.	SA	A	U	D	SD
3. I am sad about the mental and physical changes I see in my relative.	SA	A	U	D	SD
4. I miss the little things my relative and I did together in the past.	SA	A	U	D	SD
5. I am sad about losing the person I once knew.	SA	A	U	D	SD
6. I miss not being able to be spontaneous in my life because of caring for my relative.	SA	A	U	D	SD
12. I miss not having more time for other family members and/or friends.	SA	A	U	D	SD
13. I have no hope; I am clutching at straws.	SA	A	U	D	SD
18. I miss our previous social life.	SA	A	U	D	SD
19. I have no sense of joy.	SA	A	U	D	SD
24. I miss not being able to travel.	SA	A	U	D	SD
25. I wish I were free to lead a life of my own.	SA	A	U	D	SD
30. I miss having given up my job or other personal interests to take care of my family member.	SA	A	U	D	SD
31. I feel trapped by my relative's illness.	SA	A	U	D	SD
34. We had goals for the future but they just folded up because of my relative's dementia.	SA	A	U	D	SD
36. I miss my relative's sense of humor.	SA	A	U	D	SD
37. I wish I could run away.	SA	A	U	D	SD
41. I feel that the quality of my life has decreased.	SA	A	U	D	SD
7. My situation feels endless.	SA	A	U	D	SD

	SA STRONGLY AGREE	A AGREE	U UNDECIDED	D DISAGREE	SD STRONGLY DISAGREE
2. Provisional Meaning (PM)					
8. I enjoy having my relative with me: I would miss it if he/she were gone.	SA	A	U	D	SD
9. I count my blessings.	SA	A	U	D	SD
10. Caring for my relative gives me my life a purpose and a sense of meaning.	SA	A	U	D	SD
14. I cherish the past memories and experiences that my relative and I have had.	SA	A	U	D	SD
15. I am a strong person.	SA	A	U	D	SD
16. Caregiving makes me feel good that I am helping.	SA	A	U	D	SD
20. The hugs and "I love you" from my relative make it worth it all.	SA	A	U	D	SD
21. I'm a fighter.	SA	A	U	D	SD
22. I am glad I am here to care for my relative.	SA	A	U	D	SD
26. Talking with others who are close to me restores my faith in my own abilities.	SA	A	U	D	SD
27. Even though there are difficult things in my life, I look forward to the future.	SA	A	U	D	SD
28. Caregiving has helped me learn new things about myself.	SA	A	U	D	SD
32. Each year, regardless of the quality, is a blessing.	SA	A	U	D	SD
33. I would not have chosen the situation I'm in, but I get satisfaction out of providing care.	SA	A	U	D	SD
38. Every day is blessing.	SA	A	U	D	SD
39. This is my place: I have to make the best out of it.	SA	A	U	D	SD
40. I am much stronger than I think.	SA	A	U	D	SD
42. I start each day knowing we will have a beautiful day together.	SA	A	U	D	SD
43. Caregiving has made me a stronger and better person.	SA	A	U	D	SD
3. Ultimate Meaning (UM)					
11. The Lord won't give you more than you can handle.	SA	A	U	D	SD
17. I believe in the power of prayer: without it I couldn't do this.	SA	A	U	D	SD
23. I believe that the Lord will provide.	SA	A	U	D	SD
29. I have faith that the good Lord has reasons for this.	SA	A	U	D	SD
35. God is good.	SA	A	U	D	SD

Farran, C., Miller, B., Kaufman, J., Donner, D., & Fogg, L. (1999). Finding meaning through caregiving: Development of an instrument for family caregivers of persons with Alzheimer's disease. *Journal of Clinical Psychology, 55*(9), 1107-1125. Reprinted with permission of John Wiley & Sons, Inc.

Part 2: INTERVENTION

This final section of this workbook suggests items to organize your intervention plan based on the assessment of functional capacity of the care recipient. Use Table 12 to establish the extent of care needed.

Reading to facilitate the completion of this section includes:

Greene, R. R. (2000). *Social work with the aged and their families*. New York: Aldine De Gruyter. Chapters 8, 9, & 10.

Not only can today's social workers draw on systems and ecological practice strategies, the increase in caregiving families has brought about an intensified interest in techniques that promote the positive aspects across the life course. Theorists have addressed the topic of wellness from a number of vantage points. For example, Walsh (1998; 1999) has pointed out that studies of adult development and family functioning reveal that families have a variety of adaptive mechanisms to help them successfully meet the challenges of later life. She indicated that flexibility in family structure, roles, and reactions to developmental tasks can play a vital function in exploring new options. She prompted practitioners to foster family coping and adaptational process to enable them to better address disruptive life challenges.

Another example of a positive approach to aging was developed by Antonovsky (1998) who used the phrase *salutogenesis orientation* to encompass his study of how people naturally use their resources to strive for health. He also assumed that a family is a collective that employs its coping capacities to return to stability when faced with stressors such as chronic illness or disability. Similarly, gerontologists, such as Atchley (1999), developed continuity theory to examine how older adults adapt to changing situations. Such theorists provide practitioners with ideas about how to promote competence among older adults by tapping natural coping mechanisms. The major question is, What enables you to cope? or,

What keeps you going? Atchley was impressed with the research finding that, irrespective of changes in health, a large proportion of older adults continue to show consistency in thinking patterns, activities, living arrangements, and social relationships. He used the term *continuity strategies* to refer to the means that older adults take to maintain life satisfaction despite disability. Such continuity was attributed to a coherence in psychological, behavioral, and social patterns of aging individuals (Atchley, 1999, p. 8).

Other positive aging concepts that are increasingly being applied to older adults include successful aging and resilience (Rowe & Kahn, 1998). While successful aging has been of interest for a number of decades, the interest has been renewed by a decade of research sponsored as part of the MacArthur Foundation Studies. *Successful aging*, according to Rowe and Kahn (1998), consists of three major factors: (1) Avoiding disease by adopting a prevention orientation; (2) engaging in life by continuing social involvement; and (3) maintaining high cognitive and physical functioning through ongoing activity. This shift in paradigm suggests that social workers develop more programs that promote health and psychosocial well-being, as well as use assertive rehabilitation strategies. Moreover, Crowther et al., have expanded the conceptualization of successful aging expanded to include positive spirituality as an often forgotten component of health and well-being.

A resilience-based orientation, a theoretical advance currently underway that builds on social work's strengths perspective, examines what factors contribute to successful outcomes in the face of a crisis or how people overcome the odds. The concept of resilience has a variety of meanings, referring to the ability to recover strength, spirits, and good humor (Webster, 1983). The term is used in social work to pertain to people's ability to spring back after experiencing adverse stress or problems (Barker, 1995). Although originally applied to children and youth, the term resilience is increasingly being applied to older adults and may substitute for the associated concepts of *competence* or a person's ability to overcome stress and to perform adequately to live in one's environment– and *self-effi-cacy* a person's belief that he or she can accomplish certain tasks (Lewis & Harrell, 2002).

The resilience approach has become sufficiently sophisticated to provide ideas for highly useful intervention strategies (Fraser, Richman, & Galinsky, 1999). For example, Walsh (1998; 1999) has used the research of the last two decades and her own clinical experiences to substantiate that families are *resilient* or have the ability to overcome adversity. She has suggested that practitioners stay in tune to a family's naturally healing capacity. Social workers who foster family resilience focus on a family's intrinsic strengths and resources that allow them to better meet life crises (Carter & McGoldrick, 1999). In addition, practitioners examine the match between family strengths and the family's specific circumstances. That is,

> family resilience describes the path a family follows as it adapts and prospers in the face of stress, both in the present and over time. Resilient families respond positively to these conditions in unique ways, depending on the context, developmental level, the interactive combination of risk and protective factors, and the family's shared outlook. (Hawley & DeHaan, 1996, p. 293)

Practitioners who use a resilience orientation see every family as having the capacity for growth and the potential to engage in self-righting behavior. Moreover, such practitioners see every intervention as preventative and having the potential to reduce family stress. In this instance, the concept of resilience is important to how the family perceives and meets the stress of family caregiving. For example, the resilience perspective recognizes that, although stress puts an extra burden on family life, families are inherently prepared to maintain their equilibrium.

Activity 1

Complete Table 12 for your designated care recipient.

TABLE 12
Five Continua for the Elderly

1. Continuum of Need

Independent (Little or no need)	Moderately dependent	Dependent (Multiple needs)

2. Continuum of Services

Health promotion/ disease prevention	Screening and early detection	Diagnosis and pre-treatment evaluation	Treatment	Rehabilitation: skilled nursing services	Continuing care and hospice

3. Continuum of Service Settings

Own home, apartment, etc.	Friend or relative's home apartment, etc.	Congregate living situation	Sub-acute care facility (e.g., day hospital)	Acute care facility (e.g., hospital)	Skilled long-term care facility (e.g., nursing home)	Continuing care and hospice

4. Continuum of Service Providers

Non-service	Self-care	Family friends (support network)	Para-professionals	Professionals

5. Continuum of Professional Collaboration

Single discipline	Multidisciplinary	Interdisciplinary

Hooyman, N., Hooyman, G., & Kethley, A. (1981). The role of gerontological social work in interdisciplinary care. Paper presented at Council on Social Work Education Annual Program Meeting, Louisville, Kentucky, March. Used with permission.

Activity 2

Choose systems, ecological, resilience-enhancing interventions, and oral history to write the care plan for helping your family in caregiving situations.

TABLE 13
The Role of the Social Worker as a Change Agent

Systems theory suggests that the social worker as change agent:

- Brings the client system together to promote self-knowledge about sources of difficulty or problem-solving,
- Leads the family in an examination of structural and communications patterns,
- Points out the here-and-now behaviors that might help the family understand and solve their difficulty(ies),
- Asks questions and uses other techniques to coach the family on what behaviors may be more effective,
- Works with the family to find and access solutions and resources, and strives to help the family move to a new level of functioning.

Summarized from: Greene, R. R. (1999). General systems theory. In R. R. Greene, *Human behavior theory and social work practice* (p. 241). New York: Aldine De Gruyter.

TABLE 14
Systems Theory Guidelines
for Assessment and Intervention in Family Social Work

Assume the family is a system with a unique structure and communication patterns that can be examined. The purpose of assessment is to work with the family to determine what is bringing about its dysfunction.

Define the boundaries of the family system by working with the family to ascertain membership. Observe functions and behaviors, and be cognizant of cultural forms. Assess the properties related to relative openness or closed boundaries by observing and asking about the extent of exchange the family has with larger societal systems.

Determine how well the family system fits with its environment. Review what additional resources need to be obtained or accessed to improve the family system-environment fit.

Develop a picture of the family structure through an understanding of its organization. Explore socialization processes, how subsystems are created, the nature of their hierarchy or hierarchies, and the way in which roles are and continue to be differentiated. Learn from the family how its culture influences organizational structure.

Examine the family's communication patterns. Follow the transfer of information and resources in and between the system and its environment. Assess the relative nature of the systems feedback processes. Determine how this relates overall to patterns of interaction. Ask if the family can describe its rule. Work with the family to identify dysfunctional triangulation in communication. Ask family members about their specific cultural communication clues.

Determine how responsive the family is to stress. Work with family members to identify elements in their structure and communication patterns that contribute to entropy, synergy, or achieving a steady state. Explore ways the system can decrease stress and move to a new level of adaptation, possibly by restructuring.

Summarized from: Greene, R. R. (1999). General systems theory. In R. R. Greene, *Human behavior theory and social work practice* (p. 224). New York: Aldine De Gruyter.

TABLE 15
Guidelines for the Ecological Approach to Social Work Intervention

- View the person and environment as inseparable.
- Be an equal partner in the helping process.
- Examine transactions between the person and environment by assessing all levels of systems affecting a client's adaptiveness. Assess life situations and transactions that induce high stress levels.
- Attempt to enhance a client's personal competence through positive relationships and life experiences.
- Seek interventions that affect the goodness-of-fit among a client and his or her environment at all systems levels.
- Focus on mutually sought solutions and client empowerment.

Summarized from: Greene, R. R. (1999). Ecological perspective. In R. R. Greene, *Human behavior theory and social work practice* (pp. 259-300). New York: Aldine De Gruyter.

TABLE 16
Resilience-Enhancing Interventions

To what degree do you accept these interventions as important to your social work practice?

1. Acknowledge client loss, vulnerability, and future.
Low acceptance   1   2   3   4   5 high acceptance
2. Identify the client's source of stress.
Low acceptance   1   2   3   4   5 high acceptance
3. Recognize client stress.
Low acceptance   1   2   3   4   5 high acceptance
4. Stabilize or normalize the situation.
Low acceptance   1   2   3   4   5 high acceptance
5. Help clients take control.
Low acceptance   1   2   3   4   5 high acceptance
6. Provide resources for change.
Low acceptance   1   2   3   4   5 high acceptance
7. Promote client self-efficacy
Low acceptance   1   2   3   4   5 high acceptance
8. Collaborate in client self-change
Low acceptance   1   2   3   4   5 high acceptance
9. Strengthen a client's problem-solving abilities
Low acceptance   1   2   3   4   5 high acceptance
10. Address positive emotions
Low acceptance   1   2   3   4   5 high acceptance
11. Use Humor
Low acceptance   1   2   3   4   5 high acceptance
12. Achieve creativity
Low acceptance   1   2   3   4   5 high acceptance
13. Listen to client stories
Low acceptance   1   2   3   4   5 high acceptance
14. Make meaning of client's critical events
Low acceptance   1   2   3   4   5 high acceptance
15. Help clients find the benefits of adverse events
Low acceptance   1   2   3   4   5 high acceptance
16. Attend to client's spiritually
Low acceptance   1   2   3   4   5 high acceptance
17. Assist clients in transcending the immediate situation
Low acceptance   1   2   3   4   5 high acceptance

TABLE 17
Oral History Guideline

Oral history is the systematic collection of living people's testimony about their own experiences. Oral historians attempt to verify their findings, analyze them, and place them in an accurate historical context. Oral historians are also concerned with storage of their findings for use by later scholars. In oral history projects, an interviewee recalls an event for an interviewer who records the recollections and creates a historical record.

Sequence for Oral History Research

1. Formulate a central question or issue.
2. Plan the project. Consider such things as end products, budget, publicity, evaluation, personnel, equipment, and time frames.
3. Conduct background research.
4. Interview.
5. Process interviews.
6. Evaluate research and interviews and cycle back to step 1 or go on to step 7.
7. Organize and present results.
8. Store materials as archival documents.

How do I ask oral history questions?

1. You should have a list of topics in mind. They do not have to be specific. It is best to have a start-up list of questions to get your interviewee and yourself comfortable before you change to your topic list.
2. Do plan your topic and form of your first substantial question after you and the interviewee "settle down." Ask a question that will prompt a long answer and "get the subject going."
3. Start off with easy questions first, such as brief biographical facts. Only ask very personal or emotionally demanding questions after a rapport has developed. End with gentle lighter questions.
4. Ask questions one at a time.
5. Allow for silences. Be prepared to wait.
6. Be a good listener, look at the interviewee (when culturally appropriate), nodding, and smiling to encourage and give the message, "I am interested."
7. If necessary, use verbal encouragement such as "How interesting!" However, don't push for too much disclosure when inappropriate.
8. You may want to ask for specific examples if the interviewee gives too general a statement.
9. Ask for definitions and explanations of words that the interviewee uses and that have critical meaning for the interview.
10. Reframe and re-ask an important question several times to get the full amount of information the interviewee knows. Again be culturally-sensitive to disclosure issues.
11. Try to avoid a simple "yes" or "no" answer. Ask follow-up questions and then ask some more.
12. Be flexible. Watch for and pick up on promising topics introduced by the interviewee.

Adapted from: Moyer, J. (1999). *Step-by-Step Guide to Oral History*. Retrieved November 27, 2004 from http://www.dohistory.org/on_your_own/toolkit/oralHistory.htm#WHATIS

Clinical Intervention with Intergenerational Families Giving Care

Paper Outline

1. Introduction   1 page

Describe your care recipient and caregiver and the reason(s) the recipient needs care. Include demographic information and presenting concerns.

2. Assessment   4-5 pages

Present a biopsychosocial and spiritual assessment of the care recipient-in-situation. Include information about

- Individual and caregivers history
- Current environmental supports
- Strengths, stressors, and buffers that support and protect resilience for both care recipient and care provider
- Issues of membership in at-risk populations

3. Interventions   4-5 pages

First describe your overall care plan. Then give specifics about the interventions you believe will work best with your care recipient and care provider. Be sure to list what techniques/schools of thought you will implement and why?

4. Social worker self-analysis   1-2 pages

Use this section to examine your professional use of self. How does the need for care affect you and the helping process? For example, are you imposing your own agenda? Are some topics painful to address?

Index